PSORIASIS – A SYSTEMIC DISEASE

Edited by **Jose O'Daly**

Psoriasis – A Systemic Disease
Edited by Jose O'Daly

Published by InTech
Janeza Trdine 9, 51000 Rijeka, Croatia

Publishing Process Manager Marija Radja

Technical Editor Teodora Smiljanic

Cover Designer InTech Design Team

Additional hard copies can be obtained from orders@intechopen.com

Psoriasis – A Systemic Disease, Edited by Jose O'Daly
p. cm.
ISBN 978-953-51-0281-6

For EU product safety concerns:
IN TECH d.o.o., Prolaz Marije Krucifikse Kozulić 3, 51000 Rijeka, Croatia,
info@intechopen.com or visit our website at intechopen.com.

Meet the editor

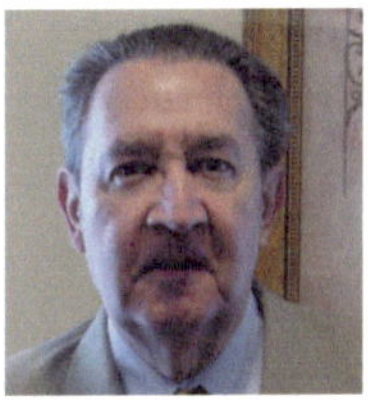

Dr Jose A. O'Daly was born in Caracas, Venezuela, BS La Salle High School in Caracas (1958), MD (1964), Doctor of Medical Sciences (1968) from the Central University of Venezuela (UCV), Caracas, PhD from Johns Hopkins University, Baltimore, Maryland USA (1971).

Contents

Preface

The purpose of this book is to present a comprehensive analysis of Psoriasis, a disease that affects approximately 2-3% of humanity in all countries. Psoriasis existence is surveyed since the clay tablets of Assyrians and Babylonians 3.000-5.000 years ago, thru the middle ages, the renaissance, XIX and XX centuries. In the first and second part of the XX century clinical forms were described, as well as the role of keratinocytes, multifactorial genes, T lymphocytes, mast cells, natural killer cells, nerve growth factor, psychosomatics, neuropeptides and environmental factors triggering the disease. Treatment of psoriasis is detailed thru history from old ointments in the XVIII and XIX centuries, up to UVA irradiation, new immunosuppressive and immunomodulatory drugs as parasite vaccines in the XX and XXI centuries. Epidemiology of psoriasis, a disease that affects around 125 million people (mainly Caucasians), is described. Psoriasis is less common in Chinese, Eskimos, West Africans and African-Americans. The course and evolution of psoriasis is very hard to predict. A description of the wide clinical spectra is presented, considering psoriasis as a systemic disease a better concept to explain its pathogenesis, with manifestations in skin, nails, tendons, ligaments, spinal cord, joints and ophthalmic complications easily missed. The balance between angiogenic and antiangiogenic factors are proposed to explain the pathogenesis in psoriatic skin. Psoriasis and atherosclerosis are interrelated; pathogenic mechanisms are shared between the two diseases inducing inflammation.

Histological characteristics are discussed in depth in plaque psoriasis describing cells and cytokines involved in the process as well as the genes responsible for inflammation. Assessment of psoriasis severity is explained in an easy way useful for the clinician and researcher working in psoriasis. The role of streptococcal infections and fungal infections as well as Malassezia species and lipophilic yeast are presented as well as antifungal treatments for control of psoriasis.

Synovitis, acne, pustulosis hyperostosis, and osteitis (SAPHO syndrome) are discussed in its relation with psoriasis with many features in common with ankylosing spondilytis and psoriatic arthritis. Peptidylarginine deiminases are discussed concerning their expression in keratinocytes, their association with skin diseases and as therapeutics and prophylactic targets in severe psoriasis.

We would like to acknowledge to the contributors to the several chapters as follows:

Ines Brajac and Franjo Gruber
Department of Dermatovenerology, University Hospital Centre Rijeka Croatia

Susana Coimbra[1,2], Hugo Oliveira[3], Américo Figueiredo[3],
Petronila Rocha-Pereira[1,4] and Alice Santos-Silva[1,5]
[1]*Instituto de Biologia Molecular e Celular (IBMC), Universidade do Porto, Porto, Portugal*
[2]*Centro de Investigação das Tecnologias da Saúde (CITS) – Instituto Politécnico da Saúde Norte, CESPU, Gandra-Paredes, Portugal*
[3]*Serviço de Dermatologia, Hospitais da Universidade de Coimbra, Coimbra, Portugal*
[4]*Centro de Investigação em Ciências da Saúde (CICS), Universidade da Beira Interior, Covilhã, Portugal*
[5]*Departamento de Ciências Biológicas, Laboratório de Bioquímica, Faculdade de Farmácia, Universidade do Porto, Porto, Portugal*

Asja Prohić
Department of Dermatovenerology, University Clinical Center of Sarajevo
Bosnia and Herzegovina

Gunter Assmann
University Medical School of Saarland, Germany

Shibo Ying[1], Michel Simon[2], Guy Serre[3] and Hidenari Takahara[1]
[1]*Ibaraki University, Japan*
[2]*CNRS-University of Toulouse III, France*

Jose O'Daly
Astralis Ltd, Irvington, NJ
USA

1

Psoriasis, a Systemic Disease Beyond the Skin, as Evidenced by Psoriatic Arthritis and Many Comorbities – Clinical Remission with a Leishmania Amastigotes Vaccine, a Serendipity Finding

J.A. O'Daly
Astralis Ltd, Irvington, NJ
USA

1. Introduction

Psoriasis is a systemic chronic, relapsing inflammatory skin disorder, with worldwide distribution, affects 1–3% of the world population, prevalence varies according to race, geographic location, and environmental factors (Chandran & Raychaudhuri, 2010; Christophers & Mrowietz, 2003; Farber & Nall, 1974). In Germany, 33,981 from 1,344,071 continuously insured persons in 2005 were diagnosed with psoriasis; thus the one year prevalence was 2.53% in the study group. Up to the age of 80 years the prevalence rate (range: 3.99-4.18%) was increasing with increasing age and highest for the age groups from 50 to 79 years The total rate of psoriasis in children younger than 18 years was 0.71%. The prevalence rates increased in an approximately linear manner from 0.12% at the age of 1 year to 1.2% at the age of 18 years (Schäfer et al., 2011). In France, a case-control study in 6,887 persons, 356 cases were identified (5.16%), who declared having had psoriasis during the previous 12 months (Wolkenstein et al., 2009). The prevalence of psoriasis analyzed across Italy showed that 2.9% of Italians declared suffering from psoriasis (regional range: 0.8-4.5%) in a total of 4109 individuals (Saraceno et al., 2008). The overall rate of comorbidity in subjects with psoriasis aged less than 20 years was twice as high as in subjects without psoriasis. Juvenile psoriasis was associated with increased rates of hyperlipidaemia, obesity, hypertension, diabetes mellitus, Crohn disease and rheumatoid arthritis. The best-known noncutaneous condition associated with psoriasis is joint disease, mostly expressed as Psoriatic arthritis (PsA), (Mrowietz et al., 2007). Palmoplantar psoriasis is associated with significant quality-of-life issues. In 150 patients with palmoplantar psoriasis, 78 (52%) patients displayed predominantly hyperkeratotic palmoplantar lesions, 24 (16%) pustular, 18 (12%) combination, and 30 (20%) had an indeterminate phenotype. In 27 (18%) patients, lesions were confined to the palms and soles. In all, 27 (18%) had mild, 72 (48%) moderate, and 51 (34%) severe disease involvement (Farley et al., 2009).

2. Psoriasis in the clinic

The disease has wide clinical spectra that range from epidermal (scaly) and vascular (thickened, erythematous) involvements of the skin, to the malignant form known as generalized erythrodermia. Skin involvement is characterized by symmetrically distributed, well-demarcated plaques, its most common form named psoriasis vulgaris or plaque-type psoriasis. Two forms of psoriasis can be recognized: Type I psoriasis, characterized by been hereditary, dominant autosomic (60% penetration), onset: 16 years females, 22 years males; HLA-Cw6 positive (73.8% vs. 20.4 % in normal subjects). Type II psoriasis, characterized by been sporadic, major incidence 57-60 years, poor correlation with HLA-CW6 (27.3% vs. 10.1% in controls). Psoriasis plaques with silvery scales present the Auspitz sign a pinpoint capillary bleeding when the scales are gently scraped away with a spatula or fingernail (Mrowietz, et al., 2007, 2009; Naldi & Mercuri, 2010). Psoriasis may also attack nails, (Augustin et al., 2010b; Farber, & Nall , 1974), tendons, ligaments, fascia, and spinal or peripheral joints as the clinical form, inflammatory PsA similar to rheumatoid arthritis, but no rheumatoid factor present in the blood. PsA can be severely disabling, occurring in up to 10–30% of patients with psoriasis, and is associated with HLA-B27 MHC Class I marker (Mrowietz et al., 2007). Psoriatic plaques induce pain and pruritus, generating discomfort and persistent insomnia. Quality of life decreases considerably because it is a physically disfiguring illness that disrupts social life, induces constant psychological stress, lowered self-esteem, and feelings of being socially ostracized. Common among many patients are the use of tranquilizers, sleeping pills, antidepressants, consumption of alcohol, and cigarette smoking (Choi & Koo 2003, Zeljko-Penavi´c et al. 2010, Wu et al., 2009, Van Voorhees & Fried 2009). Pruritus is an important symptom in psoriasis vulgaris may be severe and seriously affect the quality of life. 85% of psoriatic patients suffered from itching; the frequency of pruritus was daily and mean intensity was moderate. The results confirmed the need for a global study of psoriasis with regard to both the cutaneous manifestations and the itch symptom (Prignano et al., 2009). Ophthalmic complications of psoriasis are numerous and affect almost any part of the eye; however, they may be easily missed. Complications include direct cutaneous effects such as eyelid involvement and blepharitis, and immune mediated conditions such as uveitis (Rehal et al., 2011). In Spain, between January 2007 and December 2009 of a total of 661 patients included, 47.4% were diagnosed with nail psoriasis, which was 13.5% more prevalent in men. The group of patients with nail disease had more severe psoriasis (12.82 vs 8.22 points on PASI) and a longer disease duration (20.30 vs 13.94 years), and included a larger percentage of patients with psoriatic arthritis (29.7% vs 11.5%), a positive family history of the disease (53.7% vs 42.8%), and a body mass index greater than 30 (31.6% vs 23.9%). A larger percentage of the patients with nail disease had early-onset psoriasis (74.1% vs 65.5%) and fewer were carriers of the human lymphocyte antigen Cw0602 allele (33% vs 50.3%). Nail disease is frequent in psoriasis and is associated with greater severity of psoriasis and a larger number of comorbidities (Armesto et al., 2011).

3. Psoriasis pathogenesis

3.1 General concepts

The introduction of the new concept of psoriatic disease represents a novel opportunity to better understand the pathogenesis of psoriasis and comorbidities (Scarpa et al., 2010). The disease is genetically determined with the involvement of multiple genes that interact with each other and with environmental factors (Elder, 2009). Analysis of patients demonstrated a strong association between psoriasis and all components of metabolic syndrome, which also explains comorbidities (Boehncke & Sterry, 2009). In early lesions, macrophages are present in the epidermis followed by monocytes, lymphocytes, and granulocytes with formation of spongiform micro abscesses (Munro abscesses), more pronounced with disease activity, a hallmark of psoriasis. Physical trauma to the skin, results in a psoriatic lesion (Koebner phenomenon), which increases when the disease is active (Farber & Nall, 1974). The inflammatory process is immune mediated by unknown antigens through binding and specific activation and costimulation of T cells by antigen-presenting cells (APC), dendritic cells (DC), and macrophages in epidermis and dermis. A multimolecular complex is formed between APC and T cells: the immunological synapse, structured by major histocompatibility complex (MHC) receptors and T-cell receptors (TCR), with the following costimulatory molecules: lymphocyte functional antigen (LFA-1 and LFA-3), intercellular adhesion molecule (ICAM- 1), cluster of differentiation CD2, CD28, CD80, (Mrowietz, & Reich, 2009). Epidermal keratinocytes are highly active immunological cells, controlling the acute and the chronic phase of skin inflammation by cytokine/chemokine production and surface molecule expression, which lead to inflammatory infiltrate in the whole skin including the upper layers of the epidermis, perpetuating the skin disorder (Albanesi & Pastore, 2010). Dendritic cells and effector T-cells are central in the development of the psoriastic lesion, and cytokines produced by these cells stimulate keratinocytes to proliferate and increase the migration of inflammatory cells into the skin, promoting epidermal hyperplasia and inflammation (Monteleone et al., 2011). Psoriasis is a common chronic inflammatory disease of the skin and joints. Autoantibodies have been reported in psoriasis patients. Anti-nuclear antibody and antibody to double-stranded deoxyribonucleic acid, rheumatoid factor, anti-thyroid microsomal antibody (anti-TMA) were studied. About 28.8% of psoriasis cases were positive for at least one autoantibody. Age of onset and types of psoriasis had significant association with gender. Anti-double-stranded deoxyribonucleic acid and anti-thyroid microsomal antibody had significant association with types of psoriasis. Gender wise distribution of psoriasis in age group had significant association with anti-TMA. Autoantibodies are found to be present in psoriasis patients or latent autoimmune diseases develop in psoriasis patients without any clinical symptoms (Singh et al., 2010).

3.2 Blood vessels in psoriasis pathogenesis

Angiogenesis is essential for embryo development as well as for wound healing and progression of a number of diseases such as cancer, inflammatory conditions, eye diseases, psoriasis, and rheumatoid arthritis (RA) in the adult. Current paradigms explain blood vessel growth entirely by sprouting angiogenesis or by vessel splitting through so called intussusceptive angiogenesis. However, these mechanisms are mainly derived from experiments on the developing embryo while less is known about angiogenesis in the adult during, e.g., wound healing, tumor growth, and inflammation. Blood vessel growth in the adult can be induced and directed by mechanical forces that naturally develop during healing or remodeling of tissues (Kilarski & Gerwins, 2009). It is regulated by pro- and anti-angiogenic molecules, and was only implicated in few diseases, such as, cancer, arthritis, and psoriasis, now its research offers a potential to cure a variety of diseases such as Alzheimer's and AIDS. Angiogenesis may have an impact similar to that of antibiotics had in the twentieth century (Bisht et al., 2010). Angiogenic factors, such as vascular endothelial growth factor (VEGF), may dominate the activity of anti-angiogenic factors and accelerate angiogenesis in psoriatic skin. Small peptides with homologies to pigment epithelium derived factor (PEDF) show anti-angiogenic potential for the topical treatment for psoriasis. The specific low-molecular weight peptides (MW<850 Da) penetrated the skin and showed significant anti-angiogenic activity in vitro. Topical application of these peptides in a severe combined immunodeficient mouse model of psoriatic disease led to reduced angiogenesis and epidermal thickness (Abe et al., 2010). VEGF is overexpressed in lesional psoriatic skin and its serum levels are significantly elevated in patients with moderate to severe disease. Thirty patients with moderate to severe psoriasis and 10 healthy controls were subjected to baseline evaluation of VEGF. Patients were divided into three groups according to the received treatment: psoralen plus ultraviolet A (PUVA) thrice weekly (group 1), acitretin 50 mg daily (group 2), and combined PUVA twice weekly and acitretin 25 mg daily (group 3). Treatment continued for 16 weeks or up to clinical cure. Every patient was subjected to severity evaluation by PASI and measurement of serum VEGF before and after treatment. Mean serum levels of VEGF were significantly elevated in patients (327 ± 66.2 pg/mL) than control subjects (178 ± 83.4 pg/mL). A highly significant correlation was found between VEGF and PASI score. VEGF is important in the pathogenesis of psoriasis, and could serve as a good indicator of disease severity and control (Nofal et al., 2009).

3.3 T cells and cytokines in psoriasis

The chemokine/chemokine receptor network is an integral element of the complex system of homeostasis and immunosurveillance. Initially studied because of their role in coordinating tissue-specific migration and activation of leucocytes, chemokines have been implicated in the pathogenesis of various malignancies and diseases with strong inflammatory components. There is a critical involvement of chemokine receptor interactions in the immunopathogenesis of classical inflammatory skin disorders such as psoriasis and atopic dermatitis, as well as neoplastic diseases with a T-cell origin, such as mycosis fungoides (Lonsdorf et al., 2009). In psoriasis, leukocytes that infiltrate skin lesions have been shown to be involved in the pathogenesis of this disease. The presence of CXCR3+ T lymphocytes in psoriatic lesional skin, have suggested a role of this receptor in the recruitment of T cells into the lesion. The mRNA levels of CXCR3 and its ligands, CXCL9-11, were significantly elevated by real-time reverse transcriptase-polymerase chain reaction in psoriatic lesions, as compared to non-lesional samples. The number of CXCR3+ cells was low in non-lesional tissues, wile the number of both epidermal and dermal CXCR3+ cells increased in lesional compared with non-lesional tissues. The majority of CXCR3+ cells were located in the dermis of the lesional skin and 74% were CD3+ T lymphocytes. A small number of CXCR3+ cells were CD68+ myeloid cells and all BDCA-2+ plasmacytoid dendritic cells were CXCR3+ (Chen et al., 2010).

Psoriasis is associated with chronic inflammation and it often coexists with inflammatory arthritis (Nestle et al., 2009) in which IL-33 has been implicated (Xu et al., 2008). IL-33 is one of the newest members of the IL-1 family of inflammatory cytokines (Castellani et al., 2009) and can mediate IgE-induced anaphylaxis in mice (Pushparaj et al., 2009). IL-33 also induces release of IL-6 from mouse bone marrow-derived cultured mast cells (Moulin et al., 2007) and IL-8 (Iikura et al., 2007). IL-33 augments SP-stimulated VEGF release from human mast cells and IL-33 gene expression is increased in lesional skin from patients with psoriasis (Theoharides et al., 2010b). Mast cells may, therefore, be involved in the pathogenesis of psoriasis and other inflammatory skin diseases. Macrophage migration inhibitory factor (MIF) is implicated in a range of pathological conditions, including asthma, rheumatoid arthritis, atherosclerosis, inflammatory bowel disease and cancer. In the field of dermatology, MIF is believed to be a detrimental factor in diseases such as systemic sclerosis, atopic dermatitis, psoriasis, eczema and UV radiation damage (Gilliver et al., 2011).

CD4+ effector cells have been categorized into four types: 1)- T helper1 cells produce IFN-γ, TNF-β, lymphotoxin and IL-10; 2)- T helper2 cells produce IL-4, IL-5, IL-10, IL-13, IL-21, IL-31; 3)- T helper3, or regulatory T-cells, produce IL-10, TGF-β and IL-35; 4)- T helper-17 cell produces IL-17, IL-17A, IL-17F, IL-21, IL-26 and CCL20. By producing IL-17 and other molecules, Th17 contributes to the pathogenesis of multiple autoimmune diseases including psoriasis, allergic inflammation, rheumatoid arthritis, autoimmune gastritis, inflammatory bowel disease and multiple sclerosis. IL-17-producing CD4+ T lymphocytes (Th17) are currently considered relevant participants in the pathogenesis of psoriasis skin lesions, together with IL-17-producing CD8+ T cells, which are also present at the psoriatic plaque, and produce TNFα and IFNγ as well as IL-17, IL-21, and IL-22. These cells are refractory to Tregs but show a proliferative response to anti-CD3/CD28 stimulation that is enhanced by IL-12 and IL-15. Blocking of TNF-α activity inhibits TCR-mediated activation and IL-17 production. CD8+IL-17+ T cells are cytotoxic cells that display TCR/CD3-mediated cytotoxic abilities to kill target cells (Ortega et al., 2009). Human Th17 cells and IL-23 play an important role, in the context of Th17 cell dependent chronic inflammation in psoriasis (Di Cesare et al., 2009). Th17 cells, is now into the centre of psoriasis pathogenesis. These cells secrete interleukin (IL)-17, IL-21 and IL-22, the latter of which appears to significantly contribute to the epidermal changes observed in this disease. Differentiation and maintenance of Th17 cells depends on IL-23 and transforming growth factor (TGFβ) secreted by activated monocytes or macrophages within the dermal compartment (Kunz, 2009). Factors such as climate, physical trauma, drug, stress and infections (Streptococcus, human immunodeficiency virus) are known to trigger psoriasis. T helper (Th) 17 mechanisms of how these cells traffic into inflamed skin are unknown. By immunostaining for interleukin (IL)-17A and IL-22, it has been shown numerous cells present in psoriasis lesions that produce these cytokines. Th17 cytokines (IL-17A, IL-22, and tumor necrosis factor (TNFα) markedly increased the expression of CC chemokine ligand (CCL)-20, a CC chemokine receptor (CCR)6 ligand, in human keratinocyte monolayer and raft cultures in a dose- and time-dependent manner. In mice that subcutaneous injection with recombinant IL-17A, IL-22, or TNF-α led to the upregulation of both CCL20 and CCR6 expression in skin as well as cutaneous T-cell infiltration. Taken together, these data show that Th17 cytokines stimulate CCL20 production in vitro and in vivo, and thus provide a potential explanation of how CCR6-positive Th17 cells maintain their continual presence in psoriasis through a positive chemotactic feedback loop (Harper et al., 2009).

The skin harbors a complex and unique immune system that protects against various pathologies, such as infection and cancer. Several cell populations are involved in this immune regulatory function, including CD4+ T cells that coexpress the transcription factor Foxp3, known as Tregs, and cells with immune-regulatory function known as myeloid-derived suppressor cells (MDSCs). Although their depletion may serve to augment immunity, expansion of these cells may be used to suppress excessive immune reactions (Ilkovitch, 2011).

Production and uptake of inducible HSP70 by keratinocytes may critically influence the chronic course of inflammatory skin diseases. Human keratinocytes release high levels of inducible heat shock protein (HSP)-70 that enhances peptide uptake. The stress-inducible chaperone HSP70 is considered a 'danger signal' if released into the extracellular environment. It has been proposed to play a role in the pathogenesis of skin diseases such as psoriasis and lupus erythematosus (LE). Living keratinocytes are an important source of HSP70 in the skin and release more HSP70 than fibroblasts, macrophages or lymphocytes. Keratinocytes also bind and internalize HSP70 / HSP70-peptide complexes a process enhanced by TNFα and IL-27. No difference with regard to HSP70 release or uptake was observable between keratinocytes from healthy donors or patients with cutaneous LE. Keratinocytes pulsed with HSP70-peptide complexes significantly increased IFNγ production by autologous T cells which influence the chronic course of inflammatory skin diseases (Wang et al., 2011).

3.4 Mast cells and natural killer cells in plaque psoriasis

Psoriasis is a common inflammatory skin disease triggered by dysregulated immune response and characterized by hyperproliferation and altered differentiation of keratinocytes, as well as mast cell accumulation and activation (Harvima et al., 2008). Mast cells are increased in lesional psoriatic skin (Özdamar et al., 1996), and have important functions as sensors of environmental and emotional stress (Paus et al., 2006; Harvima et al., 1993) possibly due to direct activation by corticotrophin release hormone (CRH) and related peptides secreted under stress (Theoharides et al., 2004; Katsarou-Katsari et al., 1999; Church & Clough 1999; Theoharides et al., 2010; Harvima et al., 1993; Fortune et al., 2005; Harvima et al., 1996). Psoriasis is associated with increased serum CRH and decreased lesional skin CRHR-1 gene expression (Tagen et al., 2007). Formation of psoriatic lesions is elicited by the complex cellular and cytokine network arising from the pathogenic interactions between keratinocytes and components of innate and acquired immune system. Natural killer T (NKT) cells are a heterogenous T-cell lineage that has been implicated in the pathogenesis of various autoimmune diseases including psoriasis. Due to the numerous functions of NKT cells that link innate and adaptive immunity, their role in psoriasis is still elusive (Peternel & Kastelan, 2009). NKT cells are best known for their ability to recognize and kill tumor cells and virally infected cells and by production of large amounts of some cytokines, such as IFNγ. In addition to the functions in cancer and autoimmunity, contributions from NK cells to allergies and various skin diseases have emerged. In patients with allergic diseases, the production of TH2 cytokines by NKT cells contributes to the known immune deviation. In patients with psoriasis, their pathophysiologic role seems to be especially the production of IFNγ. NK cell overactivation can be found in patients with alopecia areata and pemphigus vulgaris (von Bubnoff et al., 2010).

3.5 Psychosomatics, neuropeptides, central and peripheral nervous system, nerve growth factor, and skin

In the central nervous system (CNS), neuroinflammation is due to local production of IL-17 in the brain. Inflammation in various tissues is achieved by secreted IL-17, IL-17A, and IL-17 F due to their proinflammatory effects on cellular targets, which include endothelial cells, epithelial cells, fibroblasts, keratinocytes, monocytes/macrophages and osteoclasts. Under CNS inflammatory conditions, microglia, which act as antigen presenting cells, produce IL-1b and IL-23. Acting in an autocrine manner, these cytokines may further induce IL-17 expression in microglia, contributing to neuroimmune disorders. Another inflammatory pathway involving IL-17 is the IL-17-induced activation of MMP-3, which recruits neutrophils to the site of inflammation (Vojdani &, Lambert, 2009).

Outpatients experiencing exacerbation of psoriasis in the last 6 months (n = 110) were compared with outpatients affected by skin conditions in which psychosomatic factors are believed to play a minor role (n = 200). In comparison with controls the patients with psoriasis reported more stressful life events. Also, patients with psoriasis were more likely to score higher on both anxiety and avoidance attachment scale and perceived less support from their social network than did the comparison subjects (Janković et al., 2009). 32 consecutive outpatients (9 males and 23 females), age M = 43.9 with psoriasis were examined by a team of dermatologists, psychiatrists and a psychologist using a standard set of methods. In addition, 32 patients with other chronically occurring skin diseases, including 11 males and 21 females, age M = 31.6, were also examined and formed the control group. The point prevalence of mental disorders was significantly higher in the psoriatic group: 20 (62.5%) versus 5 (15.62%) in the control group. In all of the cases, affective disorders were diagnosed. Mild anxiety disorders were additionally found in 10 psoriatic patients (31.25%) and in 2 controls (6.25%). The level of depression was much higher in the study group than in the control group. Neurotic symptoms were also significantly more intense in the psoriatic group (54.37± 40.99) than in the control group (35.28±23.96). The results imply the need for the careful examination of the mental state of patients with psoriasis in order to offer and provide treatment of any concomitant psychiatric conditions (Parafianowicz et al., 2010).

Neuropeptides (Saraceno et al., 2006) especially substance P (SP) (Remröd et al., 2007) are involved in the pathogenesis of psoriasis. In particular, SP reactive fibers are localized close to mast cells (Naukkarinen et al., 1996). SP can stimulate mast cells (Kawana et al., 2006; Kandere-Grzybowska et al., 2003) and contributes to inflammation (Leeman & Ferguson, 2000; O'Connor et al., 2004). SP-positive nerve fibers are denser in psoriatic lesions and have an increased number of mast cell contacts compared to normal skin (Chan et al., 1997; Al'Abadie et al., 1995). The nervous system contributes to inflammatory skin diseases. The neuronal contribution to psoriasis at the remission and exacerbation phases were analyzed by the expression of the neuronal markers protein gene product 9.5 (PGP 9.5), growth-associatedprotein-43 (GAP-43) and substance P, in addition to its receptor (R), neurokinin-1R (NK-1R) in psoriatic skin from seven female patients at remission and exacerbation, using immunohistochemistry. The number of epidermal PGP 9.5 immunoreactive nerve fibres in the involved skin during exacerbation was decreased compared to involved skin at remission and non-involved skin at the exacerbation phase. GAP-43-positive nerve fibres were decreased in the involved skin in contrast to non-involved skin, during exacerbation. Substance P expression was seen on both immunoreactive nerve fibres and cells with a down-regulation in the number of positive nerve fibres in the involved skin compared to non-involved skin, at the exacerbation phase. The number of substance P-positive cells was slightly lower in the involved skin at exacerbation than at remission. The number of NK-1R immunoreactive cells was increased in the involved skin in contrast to non-involved skin, at the exacerbation phase. These findings suggest a crosstalk between the nervous system and inflammation during psoriasis exacerbation in the form of an altered expression of nerve fibres, substance P and its NK-1R(El-Nouretal.,2009). A contributing role of nerve growth factor (NGF) mediated neuroimmunologic mechanisms has provided a new dimension in the understanding of various cutaneous and systemic inflammatory diseases and comorbidities. Recent evidence implicates NGF as a key mediator of inflammation and pain.

NGF influences an inflammatory reaction by regulating neuropeptides, angiogenesis, cell trafficking molecules, and T cell activation. The recognition of a pathologic role of NGF and its receptor system has provided an attractive opportunity to develop a novel class of therapeutics for inflammatory diseases and chronic pain syndromes (Raychaudhuri SK, & Raychaudhuri SP , 2009). Psoriasis is characterized by keratinocyte hyperproliferation and reduced apoptosis, leading to an increased epidermal turnover. Interestingly, NGF that is both a mitogen and a survival factor for keratinocytes, is overexpressed in psoriatic lesions as well as in psoriatic keratinocytes, (Fantini et al., 1995; Raychaudhuri et al., 1998) and its high-affinity receptor TrkA, that is located only in basal keratinocytes in healthy skin, is expressed throughout all epidermal layers in psoriasis (Pincelli, 2000). On the other hand, P75NTR that plays a proapoptotic role in keratinocytes, is absent in psoriatic keratinocytes. The rate of apoptosis in psoriatic transit amplifying (TA) cells is significantly lower as compared to TA cells from normal epidermis. On the contrary, in psoriasis, NGF and Trk upregulation associated with reduced P75NTR expression result in increased keratinocyte proliferation and reduced apoptosis, thus favoring epidermal thickness, a typical feature of this dermatosis (Truzzi et al., 2011). The question of lymphocyte being an initiator of psoriatic events remains open. Plaque symmetry, stress-induced onset or exacerbations, pruritus, and possibility of generalization, suggest a role of the nervous system and neurogenic inflammation in pathogenesis. A key to understanding the role of melanocyte in psoriasis is their ability to act as regulatory cell in maintaining epidermal homeostasis. It has been suggested melanocyte, acting as a local "stress sensor", provide communicatory link between CNS and skin. The disease probably begins with so far unknown signal directed through neuronal network to the melanocyte, placed in the center of epidermal unit. That signal governs keratinocyte cellular activities and lead to reactive abnormal epidermal differentiation and hyperproliferation. Increased proliferation of basal keratinocytes and high metabolic demands creates angiogenesis in papillary dermis and elongation of dermal papillae. Stimulated melanocytes and basal keratinocytes become an important source of proinflammatory cytokines that attract lymphocytes into the dermis (Brajac et al., 2009). Pruritus involves skin surface receptors, peripheral and central nerves and specific brain regions. Peripheral unmyelinated C nerve fibres are stimulated. These nerves relay the itch signal to an ipsilateral spinal nucleus. At the same spinal level, involved nerve fibres carry the signal to the thalamus while giving off fibres to the cerebral aqueduct; the thalamus relays the signal to the somatosensory cortex. Psoriasis, has been named as the itch that scales; its importance is shown by the observation that sensory denervation leads to plaque resolution. Characteristic areas of psoriatic itch are the buttocks, extensor surfaces of the knees and elbows, and the ears and scalp. In psoriasis, 41–80% of patients have daily itch. Neuropeptide Y is inhibitory with respect to itch and decreased levels are seen in patients with psoriasis, which may explain the increased pruritus in psoriasis. Itch description varies in patients with psoriasis, ranging from stinging to burning to itch that affects sleep (Langner & Maibach, 2009)

3.5.1 Oxidative stress in skin disorders

The involvement of oxidative stress in the pathogenesis of various skin disorders has been suggested for decades. However, few clinical studies have assessed oxidative stress in skin diseases. The easiest and least invasive method to assess oxidative stress in patients may be the measurement of oxidation products in urine. Nitrate as a metabolite of nitric oxide, malondialdehyde as a major lipid oxidation product, and 8-hydroxydeoxyguanosine (8-OHdG) as a DNAoxidation marker. Urinary nitrate and 8-OHdG levels, but not malondialdehyde, were significantly higher in psoriasis patients than those in healthy controls. The severity and extent of both psoriasis and atopic dermatitis significantly correlated with urinary nitrate level and malondialdehyde level, but it did not correlate with urinary 8-OHdG level (Nakai et al., 2009). Psoriatic keratinocytes are poorly differentiated and hyperproliferative. Low concentrations of nitric oxide (NO) induce keratinocyte proliferation, while high concentrations induce differentiation. The NO-producing enzyme inducible NO synthase is overexpressed in psoriatic skin, but so is arginase. The overexpressed arginase competes for arginine, the common substrate for both enzymes, and may reduce NO production. Arginase is overactive in psoriatic skin, leading to a relative increase in the consumption of arginine (Abeyakirthi et al., 2010). Oxidative stress (OS) and increased free-radical generation have been linked to skin inflammation in psoriasis (Rashmi et al., 2009). Skin is a major target of oxidative stress mainly due to reactive oxygen species (ROS) originating from the environment and skin metabolism itself. Although endogenous antioxidants attenuate the harmful effects of ROS, increased or prolonged presence of free radicals can override ROS defense mechanisms and mediate numerous cellular responses that contribute to the development of a variety of skin disorders, including psoriasis. The cellular signaling pathways such as mitogen-activated protein kinase/activator protein 1, nuclear factor κB, and Janus kinase–signal transducers and activators of transcription are known to be redox sensitive and proven to be involved in the progress of psoriasis (Zhou et al., 2009). The skin is permanently exposed to physical, chemical, and biological aggression by the environment, and chronic inflammatory events taking place in the skin are accompanied by abnormal release of pro-oxidative mediators. Homeostatic systems are active in the skin to maintain the redox balance and also to counteract abnormal oxidative stress. There is evidence that a local and systemic redox dysregulation accompanies the chronic inflammatory disorder events associated to psoriasis, contact dermatitis, and atopic dermatitis. Several treatments for the therapy of chronic inflammatory skin disorders are based on the application of strong physical or chemical oxidants onto the skin, indicating that, in selected conditions, a further increase of the oxidative imbalance may lead to a beneficial outcome (Pastore & Korkina, 2010).

3.6 Genetics in skin psoriasis

Psoriasis is a complex inflammatory skin pathology probably of autoimmune origin. Several cell types are perturbed in this pathology, and underlying signaling events are complex and still poorly understood. Network-based analysis revealed similarities in regulation at both proteomics and transcriptomics level. A group of transcription factors are responsible for overexpression of psoriasis genes and a number of previously unknown signaling pathways may play a role in this process. Investigation of proteomics and transcriptomics data sets on psoriasis revealed versatility in regulatory machinery underlying pathology and showed complementarities between two levels of cellular organization (Piruzian et al., 2010). The linkage analysis has been used to identify multiple loci and alleles that confer risk of the disease. Some other studies have focused upon single nucleotide polymorphisms (SNPs) for mapping of probable causal variants. Other studies, using genome-wide analytical techniques, tried to link the disease to copy number variants (CNVs) that are segments of

DNA ranging in size from kilobases to megabases that vary in copy number, an important element of genomic polymorphism, predisposing to a variety of human genetic diseases. Genotyping of single nucleotide polymorphisms, copy number variations and statistical tools have become extremely important to researchers for understanding the pathogenesis and molecular mechanism of psoriasis. Microarray analysis of psoriasis patients highlights the variability in gene expression occurring between individual patients, probably on the basis of their age, ethnicity, sex, genetics, skin types and environmental influences. The gene expression data and their analyses have suggested that psoriasis is a chronic interferon-γ and T cell mediated immune disease of the skin with imbalances in epidermal cellular structures (Al Robaee, 2010). Psoriasis is a systemic disease of the skin, nails, and joints, with an acknowledged but complex genetic basis. Early genome-wide linkage studies of psoriasis focused on segregation of microsatellite markers in families; however, the only locus consistently identified resided in the MHC. Subsequently, several groups mapped this locus to the vicinity of HLA-C, and two groups have reported HLA-Cw6 itself to be the major susceptibility allele. The development of millions of SNP, coupled with the development of high-throughput genotyping platforms and a comprehensive map of human haplotypes, has made possible a genome-wide association approach using cases and controls rather than families. A collaborative genome-wide association study of psoriasis involving thousands of cases and controls revealed association between psoriasis and seven genetic loci: HLA-C, IL12B, IL23R, IL23A, IL4/IL13, TNFAIP3, and TNIP1 (Elder et al., 2010).

3.7 Infections and psoriasis

Invasive streptococcal infections may have been a factor in psoriasis becoming a common skin disease in some parts of the world. Many of the candidate genes linked to psoriasis are associated with the acquired or innate immune system, which are also important in host defence to invasive streptococcal infections. High rates of positive streptococcal throat swabs among patients with chronic plaque psoriasis suggest that they are efficient at internalizing/carrying beta-haemolytic streptococci. Internalization of streptococci in the throat is dependent upon the transforming growth factor (TGF)-β/fibronectin/α-5 β-1 integrin pathway that also appear to be operative in psoriasis. It has been postulated that some of the genotypic/phenotypic changes in different immunological pathways in psoriasis, including the acquired T-cell response, the innate immune response, the TGF-β/fibronectin/α-5 β-1 integrin pathway and the Th17 cell system, confer protection against mortality during epidemics of invasive streptococcal infections, heightened efficiency in internalizing and allowing carriage of streptococci as well as predisposition to the development of psoriasis (McFadden et al., 2009).

4. Psoriatic comorbidities

Psoriasis has been associated with a number of behavioral and systemic comorbidities, including psoriatic arthritis, anxiety, depression, obesity, hypertension, diabetes mellitus, hyperlipidemia, metabolic syndrome, smoking, cardiovascular disease, alcoholism, Crohn's disease, lymphoma, and multiple sclerosis. Many of these conditions have a similar immunologic pathogeneses. Canadian and international studies have not only confirmed the presence of these comorbidities but also have demonstrated that patients with psoriasis have a significantly reduced life span. Given that patients with psoriasis are often unaware of their comorbidities, they should be screened for these conditions and treated if required by their dermatologist and/or primary care physician. It is important to keep in mind that the comorbidities and drugs used to treat them have an impact on the choice of antipsoriatic treatment. In addition, comorbidities often preclude the use of traditional systemic agents. Recent studies have demonstrated that patients with preexisting comorbidities can be safely and effectively treated with biologic therapy. Furthermore, literature is evolving to suggest that better control of psoriasis might decrease cardiovascular mortality and prolong life (Guenther & Gulliver, 2009). In Taiwan, 51,800 psoriasis cases were identified (prevalence: 0.235%) and 17.5% of cases were severe psoriasis type. Psoriasis was associated with a significantly increased prevalence ratio (RR) for hypertension (1.51), diabetes (1.64), hyperglyceridaemia (1.61), heart disease (1.32), hepatitis B viral infection (1.73), hepatitis C viral infection (2.02), rheumatoid arthritis (3.02), systemic lupus erythematosus (6.16), vitiligo (5.94), pemphigoid (14.75), pemphigus (41.81), alopecia areata (4.71), lip, oral cavity and pharynx cancer (1.49), digestive organs and peritoneum cancer (1.57), depression (1.50), fatty liver (2.27), chronic airways obstruction (1.47), sleep disorder (3.89), asthma (1.29), and allergic rhinitis (1.25). Conversely, psoriasis was not associated with an increased risk of Crohn's disease. Psoriasis was associated with a significantly increased risk of comorbidities, especially for those patients with moderate to severe disease (Tsai et al., 2011).

Epidemiological studies have shown that, in patients with psoriasis, associated disorders may occur more frequently than expected. Such comorbidities include PsA, inflammatory bowel disease, obesity, diabetes, and cardiovascular disease (CVD), several cancer types, and depression. Comorbidities often become clinically manifest years after onset of psoriasis and tend to be more frequently seen in severe disease (Naldi & Mercuri, 2010). In particular, nonalcoholic fatty liver disease affects about 50%, Crohn's disease 0.5% and celiac disease 0.2 to 4.3% of patients with psoriasis. The presence of comorbidities has important implications in the global approach to patients. In particular, traditional systemic antipsoriatic agents could negatively affect cardio-metabolic comorbidities as well as nonalcoholic fatty liver disease and may have important interactions with drugs commonly used by psoriasis patients. Moreover, patients with psoriasis should be encouraged to drastically correct their modifiable cardiovascular and liver risk factors, in particular obesity, alcohol consumption, and smoking habit, because this could positively affect psoriasis, PsA and their life expectance (Gisondi et al., 2010). Clinical measures of disease activity were related to fatigue over time; however, these relationships disappeared in the context of patient reported physical disability and pain. Patient reported measures of physical disability, pain, and psychological distress were most closely related to higher "Modified Fatigue Severity Scale" (mFSS) scores (greater fatigue) across clinic assessments. Fatigue was found to vary over time, at least when assessed at yearly intervals. In general, measures of clinical and functional status at the current visit were more predictive of change in mFSS scores in between previous and current visits than change scores between visits. Comorbid fibromyalgia and hypertension were also associated with greater fatigue across multiple visits and with change in fatigue between visits. A combination of factors is associated with fatigue in PsA (Husted et al., 2010) .

Higher percentage frequency in PsA than psoriasis patients was found in hypertension, vascular diseases, intestinal diseases, infections, gastritis, cardiac arrhythmia, gallstones in gallbladder, osteoporosis, hyperuricemia and epilepsy. Up to 7-8 comorbidities were found in both psoriasis and PsA patients together in the same subject, thus, psoriasis is a systemic disease, induced by cytokines in all body organs, being expressed in each tissue according to genetic and environmental factors due to shared inflammatory pathways. Development of psoriasis and PsA is centered in the blood vessels behavior. Both diseases start by proliferation of blood vessels after up-regulation of VEGF, TGFβ and other angiogenic factors. Clinical remission in psoriatic lesions also starts by decrease proliferation of blood vessels, after treatment with leishmania antigens (O'Daly, 2011, manuscript in press).

4.1 Cardiovascular disease

Psoriasis and atherosclerosis are interrelated; pathogenic mechanisms are shared between the two diseases inducing inflammation. Within the lymph nodes, antigen-presenting cells activate naive T-cells to increase expression of LFA-1 following which activated T-cells migrate to blood vessel and adhere to endothelium. Extravasation occurs mediated by LFA-1, LFA-3 and ICAM-1 or CD2. Activated T-cells interact with dendritic cells, macrophages and keratinocytes in psoriasis or with smooth muscle cells in blood vessels, in atherosclerosis. These cells further secrete chemokines and cytokines that contribute to the inflammatory environment, resulting in the formation of psoriatic plaque or atherosclerotic plaque (Ghazizadeh et al., 2010). Patients with psoriasis are at increased risk for severe vascular disease (Shelling *et al.*, 2008). This increased risk is imparted by both a predilection for patients with psoriasis to have traditional vascular disease risk factors like diabetes, hypertension, smoking, dyslipidemia (Federman *et al.*, 2009) and the recognition that psoriasis itself is an independent risk factor for vascular disease (Gelfand *et al.*, 2011). The latter is probably mediated by systemic inflammation associated with psoriasis, similar to that observed in patients with rheumatoid arthritis. Patients whose psoriasis develops at a young age and those with more severe disease are at the greatest risk (Gelfand *et al.*, 2011). Initial psoriasis comorbidity studies focused on cardiovascular disease, but atherosclerosis is a systemic disease (Prodanovich *et al.*, 2009). It is reasonable to postulate that if the likelihood of myocardial infarction is increased in patients with psoriasis, other manifestations of atherosclerosis, such as stroke, might also be more common in these patients. Stroke is a leading cause of mortality, and many who survive experience functional disability, with up to 30% being permanently disabled and 20% requiring institutional care (Rosamond *et al.*, 2008; Rico et al., 2009). A cohort study of patient's ≥18 years from 1987 to 2002, were analyzed. Patients with a psoriasis code and a history of systemic therapy consistent with severe psoriasis (n=3603) were compared with patients with no history of psoriasis (n=14,330). Patients with severe psoriasis were at increased risk of death from cardiovascular disease hazard ratio (HR) (1.57), malignancies (1.41), chronic lower respiratory disease (2.08), diabetes (2.86), dementia (3.64), infection (1.65), kidney disease (4.37), and unknown/missing causes (1.43). The absolute and excess risk of death was highest for cardiovascular disease (61.9 and 3.5 deaths per 1000 patient-years, respectively). Severe psoriasis is associated with an increased risk of death from a variety of causes, with cardiovascular death being the most common aetiology (Abuabara et al., 2010).

Psoriasis patients of a health-maintenance organization were compared with enrollees without psoriasis regarding the prevalence of hypertension in a case-control study. The study included 12,502 psoriasis patients over the age of 20 years and 24,285 age- and sex-frequency-matched controls. The prevalence of hypertension was significantly higher in psoriasis patients than controls (38.8% vs. 29.1%, respectively). In a multivariate analysis, hypertension was associated with psoriasis after controlling for age, sex, smoking status, obesity, diabetes, non-steroidal anti-inflammatory drugs (NSAIDs) and use of Cox-2 inhibitors (odds ratio: 1.37). The results of this study support the previously noted association between psoriasis and hypertension (Cohen et al., 2010).

Treatment with multiple anti-hypertensives was significantly associated with the presence of psoriasis using univariate and multivariable analysis, after adjusting for diabetes, hyperlipidemia, and race. Compared to hypertensive patients without psoriasis, psoriasis patients with hypertension were 5 times more likely to be on a monotherapy antihypertensive regimen, 9.5 times more likely to be on dual antihypertensive therapy, 16.5 times more likely to be on triple antihypertensive regimen, and 19.9 times more likely to be on quadruple therapy or centrally-acting agent in multivariable analysis, after adjusting for traditional cardiac risk factors. Psoriasis patients appear to have more difficult-to-control hypertension compared to non-psoriatic, hypertensive patients (Armstrong et al., 2011).

The cardiovascular risk factors in patients with psoriasis and the association between psoriasis and coronary artery, cerebrovascular, and peripheral vascular diseases was examined. Similar to previous studies, it was found higher prevalence of diabetes mellitus, hypertension, dyslipidemia, and smoking in patients with psoriasis. After controlling for these variables, a higher prevalence not only of ischemic heart disease but also of cerebrovascular and peripheral vascular diseases in patients with psoriasis compared with controls. Psoriasis was also found to be an independent risk factor for mortality. Psoriasis is associated with atherosclerosis. This association applies to coronary artery, cerebrovascular, and peripheral vascular diseases and results in increased mortality (Prodanovich et al., 2009). Patients with psoriasis (N = 4752) between 1999 and 2001 and patients without a diagnosis of psoriasis (N = 23,760) who were matched by age and sex to the patients with psoriasis were analyzed. Of the total sample, 70 patients (0.2%) had acute myocardial infarct (AMI) during the 5-year follow-up period: 22 (0.5% of the patients with psoriasis) from the study cohort and 48 (0.2%) from the comparison cohort. The hazard of AMI during the 5-year follow-up period was 2.10 times greater for patients with psoriasis than for comparison patients (Lin et al., 2011).The event rates and rate ratios (RRs) of cardiovascular death, myocardial infarct (MI), coronary revascularization, stroke and a composite of MI, stroke and cardiovascular death were increased in patients with psoriasis. The RRs increased with disease severity and decreased with age of onset. The risk was similar in patients with severe skin affection alone and those with PsA (Ahlehoff et al., 2010). Patients with psoriasis have an increased prevalence of major cardiovascular (CV) risk factors and a clinically significant increased risk of myocardial infarction, stroke, and CV death that is independent of conventional risk factors (Gelfand *et al.*, 2011). These epidemiological studies have led to the recognition that psoriasis may be a systemic inflammatory disorder (Davidovici *et al.*, 2010). Two recent studies have added to this previously summarized literature. First, Ahlehoff *et al.* (2010), in a nationwide Danish study of 34,371 people with mild psoriasis and 2,621 with severe psoriasis, demonstrated independent risk ratios (RRs) for CV death of 1.14 and 1.57 respectively, with the greatest increase in young people ages 18–50, RR 2.98, with severe disease. The authors also compared CV risks in patients with severe psoriasis with the risks in patients with diabetes mellitus and found comparable increases in major adverse CV events and CV deaths in these groups, demonstrating the clinical importance of the risk of CV disease attributable to psoriasis. Other recent studies have investigated the clinical significance of CV risk in patients with severe psoriasis, demonstrating that these patients have about a 6-year reduction in life expectancy and that excess risk of CV death is the largest contributor to this premature mortality (Abuabara *et al.*, 2010; Gelfand et al., 2011)

4.2 Metabolic syndrome

Psoriasis is associated with metabolic syndrome, cardiovascular disease, and osteoporosis and may be considered a systemic disease (Nijsten & Wakkee, 2009). The metabolic syndrome is the constellation of abdominal obesity, dyslipidemia, hypertension and insulin resistance. Presence of the metabolic syndrome significantly increases a patient's risk for cardiovascular disease, stroke and type II diabetes. Recent studies have found that psoriasis patients are at increased risk for metabolic syndrome as well as the individual components of metabolic syndrome, and the two diseases appear linked through a common mechanism of inflammation. Psoriasis treatments have been shown to reduce the risk of developing metabolic syndrome components and comorbidities (Alsufyani et al., 2010). The prevalence of obesity in psoriatic patients within the "Utah Psoriasis Initiative" (UPI) population was higher than that in the general Utah population. Obesity appears to be the consequence of psoriasis and not a risk factor for onset of disease. It was not observed an increased risk for PsA in patients with obesity; furthermore, obesity did not affect the response or adverse effects of topical corticosteroids, light based treatments, and systemic medications. The prevalence of smoking in the UPI population was higher than in the general Utah population and higher than in the non-psoriatic population. It was found a higher prevalence of smokers in the obese population within the UPI than in the obese population within the Utah population (Herron et al., 2005)

5. Psoriasis treatments

Psoriasis is an inflammatory skin disease with a chronic relapsing course. In about 20%–30% of psoriatic patients, disease severity requires systemic treatment, which carries a huge economic and management burden for the healthcare system. The decision to employ systemic treatment, reserved for severe or extensive forms, needs to be weighed carefully and is influenced by factors from the host. Traditional treatments like: photochemotherapy, cyclosporin A, methotrexate, and acitretin, should be evaluated for each specific clinical condition (Altomare et al., 2009). Psoriasis is important to the clinician because it is common and has treatment implications beyond the care of skin lesions. It is important to the physician-scientist because it serves as a model for studies of mechanisms of chronic inflammation. It is important to the clinical-trial investigator because it is increasingly a first-choice disease indication for proof-of-principle studies of new pathogenesis-based therapeutic strategies. In recent years, advances have been made in elucidating the molecular mechanisms of psoriasis. However, major issues remain unresolved, including the primary nature of the disease as an epithelial or immunologic disorder, the autoimmune cause of the inflammatory process, the relevance of cutaneous versus systemic factors, and the role of genetic versus environmental influences on disease initiation, progression, and response to therapy. (Nestle et al., 2009). Psoriasis may lead to disability and significant effects on patients' quality of life. A challenge in psoriasis management is to use an effective therapy early in the disease course in order to achieve a safe and well tolerated maintenance of remission with an improvement of both skin and joint manifestations. Recent advances in knowledge of the pathogenesis of psoriasis helped develop targeted treatment options that may be effective and well tolerated over long periods of administration, thus improving the patient's quality of life. These biologic agents specifically target tumor necrosis factor-α (infliximab, etanercept, and adalimumab) or T cells (efalizumab) (de Felice et al., 2009).

Immune modulating therapies gain increasing importance in treatment of patients with autoimmune diseases such as psoriasis. None of the currently applied biologics achieves significant clinical improvement in all treated patients. In an open label study, 20 psoriasis patients were treated weekly with Alefacept over 12 wk. Transcription of the tolerance-associated gene (TOAG-1) is significantly up-regulated whereas receptor for hyaluronic acid mediated migration (RHAMM) transcription is down-regulated in PBMCs of responding patients before clinical improvement. TOAG-1 is exclusively localized within mitochondria. Overexpression of TOAG-1 in murine T cells leads to increased susceptibility to apoptosis. Addition of Alefacept to stimulated human T cells in vitro resulted in reduced frequencies of activated CD137+ cells, increased TOAG-1 but reduced RHAMM expression. This was accompanied by reduced proliferation and enhanced apoptosis. Inhibition of proliferation was dependent on enhanced PDL1 expression of APCs. Thus, peripheral changes of TOAG-1 and RHAMM expression can be used to predict clinical response to Alefacept treatment in psoriasis patients. In the presence of APCs Alefacept can inhibit T cell activation and survival by increasing expression of TOAG-1 on T cells and PDL1 on APCs (Keeren et al., 2009).

People with mild to moderate chronic plaque psoriasis after 3 months had no significant difference in the reduction PASI score between classic acupuncture vs. sham acupuncture (Jerner et al., 1997). Significantly more people (64%) having a thermal bath (bicarbonate, calcium, and magnesium rich water) had improvement in PASI score at 3 months compared with people (11%) having tap water bath (Zumiani et al., 2000).

All the data from here on have been referenced in a deep analysis of treatments for psoriasis performed in an excellent review by Naldi & Rzany, 2009, a summary follows: Fish oil and effects of psychotherapy reported inconclusive results with chronic plaque psoriasis. Tazarotene, a topical retinoid, may be more effective in the short term (6–12 weeks) at improving symptoms of mild to moderate chronic plaque psoriasis. Vitamin D derivatives (topical) were more effective at improving psoriasis severity scores at 3–8 weeks. Different types of vitamin D derivatives compared with each other revealed Calcipotriol may be more effective than tacalcitol and calcitriol at reducing psoriasis severity scores at 8 weeks. Calcipotriol may be more effective at prolonging time to relapse in people with stable psoriasis for at least 3 months after prior treatment with methotrexate for 6 months. Dithranol may be more effective at improving psoriasis severity scores at 4–8 weeks. Emollients plus UVB radiation compared with UVB alone and oil-in-water emollient plus UVB radiation may temporarily be more effective at improving psoriasis at 12 weeks. There is consensus that they are effective, and are mostly used initially or as adjunctive treatment in people with chronic plaque psoriasis. Salicylic acid may be no more effective at improving psoriasis severity scores at 3 weeks. There is consensus that keratolytics are a useful adjunct to other treatments for psoriasis Topical corticosteroids applied less frequently may be more effective at maintaining clear or nearly cleared areas at 6 months but they may cause striae and atrophy, which increase with potency and use of occlusive dressings. Continuous use may lead to adrenocortical suppression, and case reports suggest that severe flares of the disease may occur on withdrawal. Coal tar plus fatty acids is no more effective at 8 weeks at improving composite scores for erythema, desquamation, and infiltration in people with mild to moderate chronic plaque psoriasis. Goeckerman treatment compared with UVB irradiation alone. Goeckerman treatment (daily application of coal tar followed by UVB irradiation) may be no more effective at improving response rates in people with chronic plaque psoriasis. Compared with no intervention Heliotherapy may be more effective at improving symptom severity scores at 1 year in people with all forms of chronic plaque psoriasis severities. There is consensus that heliotherapy is an effective option for most people with chronic plaque psoriasis. Different doses of psoralen in PUVA regimens compared with each other. Higher doses of psoralen are more effective at increasing clearance of lesions in people with severe psoriasis. Maintenance treatment with PUVA is more effective at reducing relapses at 18 months in people whose psoriasis has been cleared with prior PUVA treatment. Long-term adverse effects of PUVA treatment include photoaging and skin cancer, mainly squamous cell carcinoma. Narrowband UVB and broadband UVB may be equally effective at increasing clearance rates. Twice-weekly and three times-weekly administration of ultraviolet light are equally effective at increasing clearance rates, but twice-weekly treatment prolongs the time to reach clearance in people with mild to moderate psoriasis. Compared with placebo UVA sun bed treatment may be more effective than visible light at improving psoriasis severity scores in people with mild to moderate chronic stable plaque psoriasis. Alefacept is more effective at increasing the proportion of people with a reduction in psoriasis severity scores at 12 weeks. The FDA issued a Medical Product Safety Alert to inform people that alefacept reduces CD4+ T lymphocyte counts and should not be given to people with HIV. Efalizumab is more effective at increasing the proportion of people who achieve an improvement in psoriasis severity scores at 12 weeks in moderate to severe psoriasis. The FDA issued a warning about Raptiva (efalizumab) to healthcare professionals and patients about reports of immune mediated haemolytic anaemia, and warnings regarding post-marketing reports of thrombocytopenia and serious infections including necrotising fasciitis, tuberculous pneumonia, bacterial sepsis with seeding of distant sites, severe pneumonia with neutropenia, and worsening of infection (e.g. cellulitis, pneumonia) despite antimicrobial treatment. Raptiva (efalizumab) has a potential risk of developing progressive multifocal leukoencephalopathy. Efalizumab is a humanised monoclonal antibody which targets the CD11a component of lymphocyte function-associated antigen-1. It is a relatively new drug for the treatment of psoriasis. Efalizumab has been associated in some cases with fatal brain infections and has been withdrawn from the market (Major, 2010). Etanercept is more effective at increasing the proportion of people with improved psoriasis severity scores at 12–24 weeks in people with moderate to severe psoriasis. A drug safety alert has been issued on the risk of opportunistic fungal infections of lymphoma and other malignancies in children and adolescents associated with TNF-α blockers, which could be fatal. Etanercept is a recombinant molecule consisting of the human TNF-α p75 receptor fused to the Fc portion of the human immunoglobulin G1 molecule.

Infliximab is more effective at increasing the proportion of people who achieve an improvement in psoriasis severity scores at 10 weeks in people with moderate to severe psoriasis. A drug safety alert has been issued on the risk of opportunistic fungal infection of lymphoma and other malignancies in children and adolescents, and the risks of leukaemia and new onset psoriasis. Infliximab is a monoclonal antibody that binds to and inhibits the activity of TNF-α. Compared with placebo Adalimumab is more effective at increasing the proportion of people with moderate to severe psoriasis who achieve an improvement in severity scores at 12 weeks. Drug safety alerts have been issued on the risk of hepatosplenic T-cell lymphoma associated with adalimumab and the risk of opportunistic fungal infections associated with TNF-α which could be fatal. A drug safety alert has been issued on the increased risk of lymphoma and other malignancies in children and adolescents, and the risks of leukaemia and new onset psoriasis, associated with TNF-α blockers. Ciclosporin may be more effective at 10 weeks at increasing lesion clearance and at reducing psoriasis severity scores in people with severe psoriasis. Conventional oil-based ciclosporin and microemulsion preconcentrate are equally effective at increasing the proportion of people achieving a marked response. Ciclosporin is more effective at increasing the proportion of people who remain in remission. Ciclosporin has been associated with hypertension, renal dysfunction and increased risk of malignancies for up to 5 years. Ciclosporin is an established treatment option for moderate to severe psoriasis. Relapses are often seen on withdrawal, and long-term treatment is limited by adverse effects. Dimethylfumaric acid alone or mixed with monoethyl fumaric acid may be more effective at 16 weeks at reducing psoriasis severity scores in people with severe psoriasis. Oral fumaric acid plus calcipotriol may be more effective at improving psoriasis scores at 13 weeks in people with severe chronic plaque psoriasis. Fumaric acid esters have been associated with flushing and with gastrointestinal symptoms.

Methotrexate may be more effective at reducing the surface area of psoriasis at 12 weeks in people with psoriatic arthritis, but has been associated with acute myelosuppression. Long-term methotrexate carries the risk of hepatic fibrosis and cirrhosis, which is related to the dose regimen employed. People using methotrexate are closely monitored for liver toxicity and are advised to limit their consumption of alcohol. The most reliable test of liver damage remains needle biopsy of the liver. When treatment was stopped, 45% of people experienced a full relapse within 6 months. Acitretin and etretinate are equally effective at increasing the proportion of people who achieve a marked improvement as measured by a reduction in psoriasis severity scores. Teratogenicity renders oral retinoids less acceptable. Etretinate is no longer available in many countries. Leflunomide may be more effective in people with psoriatic arthritis at increasing the proportion of people with a reduction in psoriasis symptom severity scores at 24 weeks. Leflunomide significantly increased the proportion of people with at least a 75% improvement in PASI but had diarrhoea (24% with leflunomide vs. 13% with placebo). More people taking leflunomide had increased liver enzymes and tiredness lethargy (alanine transaminase increase of at least 2 times the upper limit of normal:12% with leflunomide v 5% with placebo; tiredness/lethargy: 6% with leflunomide vs. 1% with placebo). Pimecrolimus significantly improved PASI at 12 weeks, but with higher rates of gastrointestinal disorders, pruritus, and paraesthesia in the pimecrolimus groups compared with the placebo group (Naldi & Rzany, 2009).

5.1 Treatment with drug product Leismania amastigotes vaccine

While treating subjects in Venezuela with a vaccine containing *Leishmania* amastigotes antigens for prevention of cutaneous leishmaniasis (CL), (O'Daly et al., 1995a, 1995b) we observed 100% clinical remission of a psoriatic lesion in one subject, a natural double blind serendipity finding. A first generation polyvalent vaccine (AS100-1) was manufactured with protein from four cultured *Leishmania* species: *L(L)amazonensis, L(V)brasiliensis, L(L)chagasi and L(L)venezuelensis* (O'Daly et al., 2009a).

5.2 Characterization of the amastigotes drug product

Protein test samples from the amastigote extracts of the four *Leishmania* spp. present in AS100-1 were tested for the presence of Leishmania DNA. PCR reactions for amplification of the variable regions of kDNA minicircles of Leishmania were performed to confirm the absence or presence of parasite DNA in the polyvalent AS100-1 final drug product. DNA isolated from Leishmania amastigote parasites were used as positive controls. No PCR product was detected in the AS100-1 protein samples. As expected, agarose gel electrophoresis of the 610 and 116pb fragments showed presence of DNA in the positive controls. Additional PCR sequencing from the positive controls showed 92% identity with the kinetoplast DNA minicircles. Lipophosphoglycan (LPG) is a glycoconjugate present on metacyclic promastigotes, which functions as a virulence factor in all *Leishmania* spp. The final product of amastigotes extracts after TLCK treatment and NP40 surface antigen extraction, had 10 ng/m or less of LPG. The acceptable endotoxin limit for the drug substance was 700 EU/ml. A sample of the drug substance was screened for endotoxin content with results <50 EU/ml but >25 EU/ml. well below the acceptable limit. BSA was between 12.5 and 25.0 ng/ml, evidence that no fetal bovine serum (FBS) proteins from the culture medium were present. SDS acrylamide gels of AS100-1 drug product under reducing conditions exhibited 23-30 bands from 112.0 to 10.0 kDa molecular weight in the four *Leishmania* spp.; 21 bands (70%) with similar molecular weights (value variations 1% or less) in all lots. The percent homology between lots of the same specie was *L(L)amazonensis* 96.6%; *L(V)brasiliensis* 86.7%; *L(L)chagasi* 95.8%; *L(L)venezuelensis* 91.3% (O'Daly et al., 2009a).

5.3 Clinical trial with amastigote antigens vaccine

A double-blind, placebo-controlled, parallel group study, of multiple doses of AS100-1 was performed on psoriatic subjects, to confirm safety and efficacy. Treatment of plaque psoriasis, was conducted in 2,770 volunteers and included plaque (79%), guttate (10%), plaque and guttate (10%), palm/plantar (0.3%), erythrodermia (1.8%), inverse (0.8%), plaque and arthritis (3.4%) and nail psoriasis (0.3%). Eficacy of AS100-1 was assessed by performing skin examinations and recording psoriasis area and severity index (PASI) parameters at each visit. The primary eficacy parameters were the percentage reduction in PASI score at each visit and the comparative proportions of subjects with 100, 75 and 50% PASI improvement in each treatment group. The lesions and the extent of body surface area involved were measured separately for the head (Ah), trunk (At), upper extremities (Au) and lower extremities (Al). The PASI combines lesion measurements of the skin erythema, (E, redness), skin induration (I, thickness) and skin desquamation (D, scaliness) of the lesions. Each sign in the lesion was quantified as follows: 0 none, 1 slight, 2 mild, 3 moderate and 4 severe. The extent of body surface area affected was evaluated as follows: 1 < 10%, 2 = 10–30%, 3 = 30–50%, 4 = 50–70%, 5 = 70–90%, 6 > 90%. For evaluation purposes, the weighted contribution of each section of the body to the total body surface area is as follows, the head 10%, the thorax 30%, the upper extremities 20% and the lower extremities 40%. To calculate disease severity, the following formula was applied: $PASI = 0.1(Eh + Ih + Dh)Ah + 0.3(Et + It +$

Dt)At +0.2(Eu + Iu + Du)Au + 0.4(El + Il + Dl)Al. PASI scores rise or fall in units of tenths (0.1) and range from 0.0 to 72.0. A score of 0.0 indicates absence of lesions, while a score of 72.0 represents the malignant form of the disease (erythrodermia). Body surface area involvement of over 10% or a PASI score greater than 10.0–12.0 is used as a criterion for severe disease. Percent PASI reduction was calculated as follows: (PASI at base line – PASI at each visit)/PASI at baseline* 100. Baseline PASI compared with post-treatment values were: PASI 100, 23%; PASI 75, 45%; PASI 50, 13%; PASI 10, 9%; <PASI 10, 3% while 7% quit treatment. Of the 648 subjects (23%) who experienced total remission of lesions, 188 (29%) had relapses of their disease after 15.4 months. The PASI values at the time of the first relapse were 7.7 units, one-third of the PASI value (21.0 units) recorded before any treatment. The new remission occurred with 7.1 doses of AS100 after 5.8 weeks, a shorter time period than initially observed in the first treatment cycle for clinical remission of lesions. In the relapsing group, 161 of the 188 subjects (85.6%) experienced new remission of lesions after six to seven doses of AS100 (O'Daly et al., 2009a).

There were no serious adverse events attributed to the treatment drug. Some patients with PsA benefited after treatment (see below). Of the 2,770 subjects treated in the open label psoriasis study, a random group of 108 subjects was selected for antibody screening. The test group included a positive control group with active CL, a negative control group before treatment and subgroups with one to six doses of the immunotherapeutic agent. All subjects received 500 µg/dose of AS100-1. The concurrent negative control group (n = 36) consisted of psoriatic subjects, prior to any AS100-1 treatment, with no previous history of Leishmania infection, no prior exposure to AS100-1 and with a negative delayed type hypersensitivity (DTH) to Leishmania antigens. All subgroups with one to six doses of AS100-1 in the treatment group had the same results as the negative control group, exhibiting antibody values between 30 and 87 ng/ml; well below 100 ng/ml, the cutoff value to consider a reaction as positive. It is also interesting to note that after four doses of AS100-1, all subjects had undetectable levels of antibodies (ELISA), but a positive DTH cellular response to AS100-1 after intradermic reaction (IDR) ≥10 mm in diameter with Leishmania antigens. These results suggest that the AS100-1 drug product does not induce significant humoral immunity but a strong cellular immunity. Approximately 2,289 subjects (83%) experienced at least one adverse event (AE). The most frequent AE were injection site related, and included the following, pain 43%, nodule formation 23%, heat 21% and erythema 14%. The injection sites were assessed after each administration of the study drug. Injection site related AE, were relatively short lived, lasting between 24 to 72 h. The types of systemic AE and their rates of occurrence were as follows: fever 18%, general discomfort 12%, a flulike syndrome 11%, pruritus 8%, sleepiness 8%, accidental injury 8%, cough 6%, dizziness 6%. AE attributed to the treatment drug were rated mild or moderate in severity, with none being classified as serious. The few severe adverse events that occurred were attributed to other diseases, the subjects were experiencing while participating in the study trial. There were no age or gender diferences observed for AE, and no deaths occurred during the study. All adverse events resolved without intervention, usually within 24–72 h. (O'Daly et al., 2009a).

To determine the effective factor, a single blind trial with four monovalent second generation vaccines (AS100-2) was performed. The AS100-2 trial was a single blind AS100-1 controlled trial with four treatment groups one for each AS1002 vaccine (AS1002-amazonensis, AS1002-brasiliensis, AS1002-chagasi, and AS1002-venezuelensis). The trial included 26 subjects, 58% females, average 43.8±16.4 years old, and age range 8–76 years, initial PASI 10.2± 6.6 units, time with psoriasis 12.2±13.1 years. The treatment subjects received 500 µg/ dose injections of AS100-2 and control subjects received 500 µg/dose of AS100-1. The results achieved with monovalent AS100-2 produced reductions in psoriatic lesions similar to those induced by polyvalent AS100-1. AS100-2 vaccines were further purified, resulting in seven chromatography fractions (AS200) per species. AS100-2, and AS200 final product, gave the following results for LPG and endotoxin: LPG: 10 ng/ml or less; Endotoxin: <50 EU/ml but >25 EU/ml. Parasitic DNA was absent in all products and BSA was between 12.5 and 25.0 ng/ml, basically within the same range, as previously published AS100-1 values. No carbohydrates were found in AS100-1, AS100-2 or Lb fractions by HPLC analysis or staining of gels with PAS-SCHIFF (O'Daly et al., 2009b).

Subsequently, a single-blind trial in 55 subjects treated with a third generation vaccine AS200 prepared with seven DEAE chromatography fractions from *L(V)brasiliensis* was performed. The AS200 study was a single-blind, AS100-1 controlled trial, with a seven arm treatment group, one for each AS200 (Lb) vaccine. The AS200 trial included 53 subjects, 62% females average 40.6±18.6 years old, age range 7–78 years of age, initial PASI 26.4±19.2, time with psoriasis 15.0±12 years.The treatment subjects received four 200 µg/dose injections of AS200 (Lb) and control subjects received four 500 µg/dose of AS100-1. However, treatment with the vaccine containing fraction 7 was discontinued due to general discomfort and psoriasis flare subsequent to vaccination in one subject. All subjects had PASI scores determined prior to treatment, prior to each injection, and at follow-up for 2 weeks after the last injection. All AS200 (Lb) vaccines induced PASI reductions in the same range as the active control. Protein (DEAE) fractions 2, 3, 4, and 5 had similar values and induced the highest in vitro lymphocyte stimulation index (SI) values in peripheral blood mononuclear cells (PBMC) from post-treatment PASI100% reduction subjects, with no statistical differences among them. The same fractions, from *L(V)brsiliensis* and *L(L)chagasi* species, also yielded the highest IDR diameter in DTH screenings. All leishmania DEAE fractions stimulated lymphocytes from PBMC from patients in vitro, after vaccination wit AS100-1, none were immunosuppressors, contrary to all treatment in the market today (O'Daly et al., 2009b).

Long-term heat shock proteins (Hsp) confrontation of the immune system similar in the host and invaders may convert the immune response against these host antigens and promote and/or decrease autoimmune diseases including psoriasis (Boyman et al., 2005; Rajesh Rajaiah & Moudgil, 2009; Rambukkana et al., 1993). There is evidence that recognition of self-Hsp60 can have beneficial effects in arthritis and may offer new strategies for improved control measures in the inflammatory processes by administration of peptides cross-reactive to self-determinants (Zügel & Kaufmann, 1999). Hsp60, Hsp70, Gp96 function as host-derived ligands for toll like receptors (TLR2), and have been described to play a role in the pathogenesis of RA and psoriasis (Rajesh Rajaiah & Moudgil 2009). Leishmania antigens are produced after a heat shock in promastigotes that become amastigotes in a liquid culture medium (O'Daly & Rodríguez, 1988). The molecular weight of AS200 is similar to the range of most Hsp host ligands (50–70 kDa) and could be inhibiting the symptoms of psoriasis, psoriatic arthritis and CIA by competing with peptides in the respective receptors (O'Daly et al., 2009a, 2009b, 2010a, 2011).

Two male subjects, both HIV+; 36 and 41 years of age, with plaque psoriasis for 4 years in one subject and 7 months in the other were treated with AS100-1. Both subjects had no familial history of psoriasis, and were treated with AS100-1 concurrently with their previously prescribed retroviral treatments. The AS100-1 treatment consisted of 500 μg/dose, injected in the deltoid area, every 2 weeks. Baseline PASI for one subject was 26.4 units, while the other subject presented with a baseline PASI of 32.4 units. Both subjects showed clinical remission of psoriasis after treatment with AS100-1. The hematologic values with respect to total lymphocytes (CD3, CD4, and CD8 cells) were lower than the values routinely found in healthy subjects. One subject had a relapse after the ninth dose and subsequently received a second course of treatment 3 weeks later. The second course resulted in clinical remission of the psoriatic lesions. Neither of these two subjects presented local adverse events nor did they present any systemic adverse events after vaccination (O'Daly et al., 2009b).

5.4 Cellular immunity in guinea pigs and regression of lesions in experimental Rheumatoid Arthritis model with amastigote antigens vaccine

AS200 *Leishmania* antigenic fractions induced linear DTH reactions in guinea pigs over a 1-40 μg dose range. This finding allowed us to build a potency assay for the drug product. Interestingly, RA, another autoimmune disease, shares several similarities with psoriasis and PsA. While some diseases lack acceptable animal models for adequate study, this is not the case with RA. Collagen induced arthritis (CIA) is an experimental animal model that has been used to dissect the pathogenesis of human RA. The model is dependent on activated T cells, is associated with both cell mediated and humoral immunity to collagen and can be induced upon immunization with heterologous collagen II (CII) or by monoclonal antibodies to CII combined with LPS in DBA/1 mice. When a DBA-1 mouse CIA model was used to compare AS200 treatment against: a polyvalent vaccine (AS100-1), a monovalent vaccine (AS100-2) and placebo, the AS200 treated mice had the least amount of forepaw inflammation and the lowest mean arthritis scores (O'Daly et al., 2010a).

5.5 Lympocyte subsets in peripheral blood monocuclear cells of psoriatic patients, before and after treatment with amastigote polyvalent vaccine

Peripheral blood mononuclear cells (PBMC) collected from subjects prior to treatment and post-treatment with AS100-1 were analyzed by flow cytometry. Lymphocyte subsets (LS) varied with PASI range (1-10, 11-20 and 21-72). Pretreatment absolute values of gated LS were as follows: CD4+CD8-, CD3+CD8-, CD8+CD3+, CD8+CD4- and CD8+HLA- decreased in PBMC as PASI increased, suggesting migration from the blood to the skin. Contrary to the previous finding, the following LS, CD8+HLA+, HLA+CD8-, CD8+CD4+, CD19, and membrane surface immunoglobulin IgA+, IgD+ and IgM+ increased in PBMC as PASI increased, suggesting activation and proliferation by unknown antigens in the skin lesions. After treatment with seven doses of AS100-1, the following LS, CD3+CD8-, CD8+CD3-, HLA+CD8-, CD8+HLA+ and CD4+CD8-, increased as PASI returns to normal values and psoriatic plaques disappeared, while CD8+CD3+, CD8+HLA-, CD19 and CD8+CD4+ decreased in PBMC suggesting lower sensitization in skin. Lymphocyte trafficking from blood to skin decreased significantly, stopping the vicious cycle as psoriasis lesions disappeared (O'Daly et al., 2010b). Previously we demonstrated that leishmania antigens induced T cell proliferation and absence of immunosuppression after stimulating PBMC from psoriatic patients with amastigote fractions. DTH positive reactions were found with isolated amastigote antigens in humans in vivo, after treatment with AS100-1 polyvalent vaccine. These facts of *in vivo* and *in vitro* T cells stimulation (O'Daly et al., 2009b) suggest that variations in blood LS, before and after treatment in psoriatic subjects, is a function of lymphocyte trafficking from blood to skin and vice versa, as well as T cell activation in skin plaques, not to killing of T cells as has been described with current treatments used in psoriatic patients.

6. Psoriatic arthritis

The first description of PsA is attributed to Louis Aliberti, who in 1818 first noted the relationship between psoriasis and arthritis (O'Neill & Silman, 1994). Pierre Bazin then described "Psoriasis Arthritique" in 1860, followed by Charles Bourdillon in 1888 with "Psoriasis et Arthropathies". Jeghers and Robinson in 1937, and Vilanova and Piñol in 1951 described PsA as a unique entity (Vilanova & Pinol, 1951). All studies of PsA use the criteria by Moll and Wright in their classic paper published in 1973 (Moll & Wright, 1973) summarized as follows: A- presence of psoriasis, B- inflammatory arthritis and C- negative test for rheumatoid factor. The PsA subgroups described with these criteria were: 1- Distal interphalangeal (DIP) joint disease (5%); 2- Asymmetrical oligoarthritis (70%); 3- Polyarthritis (15%); 4- Spondylitis (5%); 5- Arthritis mutilans (5%), (Wright 1956, 1959a, 1959b). Gladman expanded the five sub-groups to seven: Distal disease (DIP only affected), oligoarthritis (<4 joints), polyarthritis, spondylitis only, distal disease plus spondylitis, oligoarthritis plus spondylitis and polyarthritis plus spondylitis (Gladman et al., 1987).

6.1 Psoriasis artritis epidemiology

Psoriasis is widely diffused in the World. Its average prevalence is about 3-4%. This is probably an underestimate, for it is mostly based on self-reports. In fact, on the one hand minimal psoriasis, e.g. nail disease, could remain undiagnosed; on the other, precise classification criteria for PsA are lacking and the skin disease is often of elusive nature. The frequency of PsA may be higher than commonly believed, as suggested by recent studies reporting a prevalence of up to 0.42%. There are no major differences in the frequency of psoriasis between sexes, or specific time trends (Cimmino, 2007). Prevalence of PsA varies from 5-40% in several trials. A large study conducted in the UK, Italy, France, Spain and Germany in 2006 found 8.1% prevalence of PsA in patients with psoriasis. Survival analysis indicated that the incidence of PsA among plaque psoriasis patients remained constant at 74 per 100 person-years, while the prevalence increased with time since diagnosis of psoriasis, reaching 20.5% after 30 years (Christophers et al., 2010). A population based study in Minnesota USA, reported the annual incidence of PsA per 100,000 to be 7.2. The incidence increased from 3.6 between 1970 and 1979, to 9.8 between 1990 and 2000, providing the first evidence that the incidence of psoriasis increased during recent decades (Wilson et al., 2009). A previous study from 1982-1992 in the same community revealed an incidence rate of 6.59% per 100,000 US population (Shbeeb et al., 2000). The prevalence and incidence estimates of psoriasis and PsA show ethnic and geographic variations, being generally more common in the colder north than in the tropics. In Europe the prevalence of psoriasis varies anywhere from 0.6 to 6.5%. In the USA, the prevalence of diagnosed psoriasis is 3.15%. The prevalence in Africa varies depending on geographic location, being lowest in West Africa. Psoriasis is less prevalent in China (Chang et al., 2009), and Japan than in Europe, and has not been described in natives of the Andean region of South America (Kim et al., 2010;

Gottlieb et al., 2008). The prevalence of PsA also shows similar variation, being highest in people of European descent and lowest in the Japanese. Although, study methodology and case definition may explain some of the variations, genetic and environmental factors are important (Lotti et al., 2010).

People with psoriasis were identified from the computerized morbidity indices of 2 large UK general practices, total population 22,500. Questionnaires were mailed to all 633 patients thus identified. Of the respondents, a 50% sample was assessed clinically and a proportion had blood samples and radiographs taken. Of these 93 people, 12 were thought to have PsA clinically, all fulfilling the CASPAR criteria for PsA. Six of the 93 examined patients did not have psoriasis or a family history of psoriasis and had no historical features or clinical signs of psoriasis on interview and examination. The estimated prevalence of PsA in this population, using the CASPAR criteria, was 13.8% (Ibrahim et al., 2009). Many challenges have made it difficult to determine the prevalence of spondyloarthritis (SpA) in North America. They include the ethnic heterogeneity of the population, the lack of feasibility of applying current criteria as human leukocyte antigen-B27 testing and pelvic radiographs and magnetic resonance imaging scanning, and the transient nature of some SpA symptoms like peripheral arthritis and enthesitis. Current estimates of the prevalence of SpA in the United States range between 0.2% and 0.5% for ankylosing spondylitis, 0.1% for psoriatic arthritis, 0.065% for enteropathic peripheral arthritis, between 0.05% and 0.25% for enteropathic axial arthritis and an overall prevalence of SpA as high as >1% (Reveille, 2011). A population-based study was conducted in two regions of the Czech Republic (with a total population of 186,000 inhabitants), on condition of confirming a definite diagnosis according to existing classification criteria during the study period (1 March 2002 to 1 March 2003). The age-standardized estimates of incidence and prevalence were calculated using the European standard population. The total annual incidence of PsA in adults aged ≥ 16 years was 3.6/100000 and the prevalence of PsA was 49.1/100000. The annual incidence of ankylosing spondylitis (AS) in adults was 6.4/100000 and the prevalence of AS was 94.2/100000. The annual incidence of reactive arthritis (ReA) in adults was 9.3/100000 and the prevalence of ReA was 91.3/100000. The annual incidence and prevalence rates of PsA, AS, and ReA compared well with data reported from other countries (Hanova et al., 2010). SpA includes a group of diseases that share immunogenetic, clinical and radiologic findings, with a particular involvement of the axial skeleton and the entheses. SpA patients attending ambulatory care in 11 rheumatology services located in 6 Argentine provinces were included in a prospective, observational multicentre cohort of SpA. A total of 402 patients were included; 59% were male, with median age of 48.3 years and median disease duration of 8 years. Eighty-six patients were diagnosed with AS, 242 with PsA, 25 with ReA, 10 with SpA associated with inflammatory bowel disease, 33 with undifferentiated SpA and 6 with juvenile AS (Buschiazzo et al., 2011). A cohort of 233 SpA patients, observed in 2 centers in Guatemala City, Guatemala, and in hospitals in San Salvador, El Salvador, and San José, Costa Rica was analyzed. Guatemalan patients were either from the clinic of Guatemalan Association against Rheumatic Diseases (n = 105) or from the private clinic of AGK (n = 78). El Salvador patients (n = 17) were from Hospital Instituto Salvadoreño del Seguro Social, and Costa Rican patients (n = 33) were from Hospital Calderón Guardia, San José, Costa Rica. Except for the Costa Rican data, which were published in 2007, the patients' medical records were analyzed using standardized questionnaires. Prevalence of SpA was slightly higher in females than males (57% versus 43%, respectively). The median age was 47.5 years.

Most of the patients were diagnosed with ReA or undifferentiated arthritis (47% and 33%, respectively); 10% of patients had AS and 9% PsA (García-Kutzbach et al., 2011).

During the period of 2006 to 2007, Twenty eight university centers in Brazil used a standardized protocol of investigation to study the epidemiological, clinical and radiological variables of 1036 consecutive patients with the diagnosis of SpA. Validated translated (Portuguese) versions of the Bath Ankylosing Spondylitis (AS) Disease Activity Index and the Bath AS Functional Index were applied. Patient diagnoses were predominantly AS (72.3%), followed by PsA (13.7%), undifferentiated SpA (6.3%), ReA (3.6%), juvenile SpA (3.1%) and arthritis related to inflammatory bowel disease (1.0%). There was a predominance of male (73.6%) and white (59.5%) patients. Pure axial disease was observed in 36.7% of the patients, whereas the mixed pattern (axial, peripheral and entheseal) was observed in 47.9%. The most common extra-articular involvement was anterior uveitis (20.2%). HLA-B27 was positive in 69.5% of the tested patients (Sampaio-Barros, 2011). The mortality in a cohort of 453 patients with PsA (232 men, 221 women) was analyzed. The sudden mortality rate (SMR) for the men was 67.87%, and for the women, 97.01% and the overall SMR for the PsA cohort was 81.82%.The leading causes of death in this cohort were cardiovascular disease (38%), diseases of the respiratory system (27%), and malignancy (14%).These results suggest that mortality in the single center PsA cohort is not significantly different from the general UK population (Buckley et al., 2010).

A wide variation on the incidence and prevalence of PsA has been reported in different countries. The prevalence in China was similar to the rest of the world, whereas the incidence and prevalence of PsA was much lower in Japan. Among patients with psoriasis, 6-42% of the Caucasians were reported to have PsA, but figures were lower from Asian countries (1-9%). Divergent distribution of HLA in different ethnic groups and other genetic determinants may account for these differences in prevalence. PsA affects men and women almost equally in Chinese, Japanese and Iranians, which is similar to their Caucasian counterparts. Polyarthritis developing in the fourth decade was the commonest pattern of arthritis among Chinese, Indians, Iranians, Kuwaiti Arabs and Malays. Arthritis mutilans and eye lesions have rarely been reported in Asian countries. Chinese patients with nail disease and DIP joints involvement have a significantly higher risk of developing deformed joints. Premature atherosclerosis has been recognized as an important comorbidity in Asian patients with PsA. Increased prevalence of traditional cardiovascular risk factors associated with PsA suggested that the two conditions may share the same inflammatory pathway. Carotid intima-media thickness can identify PsA patients with subclinical atherosclerosis who may benefit from early intervention (Tam et al., 2009)

6.2 Psoriatic arthritis in the clinic

Psoriatic systemic disease encompassing skin, joint and nail involvement is an autoimmune process as evidenced from animal models, the HLA-Cw6 association in man, T cells infiltration in lesional skin and the response to T cell targeted therapies. The nails and joints are associated with inflammation at points of ligament or tendon insertion (i.e., enthesitis). It has been postulated that response to tissue stressing of the integrated nail-joint apparatus, rather than autoimmunity, is driving the inflammatory process with a relative differential involvement of adaptive and innate immunity in the psoriatic disease (McGonagle et al., 2010). Nail fold psoriasis and DIP joint arthritis were associated with nail involvement and were common in PsA patients. Nail psoriasis has been postulated to be related to the Koebner phenomenon and local inflammatory DIP joint arthritis, and probably indicative of distal phalanx enthesitis in PsA patients (Maejima et al., 2010).

PsA is classified as a SpA and characterized by synovitis, enthesitis, dactylitis, and spondylitis, usually manifesting in a person with skin and nail psoriasis. Our understanding about the PsA disease state, its genetics, pathophysiology, and comorbidities, as well as our ability to assess and treat the disease, has advanced as a result of significant collaborative efforts by rheumatologists and dermatologists (Mease, 2010a). For many years the concept of PsA as a separate disease entity was controversial, its importance has been underestimated. Dermatologists focus on psoriatic skin may overlook PsA due to its clinical heterogeneity or when only minor symptoms are present such as mild enthesitis or arthritis of DIP joints. Because skin lesions occur years before the manifestation of arthritis, however, it is likely that many patients are being seen by a dermatologist when PsA initially develops. A study among 1511 patients found 20% had PsA; in 85% of the cases, PsA was newly diagnosed. Of these patients more than 95% had active arthritis and 53% had five or more joints affected. Polyarthritis (58%) was the most common manifestation pattern, followed by oligoarthritis (31%) and arthritis mutilans (4%). DIP involvement was present in 41% and dactylitis in 23% of the patients. Compared with patients without arthritis, patients with PsA had more severe skin symptoms (mean PASI 14.3 vs. 11.5), a lower quality of life and greater impairment of productivity parameters (Reich et al., 2009). The Classification of Psoriatic Arthritis (CASPAR) study group was established for classification criteria for PsA. The CASPAR criteria comprised: 1- Evidence of psoriasis (a) Current psoriatic skin or scalp disease present today as judged by a rheumatologist or dermatologist (b) Personal history of psoriasis that may be obtained from patient (c) Family history of psoriasis in a first or second degree relative according to patient report, family doctor, dermatologist, rheumatologist or other qualified health-care provider. 2- Psoriatic nail dystrophy including onycholysis, pitting and hyperkeratosis observed on current physical examination. 3- A negative test for rheumatoid factor by any method except latex but preferably by ELISA or nephelometry. 4- Dactylitis: a) current swelling of an entire digit b) history of dactylitis recorded by a rheumatologist. 5- Radiological evidence of juxta-articular new bone formation as ill-defined ossification near joint margins (but excluding osteophyte formation) on plain X-rays of hand or foot. Using the CASPAR criteria, the combination of psoriasis and inflammatory arthritis gave 0.96 for sensitivity and 0.97 for specificity, respectively (Taylor et al., 2006; Chandran et al., 2007; Coates & Helliwell, 2008). The Toronto group evaluated the use of the CASPAR criteria in early disease and found a sensitivity of 99.1% in those patients with disease duration of less than 2.5 years and a sensitivity of 100% for those with disease duration of less than 12 months (Chandran et al., 2007). Both dactylitis and enthesitis are hallmark features of PsA, and dactylitis is a severity marker for the disease. Spinal disease in PsA is qualitatively and quantitatively different from classical AS, and a new scoring system combines elements of the "Bath Ankylosing Spondylitis Radiology Index" (BASRI) and "Modified Stoke AS Spinal Score" (mSASSS) to give a new modified index useful for definition of PsA types (Helliwell, 2009; Coates & Helliwell, 2010). The concept of SpA that comprises a group of interrelated disorders has been recognised since the early 1970s. While the European Spondyloarthropathy Study Group (ESSG) criteria and the Amor criteria have been developed to embrace the entire group of SpAs, new criteria for psoriatic arthritis have been developed recently. The CASPAR study, a large one of more than 1000 patients, led to a new set of validated classification criteria for psoriatic arthritis. Since their publication in 2006 the CASPAR criteria are widely used in clinical studies. In AS, the 1984 modified New York criteria have been used widely in clinical studies and daily practice but are not applicable in early disease when the characteristic radiographical signs of sacroiliitis are not visible but active sacroiliitis is readily detectable by magnetic resonance imaging (MRI). This led to the concept of axial SpA that includes patients with and without radiographic damage. Candidate criteria for axial SpA were developed based on proposals for a structured diagnostic approach. These criteria were validated in the "Assessment of Spondyloarthritis International Society" (ASAS) study on new classification criteria for axial SpA, a large international prospective study. In these new criteria, sacroiliitis showing up on MRI has been given as much weight as sacroiliitis on radiographs, thereby also identifying patients with early axial SpA. Both the CASPAR and the ASAS criteria for axial SpA are likely to be of use as diagnostic criteria to define PsA types (Rudwaleit & Taylor, 2010). Early PsA is a condition with a consistent risk of clinical progression. Abundant entheseal involvement is a distinctive clinical aspect that helps discriminate early PsA from RA. Today its detection, followed by a rapid therapeutic intervention, predicts a better clinical outcome (Scarpa et al., 2009). Different to RA, the joint distribution in PsA tends to be asymmetrical and oligoarticular (< five joints). Distal joints, particularly the DIP joints of the hands, are more frequently affected; joint tenderness tends to be less; and dactylitis, enthesitis and axial or spinal involvement are more frequent. Unlike seronegative SpA, 40% of patients with PsA suffer from a sacroiliitis that tends to exhibit an asymmetrical rather than a symmetrical distribution. Other features of PsA include the absence of rheumatoid nodules, of rheumatoid factor in the blood and, in some instances, the presence of iritis, mucous membrane lesions, urethritis, bowel inflammation and tendonitis. PsA is often characterized by plain film evidence of juxta-articular new bone formation and magnetic resonance imaging evidence of enthesitis. Eighty per cent of cases are associated with psoriatic nail changes such as pitting, ridging, oil spots and nail plate thickening. Although PsA is preceded by cutaneous psoriasis in 75% of cases, in 10–15% of cases the arthritis precedes the psoriasis, suggesting that the two diseases may be controlled by different mechanisms or that a common etiology, may remains dormant in the synovial compartment. The mean time to onset of arthritis among those with pre-existing cutaneous psoriasis is 10 years, but delays have been reported of up to 20 years. Few instances of PsA without psoriasis have been described because most cases resembling PsA in the absence of personal or family history of skin disease are classified as an undifferentiated SpA (Ciocon & Kimball, 2007; Garg & Gladman, 2010). Patients with clinical symptoms and signs of PsA and a family history of psoriasis can be classified as having PsA *sine* psoriasis. The clinical spectrum of PsA *sine* psoriasis is broad. It is identified by dactylitis and/or DIP arthritis, HLA-Cw6, and a family history of psoriasis following the CASPAR criteria (Olivieri et al., 2009). Outcome measurement is a key part of study design but presents particular challenges in SpA. Enthesitis and dactylitis are typical features of SpA and validated scoring systems for both are available, although the majority of enthesitis outcome measures are validated in AS only. Assessment of axial disease is well researched in AS and composite outcome measures are routinely used. However, assessment of axial disease in predominantly peripheral arthritis, such as PsA, is problematic and under-researched. Extensive research in dermatology has provided multiple outcome measures for skin psoriasis. The PASI remains the most common outcome measure used, despite the fact that significant problems exist with this scale and that newer scoring methods and modifications of the PASI show better validity. Nail psoriasis is accurately measured by detailed scoring systems but these can be time-consuming (Coates & Helliwell, 2010). The number of actively inflamed joints as measure of disease activity and the number of clinically deformed joints as measure of damage were significantly related to the "Health Assessment Questionnaire" (HAQ) score also useful for defining PsA types. Furthermore, interaction terms for illness duration with the number of actively inflamed joints were statistically significant, with or without inclusion of the erythrocyte sedimentation rate and morning stiffness in the model. The influence of disease activity on HAQ scores declines with increased disease duration (Husted et al., 2007).

Patients with psoriasis from 13 dermatological hospitals and 129 dermatological private practices and outpatient clinics in Germany revealed that nineteen per cent of the patients had PsA, including 14.8% previously confirmed and 4.2% newly diagnosed disease. Another 7.7% had intermittent but clinically unspecific joint symptoms, which could not be clearly attributed to PsA. About half (49.7%) of the patients with PsA had at least 1 swollen joint and 84.9% (n = 287) suffered from joint pain. Patients suffering from pain marked an average of 8.7 joints on a diagram as painful out of a possible 28. The mean number of swollen joints among the affected patients amounted to an average of 6.8. There are still a significant number of patients suspected of having joint involvement without ever having been diagnosed with PsA. Published data indicate that progression of joint damage and functional disability can be prevented if adequate treatment is started promptly (Radtke et al., 2009).

6.3 Psoriatic arthritis and genetics

The genes involved, in PsA are HLA genes of class I MHC alleles, on the HLA-B and HLA-C loci. Psoriasis is linked to HLA-Cw6 allele. Twenty percent of PsA patients with peripheral joint involvement displayed HLA-B27, a value that climbs to 70% in patients with PsA type spine involvement (Amherd-Hoekstra et al., 2010). The overlap in associated HLA antigens for both diseases (B13, B17, B57, Cw6, and DR7) suggests a shared genetic predisposition (Barton, 2002). Psoriasis and PsA are heritable diseases. Polymorphisms in the genes encoded in the MHC region have consistently been associated with psoriasis and PsA and account for about 30% of the genetic risk. In psoriasis, the association has been primarily with class I antigens: HLA-B13, HLA-B17, HLA-Cw6, and HLA-Cw7, the strongest association being with HLA-Cw6. Typing for HLA-Cw6 may have potential clinical utility, as it is associated with early onset of psoriasis, higher incidence of guttate or streptococcal induced disease flares, and more severe disease. PsA is also associated with multiple HLA antigens, many of which are similar to psoriasis antigens, as the two diseases are interrelated (O'Rielly & Rahman, 2010). However, specific associations do exist for the inflammatory arthritis, as HLA-B27 is associated with greater spinal involvement, and B38 and B39 with peripheral polyarthritis. HLA antigens are also prognostic factors, as HLA-B39 alone, HLA-B27 in the presence of HLA-DR7, and HLA-DQw3 in the absence of HLA-DR7 all confer an increased risk for disease progression. The RA shared epitope was found to be associated with radiologic erosions among patients with PsA. Patients with PsA carrying both HLACw6 and HLA-DRB107 alleles were determined to have a less severe course of arthritis. Recently, the results of multiple well powered genome-wide association studies have identified several loci outside the MHC region associated with psoriasis risk, including three genes involved in interleukin (IL)-23 signaling (IL-23R, IL-23A, IL-12B), two genes that regulate nuclear factor-κB signaling (TNIP1, TNFAIP3), and two genes involved in the modulation of T-helper type 2 immune responses (IL-4, IL-13) (Bowes & Barton, 2010). Genetic epidemiologic studies have shown that both diseases have a strong genetic component. Environmental risk factors including streptococcal pharyngitis, stressful life events, low humidity, drugs, HIV infection, trauma, smoking and obesity have been associated with psoriasis and PsA (Barton, 2002; Cantini et al., 2010). PsA is even more strongly influenced by genes than is cutaneous psoriasis (Moll & Wright, 1973; Chandran & Raychaudhuri 2010). Family studies continue to suggest a large genetic contribution to PsA. Using a candidate gene approach, genes confirmed to be associated with psoriasis vulgaris have also been found to be associated with PsA: HLA-Cw-0602, IL23R, and IL12B (Castelino & Barton , 2010).

6.4 Psoriatic arthritis interleukins and biomarkers

A key objective of the assessment working group of the "Group for Research and Assessment of Psoriasis and Psoriatic Arthritis" (GRAPPA) was to identify, develop, evaluate, and validate outcome measures for use in clinical trials of PsA and in clinical practice useful in defining PsA types (Mease, 2008) . Biomarkers are helpful in screening patients with psoriasis for PsA types. Patients with psoriasis satisfying CASPAR criteria for PsA were analyzed for IL-12, IL-12p40, IL-17, TNF super family members (TNFSF14), MMP-3, RANK ligand (RANKL), osteoprotegerin (OPG), cartilage oligomeric matrix protein (COMP), C-propeptide of Type II collagen (CPII), collagen fragment neoepitopes Col2-3/4 long mono (C2C), Col2-3/4short (C1-2C) and highly sensitive CRP (hsCRP). Serum levels of RANKL, TNFSF14, MMP-3 and COMP independently associated with psoriatic disease. Twenty six PsA patients (mean swollen and tender joint count: 16, swollen joint count: 5) were then compared with 26 patients who had psoriasis alone. Increased levels of hsCRP, OPG, MMP-3 and the CPII:C2C ratios were independently associated with PsA and are biomarkers for PsA in patients with psoriasis (Chandran et al., 2010).

6.5 Psoriatic arthritis and cardiovascular disease

Immune-mediated inflammatory diseases (IMIDs), including RA and SpA, are associated with increased cardiovascular morbidity and mortality, independent of the established cardiovascular risk factors. The chronic inflammatory state, a hallmark of IMIDs, is considered to be a driving force for accelerated atherogenesis. Consequently, aggressive control of disease activity has been suggested to be instrumental for cardiovascular risk reduction (Bisoendial et al., 2009).

Patients with PsA have an increased incidence of CVD and cardiovascular risk factors such as smoking, hypertension, and metabolic syndrome compared to the normal population as well as nonconventional risk factors such as raised levels of homocysteine and excessive alcohol consumption. In patients with PsA, carotid wave pulse velocity, a measure of arterial stiffness, was significantly higher. Patients with psoriasis were found to have increased coronary artery calcification in direct imaging study compared to controls. Two case control studies also demonstrated that patients with PsA had a higher prevalence of subclinical atherosclerosis as measured by arterial intima-media wall thicknes (IMT) and endothelial dysfunction without overt CVD. In patients without clinical CVD 35% had increased IMT despite having low cardiovascular risk. One hundred two patients with PsA had a higher prevalence of type II diabetes mellitus and hypertension, and an increased prevalence of HDL cholesterol, apolipoprotein A1 levels, lower total cholesterol and LDL cholesterol levels, and lower total cholesterol to HDL cholesterol ratio. Chronic inflammation has been shown to play a role in the development of atherosclerosis now considered as an inflammatory, autoimmune like disease. Both the innate immune system and T helper-1 lymphocytes appear to be involved in atherogenesis. This is similar to the pattern of immune mediated inflammation in psoriasis and PsA. It is possible that psoriasis and PsA produce chronic, systemic inflammation, with higher levels of inflammatory cells and cytokines invoking endothelial inflammation and plaque formation in the vascular system (Tobin et al., 2010). The increased risk for CVD in RA is well known and inflammation appears to play a pivotal etiological role. There is now substantial interest in whether or not PsA is also associated with an enhanced cardiovascular risk. In all patients CVD was defined as a history of myocardial infarct (MI), stroke and/or transient ischemic attack verified by written documentation of the event. The prevalence of CVD was 10% in patients with PsA compared with 12% in patients with RA (Jamnitski et al., 2010). Flow-mediated dilatation (FMD) was significantly impaired in PsA patients without traditional cardiovascular risk factors or CVD. Another study also showed a higher prevalence of subclinical atherosclerosis, as measured by carotid IMT, among PsA patients. As in RA, CVD and their risk factors including hyperlipidaemia, diabetes mellitus and hypertension were more common in PsA patients. However, mortality in patients with PsA, in a single center cohort was not significantly different from the general population in England. No increased risk of death was observed in this cohort (Buckley et al., 2010). In a population of patients with PsA 23.3% had renal abnormalities as defined by creatinine clearance below the lower cut off of normal distribution and urinary excretion of albumin more than 25 mg/24 hrs. These patients were significantly older at the time of the study, older at joint disease onset, had longer skin disease duration, increased serum levels of beta2-microglobulin, and higher incidence of increased erythrocyte sedimentation rate and C reactive protein levels (Alenius et al., 2001).

6.6 Psoriatic arthritis, metabolic syndrome and malignancies

To evaluate the prevalence of the metabolic syndrome (MetS), patients with RA, AS and PsA were recruited for a study of atherosclerotic risk factors and the MetS, defined according to the 2009 Joint Statements using the Asian criteria for central obesity. The prevalence of MetS was significantly higher in PsA (38%) than RA (20%) or AS (11%). Patients with PsA had significantly higher prevalence of impaired fasting glucose (30%), low HDL-cholesterol (33%), high triglyceride (21%), central obesity (65%) and high blood pressure (56%). Patients with PsA, but not RA or AS, have a significantly higher prevalence of the MetS syndrome compared to the general population. Among the three diseases studied, PsA has the highest prevalence of the MetS and is associated with highest cardiovascular risk (Mok et al., 2010; Papo et al., 2010)

A cohort analysis of SpA patients who were followed up prospectively from 1978 to 2004 at the University of Toronto PsA Clinic was performed. Of the 665 patients included, 68 (10.2%) developed a malignancy at an average age of 62.4 years. The most frequently seen malignancies were breast (20.6%), lung (13.2%), and prostate (8.8%) cancer. However, the incidence of malignancy in the large PsA cohort did not differ from that in the general population (Rohekar et al., 2008).

6.7 Inflammatory markers C-reactive protein (CRP) and complement 5a (C5a) in patients with psoriatic arthritis, before and after treatment with amastigote antigens

Inflammatory markers C-reactive protein (CRP) and complement 5a (C5a) assayed in two PsA patients decreased significantly in serum after treatment with 6 doses of AS200 DEAE fractions 3 + 4 Leishmania amastigotes antigens at 300 μg/dose (Fig 1). The Leishmania antigens decreased markedly the TNFα concentration in supernatants from PBMC in both patients and controls (Fig 1 to 5 adapted from O'Daly & Gleason, 2010c, by permission of the associate editor)

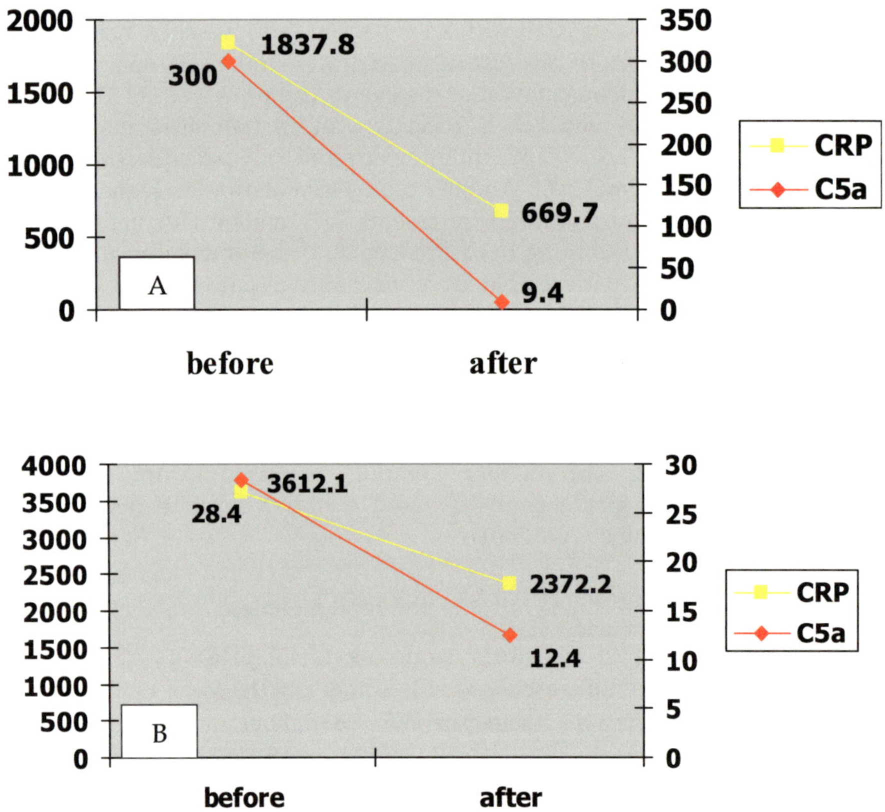

Fig. 1. Psoriatic patients (A and B) with 6 doses of AS200 at 300 μg/dose before and after treatments. Both patients had PASI reduction 61.6% and 66.4% respectively and biopsies with excellent improvement evidenced by decrease of epidermal layer and absence of inflammatory cells in epidermis and dermis in comparison to placebo (Rehydragel).

6.8 TNF-α in psoriatic patients and ConA induced hepatitis in mice

PBMC of patients and controls were stimulated with concanavalin A (ConA); ConA+AS100-2 *L(L)chagasi* antigens and compared to no treatment as control. The *Leishmania* antigens decreased markedly the TNFα concentration in supernatants from PBMC in both patients and controls (Fig 2). In mice ConA induced hepatitis, injection of 50 μg AS100-2 *L(L)chagasi* antigens subcutaneously (SC) decreased serum TNFα as compared to placebo (PBS) in 8 hours of observation (Fig 3).

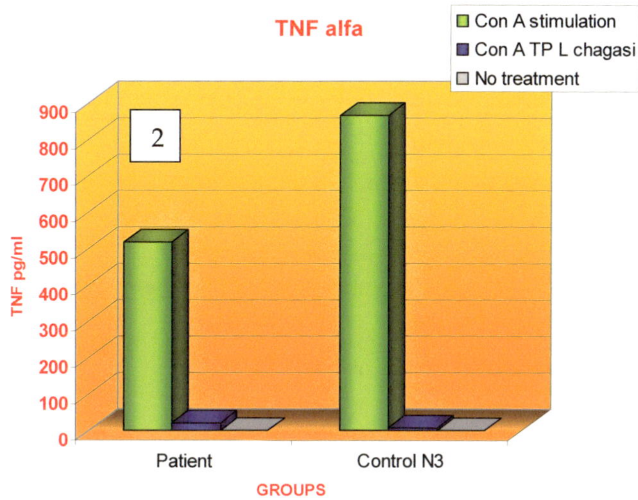

Fig. 2. PBMC of patients and controls after stimulation with concanavalin A (ConA), ConA + AS100-2 *L(L)chagasi* antigens or no treatment 3 patients and controls per group.

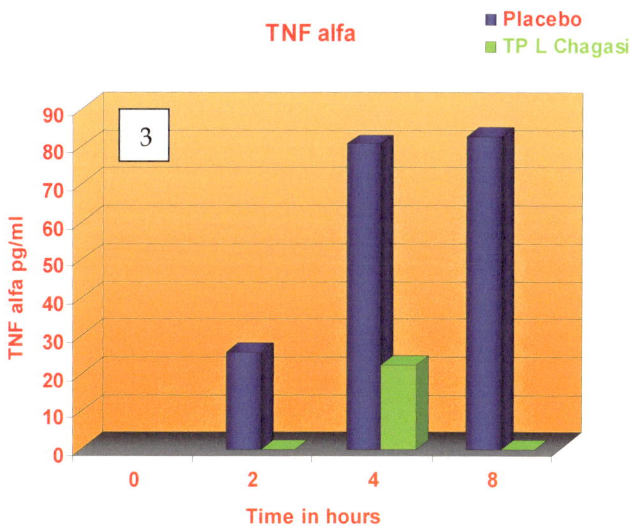

Fig. 3. Serum TNFα in ConA induced hepatitis in mice (n=3 per group). After SC injection of 50 μg AS100-2 *L. chagasi* antigens, TNFα decreased significantly as compared to placebo (PBS) at 2, 4 and 8 hours observation period. STDEV < 5% of average.

Serum IL-1β, 8 hours after SC injection of AS200 L(V)brasiliensis +RH and AS100-1+RH in mice, also decreased significantly as compared to placebo and in a range similar to the positive control dexamethasone (Fig 4). AS100-2 *L(L)chagasi* antigens decreased proliferation of cutaneous T cell lymphoma in vitro in a dose-response relationship (Fig 5).

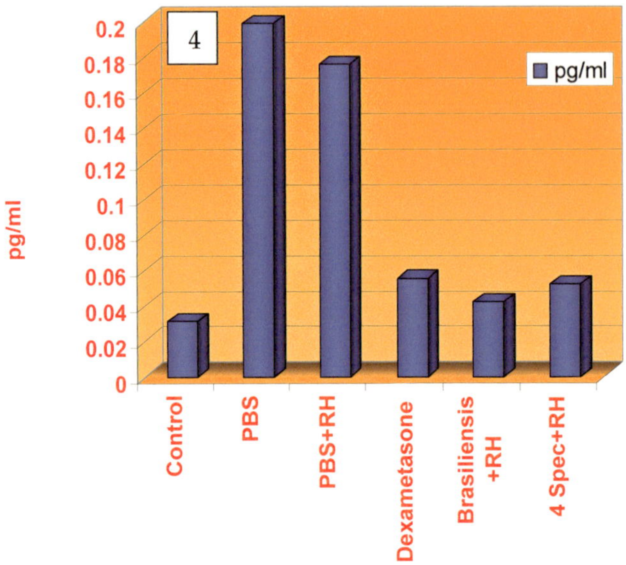

Fig. 4. Serum IL-1β in ConA induced hepatitis in mice (n=3 per group). IL-1β was determined after 8 hours of SC injection of the following products: 1- 50 μL placebo (PBS) 2- 50 μL PBS+Rehydragel (RH), 3- 50 μg/mice *L(V)brasiliensis* AS200 fraction 3 and 4 + RH, 4- AS100-1(4 species)+RH and 5- 1 mg/Kg/mice dexamethasone. Control normal mice, received no treatment. IL-1β decrease significantly after treatment with *L(V)brasiliensis* AS200 antigens 3 and 4, or polyva;ent AS100-1 vaccine, similar to dexamethasone as compared to placebos 1 and 2.

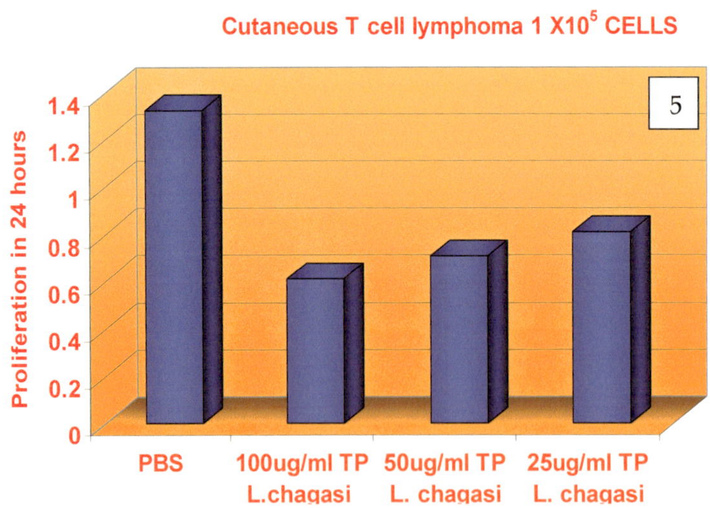

Fig. 5. In vitro proliferation of cutaneous T cell lymphoma cells at different concentrations of AS100-2 *(L) chagasi* leishmania antigens as compared to PBS after 24 hours of culture. Values are average of three different experiments. STDEV < 5% of average.

6.9 Lymphocyte subsets in patients with psoriatic arthritis

As more skin disease is present in PsA patients, more inflammation is found in the joints, suggesting a link between skin and joint inflammatory processes; since both were exacerbated in the PASI 100 and PASI 75 groups and also needed higher number of doses to achieve a lower AS, tender joints and nail changes values (O'Daly et al., 2011). Absolute values of gated LS before treatment decreased in this order: CD8+HLA-, CD8+HLA+, CD4+, CD8+CD3+, CD8+CD3 in PBMC as PASI increased, suggesting migration of CD8+ cells from the blood to the joints and skin. Contrary to the previous finding, LS: CD8+CD4-, CD3+CD8-, HLA+CD8-, CD19+, CD8+CD4+, IgA+, IgD+, IgM+, IgE+, and IgG+ increased in PBMC as PASI increased suggesting activation and proliferation by unknown antigens and subsequent migration to the blood. The LS quantification in this group of PsA patients only (n=508) were different (O'Daly et al., 2011) to the LS quantified in the psoriasis skin disease trial (n=2770, O'Daly et al., 2010b), since in PsA the majority belonged to the CD8+ phenotype, a T cell key in the PsA inflammatory process as described by many authors. In PsA patients there is also evidence of T cell recirculation before treatment and a vicious cycle with T and B cells migrating between blood and skin and joints. After treatment with nine doses of AS100-1 *Leishmania* amastigotes antigens, a dramatic decrease in LS belonging to T and B cells, in PBMC was observed, as PASI, AS, tender joint counts, and nail changes returns to normal values and the vicious cycle disappeared (O'Daly et al., 2011). AS100-1 had a cellular not humoral immune response as supported by the DTH and ELISA results in humans and guinea pigs (O'Daly et al. 2009a; O'Daly et al., 2009b; O'Daly et al., 2010a). All psoriatic patients were DTH positive after the third vaccination with AS100-1, but no ELISA antibodies were detected in serum from these volunteers up to 6 doses of vaccine (O'Daly et al., 2009a). This suggests that the immunological response to AS100-1 after TLCK treatment and NP-40 extraction was mediated by immunization of T-regulatory cells, with no antibody production, a novel mechanism that may play a role in decreasing inflammation in psoriatic skin. Amastigote peptides may induce Th3 regulatory T cells producing IL-10 that inhibits Th1 and Th2 cell cytokine production and induced peripheral cell tolerance.

6.10 Psoriatic arthritis therapies

Psoriasis is one of the most prevalent chronic inflammatory diseases with a high economic impact. The disease persists for life, and the patient has an increased risk of CVD. One out of five patients develops PsA. The clinical picture of psoriasis is highly variable with regard to lesion characteristics and the severity of disease. To improve the management of psoriasis, guidelines must be followed and all appropriate topical and systemic treatment options must be tried, with clearly defined treatment goals. The spectrum of established systemic treatments for psoriasis has been extended by the biologics (Mrowietz & Reich, 2009).

PsA is an inflammatory arthritis occurring in up to 30% of patients with psoriasis. Its clear distinction from RA has been described clinically, genetically, and immunohistologically. Therapies that target cells, such as activated T cells, proinflammatory cytokines, and TNFα, are used extensively today. A variety of items are evaluated including joints, skin, enthesium, dactylitis, spine function, quality of life, and imaging assessment of disease activity and damage (Ceponis & Kavanaugh, 2010). The performance of treatments in these various domains have being evaluated by GRAPPA, and improved measures are being developed and validated specifically for PsA. Traditional therapies for PsA like non steroidal anti-inflammatory drugs (NSAIDs), oral immunomodulatory drugs, topical creams, and light therapy have been helpful in controlling both musculoskeletal and dermatologic lesions of the disease, but may eventually show diminished benefit, and may produce severe toxicities as side effects (Mease, 2006).

The primary goals in the treatment of PsA are reduction of pain; improvement in the other signs and symptoms of disease, including skin and nail involvement; optimization of functional capacity and quality of life; and inhibition of the progression of joint damage. These goals should be achieved while minimizing potential toxicities from treatment. The management of PsA should simultaneously target arthritis, skin disease, and other manifestations of PsA, including involvement of the axial skeleton dactylitis, enthesitis, and eye inflammation. In this respect targeted biological agents, primarily TNFα inhibitors, have emerged as generally well tolerated and highly effective alternatives to traditional "Disease Modifying Anti Rheumatic Drugs" (DMARDs) (Mease, 2010b)

PsA was considered as a less damaging disease than RA. In early arthritis 50% of patients showed significant joint damage developing erosions in the first 2 years even if DMARDs were used as treatment. The treatment should aim to preserve function, prevent disability and maintain quality of life. The therapeutic approach has employed treatments to benefit both the skin and joints with minimal adverse effects, and to prevent subsequent disability and damage, inflammation i.e. synovitis which must be arrested and controlled early. In this respect combination therapy with conventional DMARDs and biologic drugs, like TNFα inhibitors, has made significant progress in the last 10 years. A remission rate of 58% of patients treated with DMARD and biologic therapy for 12 months has been achieved (Wollina et al., 2010).

Nail involvement in psoriasis is typically overlooked; it can affect up to 50% of patients with psoriasis and cause functional impact as well as psychological stress that affect quality of life. Psoriatic patients with nail disease have more severe skin lesions, and higher rate of unremitting PsA. The current management of nail psoriasis includes topical, intralesional and systemic therapies, although little clinical evidence is available on the effectiveness of conventional treatments. Biologic agents are beginning to emerge as a viable option to treat patients with both cutaneous and nail clinical manifestations of psoriasis and PsA (Vena et al., 2010).

Although they can have some beneficial effect on skin disease and peripheral arthritis, there is lack of evidence for DMARDs, such as methotrexate (MTX), Leflunomide (LEF), cyclosporine (CsA), and sulfasalazine (SSZ) in affecting dactylitis or enthesitis, and they are clearly ineffective in axial disease. Systemic glucocorticoids may cause a flare of psoriasis if treatment is stopped too quickly, and should be used with caution in PsA. In contrast, biologics, particularly TNFα inhibitors seem to be beneficial in skin psoriasis and across of all the manifestations of PsA, including arthritis, skin and nail disease, spinal disease, enthesitis and dactylitis. They also improve quality of life and inhibit joint damage. All the currently used TNFα inhibitors appear to have comparable efficacy and safety profiles in patients with PsA. They can be used as monotherapy or in combination with MTX or other traditional DMARDs. Initiation of anti-TNFα agents is recommended for patients who failed one of the traditional DMARDs or as an initial therapy in patients who have poor prognosis. Other biological agents, including alefacept and abatacept, appear to be less potent than TNFα inhibitors in PsA and their use is likely to be reserved for patients who failed or cannot be treated with TNFα inhibitors. These agents are usually used in combination with other DMARDs. The Efficacy of ustekinumab in the treatment of PsA has been recently reported and is presently under further investigation (Mease, 2009; Mease, 2010a)

Results from clinical trials of biologic anti-TNFα drugs confirmed the biological relevance of TNFα function in the pathogenesis of chronic noninfectious inflammation of joints, skin and gut. Up to April 2009, more than two million patients worldwide have received the first marketed drugs, namely the monoclonal anti-TNFα antibodies infliximab and adalimumab and the soluble TNF receptor etanercept. All three are equally effective in RA, AS, psoriasis and PsA, and only the monoclonal antibodies are effective in inflammatory bowel disease. The spectrum of efficacy with anti-TNFα therapies includes diseases such as systemic vasculitis and sight-threatening uveitis. New adverse effects are recognized, like development of new onset psoriasis. Reactivation of latent tuberculosis remains the most important safety issue of anti-TNFα therapies (Sfikakis, 2010). RA, AS and PsA are commonly thought of as inflammatory diseases that affect younger individuals. The safety profiles for etanercept, infliximab and adalimumab in patients of 65 years or more, anti-TNFα treatments for an active inflammatory disease such as RA, AS or PsA, or psoriasis were analyzed. Anti TNFα treatment is a safe option possibly leading to better disease outcome (Migliore et al., 2009).

Altogether there is sufficient reason not to dismiss traditional agents for use in PsA because of lack of evidence. Also, due consideration must be given to the considerable cost of biologic treatments versus traditional treatments. The role of combination therapy with TNFα inhibitors is an important one, especially considering that 30%–40% of patients in the TNFα inhibitor trials have been on MTX as concomitant medication (McHugh, 2009). Traditional systemic therapies for psoriasis, such as MTX, CsA, retinoids or psoralen plus ultraviolet light (PUVA) therapy, have a potential for long-term toxicity and may not always provide sufficient improvement of the disease. Biological therapies for the treatment of PsA are defined by their mode of action and can be classified into three categories: the T-cell modulating agents (alefacept and efalizumab), the TNFα blockers, (adalimumab, certolizumab, etanercept, golimumab and infliximab) and the inhibitors of interleukin IL-12 and IL-23 (ustekinumab and briakinumab) (Weger, 2010). DMARDs remain the first choice for the treatment of peripheral arthritis despite scarce evidence of their efficacy or ability to halt radiographic progression. TNFα antagonists have the greatest level of evidence for symptom control and radiographic progression. They are currently used after the failure of DMARDs to effectively treat peripheral arthritis, enthesitis, and dactylitis, and are the first choice when axial disease predominates. Despite the use of these treatments, 30% to 40% of patients will still have active disease. Among new drugs, evidence of efficacy has already been published with regard to anti-IL12/23 monoclonal antibody (ustekimumab) and golimumab (Soriano &, Rosa, 2009)

For a long time, the endothelial covering of the vessels has been considered an inert surface. On the contrary, the endothelial cells are active and dynamic elements in the interaction between blood and tissues. The control of the vessel basal tone is obtained by the complex balance between the relaxing and contracting endothelial factors. Previous clinical studies show that patients suffering from RA and other autoimmune rheumatologic pathologies are at high risk of death being prematurely affected by atherosclerosis and CVD. Blocking TNFα by biological drugs improves the endothelial function. The effects of two anti-TNFα drugs (infliximab and etanercept) on the endothelial function were evaluated by FMD, which was measured in the brachial artery before and after treatment. 36 patients were enrolled 25 with RA and 11 with PsA. They were divided into three groups: 10 patients were treated with etanercept, 13 with infliximab, and 13 with DMARDs. The carotid IMT was measured and the endothelial function was evaluated by FMD measurement in the brachial artery, before treatment, 1 h after the beginning of treatment and after 8–12 weeks. No statistically significant difference between the three groups before treatment was found for the ultrasonographic evaluation of the carotid IMT. On the contrary, the differences between FMD values before and after the treatment in the patients treated with etanercept and in the patients treated with infliximab were statistically significant. Long-term evaluation for infliximab and etanercept was performed by comparing the FMD values, 8 and 12 weeks after the first treatment. After 8 weeks, FMD value was similar to the value recorded at enrollment in the infliximab group and the FMD values in the etanercept group after 12 weeks showed a not statistically significant reduction of vasodilatating effect. Drugs in patients affected by autoimmune arthritis can modify the endothelial function, as indicated by the induced FMD changes, but the long-term effect tends to be considerably reduced (Mazzoccoli et al., 2010)

Significantly diminished values for swollen and tender joints, patients global and pain assessments, doctor's global assessment of disease activity, erythrocyte sedimentation rate, C-reactive protein, and "Health Assessment Questionnaire" (HAQ) score were observed within 3 months after commencement of both infliximab and etanercept. Values remained significantly lower throughout the 24 months of follow up. ACR20 response at 3 months was 79% (n = 22/28) for infliximab and 76% (n = 34/45) for etanercept. The first biological drug was discontinued in 16% due to lack of effectiveness and in 6% due to adverse events (Virkki et al., 2010). It is unclear if skin cancer risk is affected by the use of immunomodulatory medications in RA, psoriasis, and PsA. RA may potentiate the risk of cutaneous malignancy and therefore dermatologic screening in this population should be considered. The use of immunomodulatory therapy in RA, psoriasis, and PsA may further increase the risk of cutaneous malignancy and therefore dermatologic screening examinations are warranted in these groups. More careful recording of skin cancer development during clinical trials and cohort studies is necessary to further delineate the risks of immunomodulatory therapy (Krathen et al., 2010).

PsA provides an ideal disease model in which to investigate the bioactivities of potentially therapeutic cytokines at multiple sites of tissue inflammation. The effects of subcutaneous rhIL-10, an anti-inflammatory cytokine, was investigated for 28 days in a double-blind, placebo-controlled study in PsA patients. Synovial/skin biopsies, peripheral blood leukocytes, articular magnetic resonance images, and clinical disease activity scores were obtained sequentially. Modest, but significant clinical improvement in skin, but not articular disease activity scores with only minor adverse effects was observed. Type 1, but not Type 2 cytokine production in vitro was suppressed in human rhIL-10 treatment compared with placebo recipients. Similarly, TNFα and IL-1β, production in whole blood stimulated with LPS in vitro was reduced, whereas serum soluble TNFRII levels were elevated, indicating suppression of monocyte function. Decreased T cell and macrophage infiltration in synovial tissues was accompanied by reduced P-selectin expression. Moreover, suppressed synovial enhancement on magnetic resonance imaging and reduced α(v)β(3) integrin expression on von Willebrand factor(+) vessels were observed. Together these data demonstrate that a short course of IL-10 modulates immune responses in vivo via diverse effects on endothelial activation, leukocyte recruitment and effector functions. Such biological changes may result in clinically meaningful improvement in disease activity (McInnes et al., 2001).

Biologic agents should be considered for use solely in children with psoriasis that is refractory to conventional therapies, including children with severe, widespread, refractory pustular, plaque or PsA. Etanercept appears to have resulted in less severe side effects compared to infliximab in the juvenile RA population. Serious adverse events (including infection), have been reported in the literature and should be taken into account before beginning treatment with any biologic agent (Marji et al., 2010).

The socioeconomic scenario of PsA is similar to RA. Current treatments do not achieve remission of symptoms or prevention of the appearance of damage in the early stage of PsA nor the blocking of PsA progression in old cases. The current management of PsA includes NSAIDs, corticosteroids, DMARDs and anti-TNF-α alpha blocking agents. These biologic drugs are more effective than traditional DMARDs on inflammation, quality of life and function and can inhibit the progression of the structural joint damage. Recent advancement in the immunopathogenesis of PsA has permitted the development of novel drugs including new TNF-α blockers, IL-1, IL-6, IL-12, IL-23 and IL-17 inhibitors, co-stimulator modulation inhibitors, B-cell depleting agents, small molecules and receptor activator of NF-kappaB/receptor activator of NF-kappaB ligand inhibitors (Olivieri et al., 2010).

Baseline clinical characteristics including demographics, previous DMARDs response, tender and swollen joint counts, early morning stiffness, pain visual analogue score, patient global assessment, C reactive protein (CRP) and HAQ were collected. At 12 months remission, defined according to the disease activity score using 28 joint count and CRP (DAS28-CRP), was achieved in 58% of PsA patients compared to 44% of RA patients. DAS28 remission is possible in PsA patients at one year following anti-TNFα therapy, at higher rates than in RA patients and is predicted by baseline HAQ (Saber et al., 2010).

Therapy for inflammatory joint diseases, such as RA, AS and PsA, includes DMARDs. Conventional DMARDs are used as monotherapy or in combination and include MTX, LEF, azathioprine, CsA, hydroxychloroquine, SSZ, gold and minocycline. Biologic therapies are TNFα inhibitors, T-cell modulators and B-cell depleters. They have all been shown to have clinical efficacy and are able to retard structural damage (Vaz et al., 2009).

7. Leishmaniasis, the tropical disease root of the serendipity finding

7.1 What is Leishmaniasis?

Leishmaniasis is a globally distributed zoonosis mostly centered in the tropics and subtropics, with humans serving as accidental hosts. Due to the prevalence of the disease, one-tenth of the world's populations (600 million people) are at risk of infection. Globally, there are approximately 12 million cases and the incidence of new visceral leishmaniasis

(VL) and cutaneous (CL) infections are approximated 0.5 and 1.5 million new cases each year, respectively (World Health Organization, Leishmaniasis Control home page: http://www.who.int/ctd/html/leis.html).

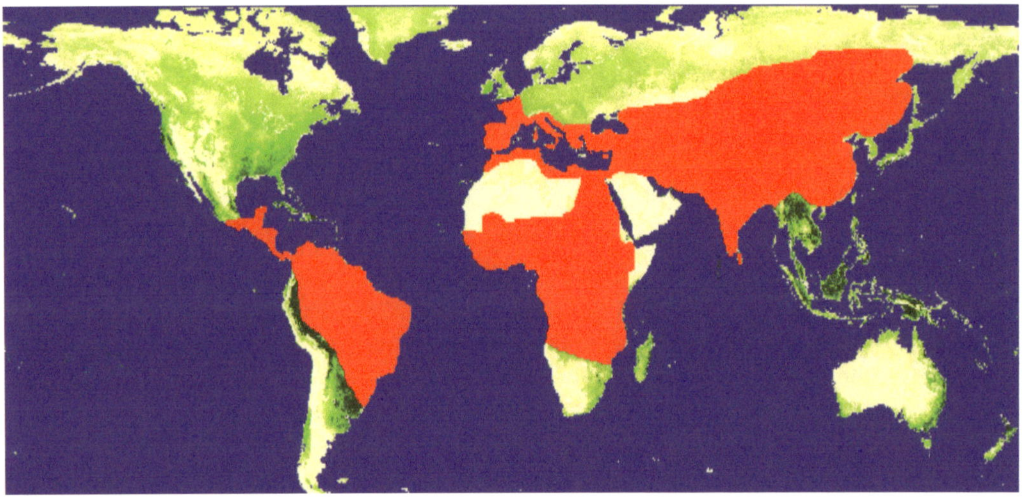

Fig. 6. Cutaneous and Visceral Leishmaniasis in our planet

7.2 Leishmania life cycle and suppression of antigen display

Extracellular procyclic promastigotes in the vector (sandfly) mature to metacyclic promastigotes (motile) that eventually evolve to amastigotes (nonmotile) once they enter cells in the vertebrate host after the insect bite. The amastigote eventually evolves back to the promastigote form in the vector, after a blood meal in infected hosts, closing the cycle. The mature infective metacyclic promastigotes have surface glycoconjugates such as glycosylinositolphopholipid (GIPL) and lipophosphoglycan (LPG), wich is a virulence factor of the mature promastigote and inhibits the action of the complement system (Okwor & Uzonna, 2009). Once inside the host, metacyclic promastigotes are taken up by macrophages through binding to complement receptors 1 and 3 or C reactive protein receptor, without leading to the activation of the macrophage. Approximately 24-72 hours after being taken up by the macrophage, the promastigotes transform into round nonmotile intracellular amastigotes with no surface GIPL or LPG. The amastigotes begin to multiply in the parasitophorous vacuole inside the macrophage (Figure 7), suppressing IFN-γ and the production of nitric oxide (NO) and superoxide (Awasthi et al., 2004; Handman, 2001). The immunological response in humans and experimental animals is induced by the amastigote form (intracellular), and not by extracellular promastigotes form, which enters the host target cell immediately after infection and is not seen by the host immune system. Amastigotes inhibit antigen presentation by repressing the expression of Class I and Class II MHC gene products, both basally and following stimulation with IFNγ (Reiner et al., 1987; Reiner det al., 1988). On the other hand, macrophages infected with *L(L)major* may express normal levels of MHC class II molecules, but inhibit antigen presentation by interfering with the loading of antigens onto the MHC class II molecule (Fruth et al., 1993). An alternative suppression technique used by several Leishmania species is to sequester the MHC II molecules and antigens within the phagolysosome (Kima et al., 1996).

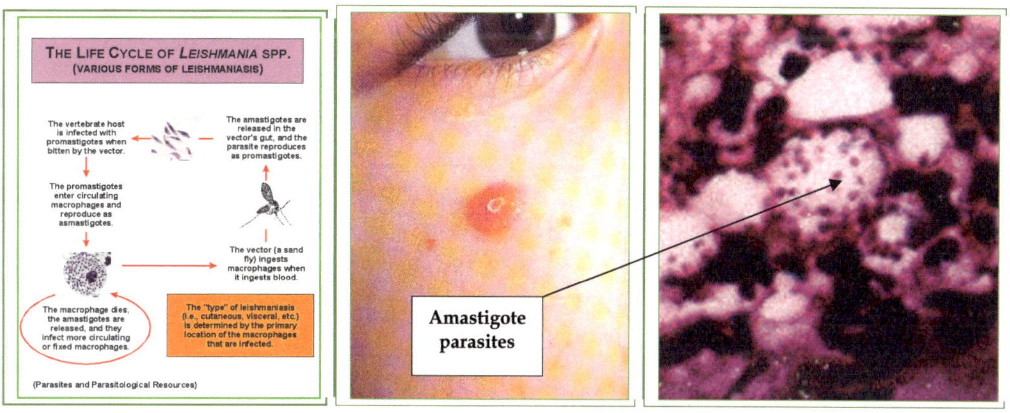

Fig. 7. Life cycle of leismania parasites and initial cutaneous lesion 2-3 weeks after bite

7.3 How do vertebrates defend against Leishmaniasis?

After being bitten, a granuloma composed of granulocytes, lymphocytes, epithelioid cells, monocytes, macrophages, and fibroblasts forms at the site of infection. In addition to killing parasites, activated macrophages produce different cytokines such as TNFα, IL-6, IL-18, IL-12, and IFNγ inducing a protective Th1-type immune response (Awasthi et al., 2004; Handman, 2001). Analyses of immune responses in natural and experimental (healthy human volunteers) infections show that the clear Th1/Th2 T cell responses to *L(L) major* seen in murine studies do not occur. Instead, a typical mixed Th1/Th2 response is observed with PBMC from patients secreting varying amounts of IFNγ, IL-10, and IL-4 depending on the clinical stage of the disease. CD4+ and CD8+ cells contribute to IFNγ and TNFα production in infected patients (Okwor & Uzonna, 2009). Residual parasites remain in the host forever and can be reactivated in the immunocompromised hosts and by AIDS (Fernandez-Guerrero et al., 1987; Rodriguez Coura et al., 1987; Rosenthal et al., 1988; Scaglia et al., 1989; Altges et al. 1991).

TNF plays a central role in the defense against intracellular infections with Leishmania, a disease that ends fatally in TNF-/- mice (Reiner et al., 1987). Resolution of an established infection is mediated by IFN-γ produced by CD4+ T cells in C57BL/6 resistant mouse strains (Reiner et al., 1988). The IFN-γ response allows macrophages to develop leishmanicidal activities as expression of inducible nitric oxide synthase (iNOS) and NO. In contrast, BALB/c susceptible strain develops IL-4- and IL-10-mediated CD4+ T cell response. Rheumatoid arthritis patients treated with TNF antagonists have reoccurrence of leishmaniasis. After blocking TNF, Leishmania donovani-infected mice were unable to resolve the infection (Körner et al., 2010). VL is characterized by abundant parasites in the spleen, liver, and bone marrow. However, the parasite only establishes chronic infection in the spleen and bone marrow because infection in the liver is self-resolving within 6–8 weeks because of a Th1-dominated granulomatous response, characterized by high IFN-γ production (Stager et al., 2010).

	Endemic area			Hyperendemic area		
Study group	**Infected**	**Noninfected**	**p**	**Infected**	**Noninfected**	**p**
Vaccinated	16	2,000		18	105	
Nonvaccinated	66	1,109	<0.001	52	50	<0.001
Protective efficacy	85.9%			71%		
95% Confidence interval	81.8- 86.1			67.9- 74.3		

Table 1. Cases of leishmaniasis according to vaccination status, protective efficacy

Neutrophils are rapidly recruited to the site of Leishmania inoculation, where they phagocytose the parasites, some of which are able to survive within these first host cells. Neutrophils can thus provide a transient safe shelter for the parasites, prior to their entry into macrophages where they will replicate (Charmoy et al., 2010).

After vaccination with 3 doses of AS100-1 at 500 µg/500 µl , one month apart in the endemic area of "Valle Arriba" and in the hyperendemic area of "La Planta" both in Guatire, Miranda State, Venezuela, (O'Daly et al., 1995a) protective efficacy were 85.9% and 71% respectively (Table 1). In the endemic area we found one person cured from plaque psoriasis one month after the third dose of vaccine. The vaccine also induced regression of leishmania lesions when used as immunotherapeutic agent as seen in Figure 8 (O'Daly et al., 1995b)

7.4 No prior sensitization required to recognize amastigote antigens

Leishmania promastigotes sonicates induced in vitro proliferation and IFNγ production in PBMC from individuals that never had contact with Leishmania parasites. The proliferating T cell population was CD2+ in a frequency <1:10,000 a response that could be abolished after depletion of CD45RO+ memory cells from the PBMC (Kemp et al., 1992). Sera from volunteers vaccinated in the Leishmaniasis trial performed in Caracas, had ELISA negative values and a similar immunoblotting band pattern before vaccination, and 1 month after 3 doses of the polyvalent vaccine using amastigote antigens from the four species present in AS100-1 (O'Daly et al., 1995a). Thus, normal CD2+ T cells (Kemp et al., 1992) and normal immunoglobulin from healthy volunteers that never experienced Leishmania infection reacted with Leishmania antigens in the immunoblotting assay. Interestingly psoriatic patients, DTH negatives to amastigote antigens, also recognized in the blastogenic assay Leishmania antigens and were distributed in two groups, low and high responders to Leishmania amastigote antigens before treatment (O'Daly et al., 2009b).

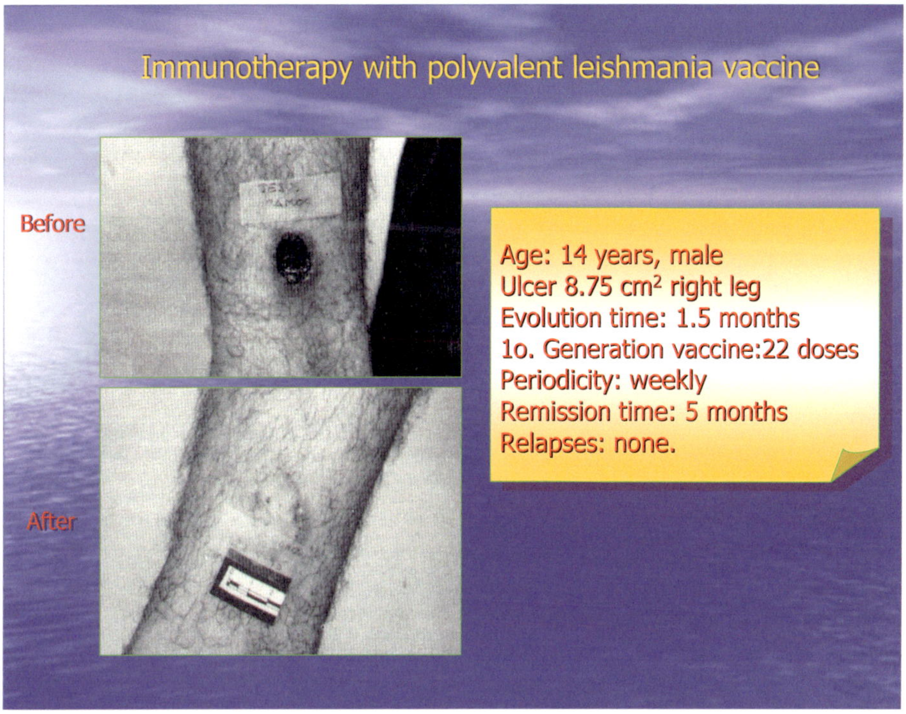

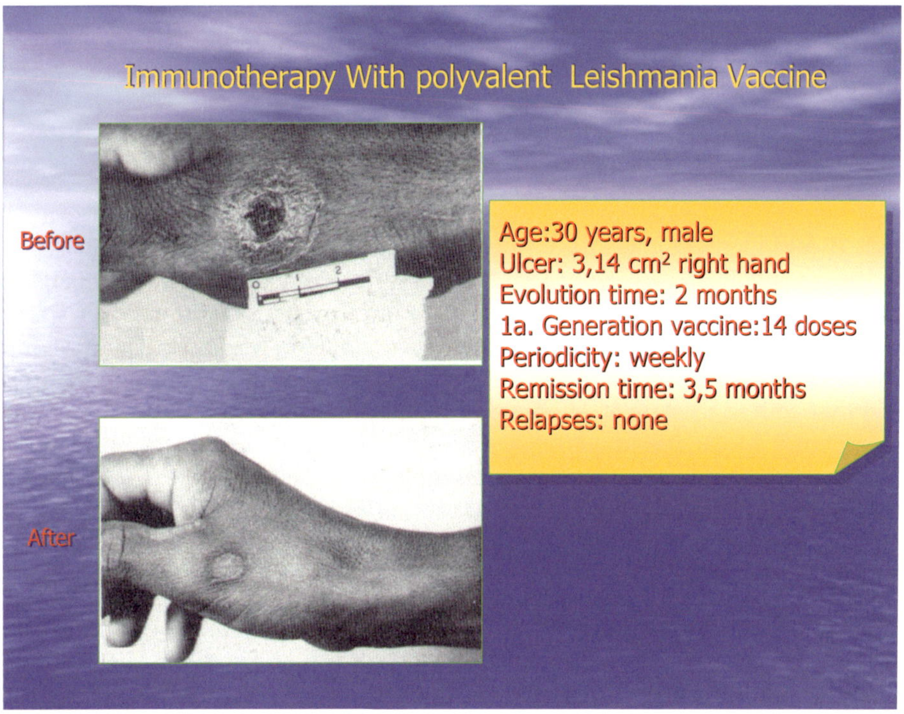

Fig. 8. Treatment with AS100-1 polyvalent vaccine as immunotherapeutic agent in infected volunteers.

Furthermore, we have demonstrated a high DTH response with *L. brasiliensis* and *L. chagasi* protein (DEAE) fractions in vivo after treatment with AS100-1 suggesting a strong T cell response after treatment and confirming the absence of immunosuppression. The SI values obtained by protein (DEAE) fractions were 50–70% lower than the values induced by intact living leishmania parasites and 90% lower than the total stimulation obtained by the T cell mitogen ConA. This suggests their stimulation potential *in vitro* appears to be selectively focus toward a particular subset of lymphocytes which may be regulatory CD8+ T cells as published (O'Daly et al. 2009a; O'Daly et al., 2009b; O'Daly et al., 2010a; O'Daly et al., 2011)

7.5 The role of IL-10 in parasitic defense and autoimmune disease

IL-10 plays an important role in many skin autoimmune diseases, and in certain parasitic infections, in humans as well as in experimental animals (Weiss et al., 2004). IL-10 stimulates NK cells cytotoxicity and IL-2 inducing IFNγ and TNFα production. In addition, IL-10 produced by Th2 cells inhibits IFNγ synthesis by Th1 cells and downregulates cellular immunity. Th3 or regulatory T cells produce IL-10 that inhibits Th1 and Th2 cell cytokine production, mediating peripheral cell tolerance (Seifert et al., 2000). Further underscoring the importance of IL-10 is its role in parasitic infections, in the persistence of *L(L)major* in the skin after healing and the therapeutic potential of anti-IL-10 receptor antibody for sterile cure. (Belkaid et al., 2001) L. donovani-infected BALB/c mice treated with anti-IL-10 receptor had accelerated granuloma formation and rapid parasite killing without excessive tissue inflammation (Murray et al., 2002). A comparison between cells, cytokines, cellular and humoral immunity in bot diseases is presented in Table 2.

7.6 Relationship between leismaniasis and psoriasis

How can we reconcile the finding that treatment with a leishmanial antigen vaccine targeted at leishmaniasis, results in clinical remission of psoriasis in subjects never exposed to Leishmania parasites? Despite some of the obvious differences between the diseases, there are some striking similarities: immunity against both diseases starts with the same cell types, and also both diseases have similar Th1cytokine patterns at least initially, both diseases respond to the Leishmania polyvalent vaccine, AS100-1. It should be noted that both trials showed evidence of cellular immunity not humoral immunity. In psoriasis, initial interaction of antigens between APC and T cells occurs in the lymph nodes. Subsequent psoriatic antigen presentation occurs in psoriatic plaques that structurally resemble a lymph node, but are found in the skin. At this stage of psoriatic disease, the cellular conformation is quite similar to the granuloma found in the skin after Leishmania infection (Table 2).

Finally, many doors have been opened with the serendipity discovery of Leishmania amastigote antigens inducing clinical remission of psoriasis as a systemic disease, which no doubt will provide new roads and answers not solved yet.

Future research and clinical efforts will illuminate many fundamental problems, encountered in those terrible illness affecting human beings in all countries on earth.

PSORIASIS	LEISHMANIASIS
Unknown etiology. Genetically determined disease, multiple genes interacting with environment involved in the inflammatory process manifested as plaques, gutatta, palm/plantar, erythrodermia, nails, and arthritic forms.	Infection by metacyclic promastigotes in vector (sandfly) that transform immediately into intracellular amastigotes in cells of vertebrate host, inducing cutaneous, mucocutaneous, diffuse and visceral clinical forms.
Starting lesions in epidermis with macrophages, monocytes, lymphocytes and neutrophiles at Munro sterile abscesses. Unknown antigen at immunological synapse structured by MHC-TCR receptors between T cells and APC with costimulatory molecules as LFA-1, ICAM-1, CD2, LFA-3 CD28, CD80. Proliferation and migration CD4+ T cells from the lymph nodes to the dermis regulated by cytokines. Dermal CD4+ and epidermal CD8+ cells contribute to plaque formation.	Neutrophiles, lymphocytes, epithelioid cells, monocytes, macrophages and fibroblasts starts at the site of infection. Leishmania antigens at similar immunological synapse MHC-TCR receptors between T cells and APC with same costimulatory molecules. CD4+ and CD8+ cells contribute to IFNγ and TNFα production in infected patients and healing of lesions. Leishmania antigens induce *in vitro* proliferation and IFNγ production in CD2+ T cells from PBMC in individuals that never had contact with parasites.
Cell-cell interactions in skin involve: keratinocytes, melanocytes, Langerhans cells, dendritic cells, mast cells, naive T cells, memory T cells expressing CLA. ICAM-1 and E-Selectin receptors on dermal endothelial cells. In the epidermis neutrophiles and CD8+ T cells with MHCII, IL-2 receptor, modulate inflammation.	Skin immunity delivered by keratinocytes, melanocytes , dendritic Langerhans cells, mast cells, tissue macrophages, neutrophils, dermal dendritic cells and fibroblasts, T cells, memory T cells expressing CLA. Similar receptors on endothelial cells. Epidermal and dermal cells cytokines modulate immune response and inflammation after infection.
TH1 cytokines increase in plaques and serum represented by TNFα, IFNγ, IL-6, IL-8, IL12, and IL-18. High levels of IFNγ, IL12, and IL-18 correlated with disease severity. Relative under expression of TH2 cytokines IL-4 and IL-10. Dilated blood vessels earliest signal within dermal papillae induced by keratinocytes pro-angiogenic cytokines.	Activated macrophages produce: TNFα, IL-6, IL-18, IFNγ and high IL-12, inducing a protective TH1 immune response in resistant mice. TH2 response with IL-4, IL-13, IL-10 and low or absent IL-12 in susceptible mice. Humans with resolving lesions have higher ratios of INFγ/IL4 compared to patients with nonhealing lesions.
Clinical response to IL-10 correlated with decreased cutaneous infiltration and decrease of IFNγ, TNFα, IL-17, IL-8 and CXCR2 in lesions. UV light exerts its therapeutic effects by stimulating keratinocytes or APC to secrete IL-10. Cutaneous IL-10 mRNA is significantly lower in psoriasis.	IL-10 promotes disease progression in cutaneous leishmaniasis. Chronic infections in humans and mice associated with generation of CD4+ T cells expressing IL-10. IL-10 responses and the generation of functionally impaired CD8+ T-cells permit parasites persistence in the host.

Table 2. Comparison of pathogenesis between Psoriasis and leishmaniasis

8. References

Abe R, Yamagishi S, Fujita Y, Hoshina D, Sasaki M, Nakamura K, Matsui T, Shimizu T, Bucala R, & Shimizu H. 2010. Topical application of anti-angiogenic peptides based on pigment epithelium-derived factor can improve psoriasis.*J Dermatol Sci.* 2010 Mar;57(3):183-91. Epub 2010 Jan 8.

Abeyakirthi S, Mowbray M, Bredenkamp N, van Overloop L, Declercq L, Davis PJ, Matsui MS, & Weller RB. 2010. Arginase is overactive in psoriatic skin. *Br J Dermatol.* 2010 Jul; 163(1):193-6. Epub 2010 Mar 10.

Abuabara K, Azfar RS, Shin DB, Neimann AL, Troxel AB, & Gelfand JM. 2010. Cause-specific mortality in patients with severe psoriasis: a population-based cohort study in the U.K. *Br J Dermatol.* 2010 Sep 163(3):586-592. doi: 10.1111/j.1365-2133.2010.09941.x.

Ahlehoff O, Gislason GH, Charlot M, Jørgensen CH, Lindhardsen J, Olesen JB, Abildstrøm SZ, Skov L, Torp-Pedersen C, & Hansen PR. 2010. Psoriasis is associated with clinically significant cardiovascular risk: a Danish nationwide cohort study. *J Intern Med.* 2010 Oct 29. doi: 10.1111/j.1365-2796.2010.02310.x.

Al Robaee AA, 2010 Molecular genetics of Psoriasis (Principles, technology, gene location, genetic polymorphism and gene expression) *International Journal of Health Sciences,* Nov 2010 4(2)/Dhu Al-Hijja 1431 H

Al'Abadie MS, Senior J, Bleehen SS, Gawkrodger DJ, Neuropeptides and general neuronal marker in psoriasis—an immunohistochemical study, *Clin. Exp. Dermatol.* 1995 20:384–389.

Albanesi, C. & Pastore, S. 2010.Pathobiology of Chronic Inflammatory Skin Diseases: Interplay Between Keratinocytes and Immune Cells as a Target for Anti-Inflammatory Drugs. *Current Drug Metabolism* Mar2010, Vol. 11 Issue 3, p210-227,

Alenius GM, Stegmayr BG, & Dahlqvist SR. 2001. Renal abnormalities in a population of patients with psoriatic arthritis. Scand J Rheumatol. 2001. 30:271-274.

Alsufyani MA, Golant AK, & Lebwohl M. Psoriasis and the metabolic syndrome. *Dermatol Ther.* 2010 Mar 23(2):137-43.

Altés J, Salas A, Riera M, Udina M, Galmés A, Balanzat J, Ballesteros A, Buades J, Salvá F, & Villalonga C. 1991. Visceral leishmaniasis: another HIV-associated opportunistic infection? Report of eight cases and review of the literature. *AIDS.* 1991 Feb;5(2):201-7.

Altomare GF, Altomare A, & Pigatto PD. 2009. Traditional systemic treatment of psoriasis. *J Rheumatol* Suppl. 2009 Aug 83:46-48. doi:10.3899/jrheum.090223

Amherd-Hoekstra A, Näher H, Lorenz HM & Enk AH. 2010. Psoriatic arthritis: a review. J Dtsch Dermatol Ges 2010. 8:332-339.

Arican O, Aral M, Sasmaz S, & Ciragil P. 2005 Serum levels of TNF-alpha, IFN-gamma, IL-6, IL-8, IL12, Il-17 and IL-18 in patients with active psoriasis and correlation with disease severity. *Mediators Inflamm.* 2005 Oct 24 2005(5):273–279.

Armesto S, Esteve A, Coto-Segura P, Drake M, Galache C, Martínez-Borra J, & Santos-Juanes J. 2011. Nail Psoriasis in Individuals With Psoriasis Vulgaris: A Study of 661 Patients. *Actas Dermosifiliogr.* 2011 Jun 102(5):365-372. Epub 2011 Apr 22.)

Armstrong AW, Lin SW, Chambers CJ, Sockolov ME, & Chin DL 2011. Psoriasis and Hypertension Severity: Results from a Case-Control Study. PLoS ONE 6(3): e18227. doi:10.1371/journal.pone.0018227

Augustin M, Glaeske G, Radtke MA, Christophers E, Reich K, & Schäfer I. 2010Epidemiology and comorbidity of psoriasis in children. *Br J Dermatol.* 2009 Nov 18, 162(3):633-636.

Augustin M, Reich K, Blome C, Schäfer I, Laass A, & Radtke MA. 2010. Nail psoriasis in Germany: epidemiology and burden of disease. *Br J Dermatol.* 2010 April 18 [Epub ahead of print].

Awasthi A, Mathur KR, & Saha B. 2004. Immune response to leishmania infection. *Indian J Med Res.* 2004. 119:238–258.

Barton AC.2002. Genetic epidemiology. Psoriatic arthritis. *Arthritis Res* 2002. 4:247-251.

Belkaid Y, Hoffmann KF, Mendez S, Kamhawi S, Udey MC, Wynn TA, Sacks DL. 2001. The role of interleukin (IL)-10 in the persistence of Leishmania major in the skin after healing and the therapeutic potential of anti-IL10 receptor antibody for sterile cure. *J Exp Med.* 2001 194:1497–1506.

Bisht M, Dhasmana DC, & Bist SS. 2010. Angiogenesis: Future of pharmacological modulation. *Indian J Pharmacol.* 2010 Feb;42(1):2-8.

Bisoendial RJ, Stroes ES, & Tak PP. 2009. Where the immune response meets the vessel wall. *Neth J Med.* 2009 Sep 67(8):328-333.

Boehncke WH, & Sterry W. 2009. Psoriasis—a systemic inflammatory disorder: clinic, pathogenesis and therapeutic perspectives. *J Dtsch Dermatol Ges.*2009;7:946–952

Bowes J, & Barton A. 2010. The genetics of psoriatic arthritis: lessons from genome-wide association studies. Discov Med. 2010. 10:177-183.

Boyman O, Conrad C, Dudli C, Kielhorn E, Nickoloff BJ, & Nestle FO. 2005. Activation of dendritic antigen-presenting cells expressing common heat shock protein receptor CD91 during induction of psoriasis. *Br J Dermatol* 152:1211–1218

Brajac I, Kastelan M, Prpić-Massari L, Perisa D, Loncarek K, & Malnar D. 2009. Melanocyte as a possible key cell in the pathogenesis of psoriasis vulgaris. *Med Hypotheses.* 2009 Aug 73(2):254-6

Buckley C, Cavill C, Taylor G, Kay H, Waldron N, Korendowych E, & McHugh N. 2010. Mortality in psoriatic arthritis - a single-center study from the UK. *J Rheumatol.* 2010 Oct 7(10):2141-2144. Epub 2010 Aug 3.

Buckley C, Cavill C, Taylor G, Kay H, Waldron N, Korendowych E, & McHugh N. 2010. Mortality in psoriatic arthritis a single center study from the UK. J Rheumatol. 37:2141-2144.

Buschiazzo E, Maldonado-Cocco JA, Arturi P, Citera G, Berman A, Nitsche A, Rillo OL; RESPONDIA Group Collaborators (7) Graf C, Alvarellos A, Wong R, Paira S, Casado G, Scherbarth H, & Barreira JC. 2011. Epidemiology of spondyloarthritis in Argentina. *Am J Med Sci.* 2011 Apr 341(4):289-292.

Cantini F, Niccoli L, Nannini C, Kaloudi O, Bertoni M, & Cassara E. 2010. Psoriatic arthritis: a systematic review. International Journal of Rheumatic Diseases 2010. 13: 300–317

Castelino M, & Barton A. 2010. Genetic susceptibility factors for psoriatic arthritis. *Curr Opin Rheumatol.* 2010 Mar 22(2):152-156.

Castellani ML, Kempuraj DJ, Salini V, Vecchiet J, Tete S, Ciampoli C, Conti F, Cerulli G, Caraffa A, Antinolfi P, Theoharides TC, De Amicis D, Perrella A, Cuccurullo C, Boscolo P, Shaik Y. 2009. The latest interleukin: IL-33 the novel IL-1-family member is a potent mast cell activator, *J. Biol. Regul. Homeost. Agents* 2009 23:11–14

Ceponis A, & Kavanaugh A. 2010. Treatment of Psoriatic Arthritis with Biological Agents. Semin Cutan Med Surg 2010. 29:56-62.

Chan J, Smoller BR, Raychauduri SP, Jiang WY, Farber EM. 1997. Intraepidermal nerve fiber expression of calcitonin gene-related peptide, vasoactive intestinal peptide and substance P in psoriasis, *Arch. Dermatol. Res.* 289 (1997) 611–616.)

Chandran V, & Raychaudhuri SP. 2010 Geoepidemiology and environmental factors of psoriasis and psoriatic arthritis. *J Autoimmunity* 34:314–321.

Chandran V, Schentag CT, & Gladman DD. 2007. Sensitivity of the classification of psoriatic arthritis criteria in early psoriatic arthritis. Arthritis Rheum 2007. 57:1560-1563

Chang YT, Chen TJ, Liu PC, Chen YC, Chen YJ, Huang YL, Jih JS, Chen CC, Lee DD, Wang WJ, Lin MW, & Liu HN. 2009. Epidemiological study of psoriasis in the national health insurance database in Taiwan. *Acta Derm Venereol* 2009. 89:262–266

Charmoy M, Auderset F, Allenbach C, & Tacchini-Cottier F. 2010. The Prominent Role of Neutrophils during the Initial Phase of Infection by Leishmania Parasites. *J Biomed Biotechnol.* 2010. 2010:719361.

Chen S, de Groot M, Kinsley D, Laverty M, McClanahan T, Arreaza M, Gustafson EL, Teunissen MBM, de Rie MA, Fine JS, & Kraan M. 2010. Expression of chemokine receptor CXCR3 by lymphocytes and plasmacytoid dendritic cells in human psoriatic lesions *Arch Dermatol Res* 2010 302:113–123.

Choi J, & Koo YM. 2003 Quality of life issues in psoriasis. *J Am Acad Dermatol.* 2003;49:S57–S61.

Christophers E, & Mrowietz U (2003) Psoriasis. In: *Fitzpatrick's dermatology in general medicine, 6th edn.*, Freedberg IM, Eisen AZ, WolV KK, Austen F, Goldsmith LA, Katz SI (eds) pp 407–427 McGraw-Hill, New York

Christophers E, Barker JN, Griffiths CE, Daudén E, Milligan G, Molta C, Sato R, & Boggs R. 2010. The risk of psoriatic arthritis remains constant following initial diagnosis of psoriasis among patients seen in European dermatology clinics. *J Eur Acad Dermatol Venereol.* 2010 May. 24(5):548-54. Epub 2009 Oct 23.

Church MK & Clough GF. 1999. Human skin mast cells: in vitro and in vivo studies, *Ann. Allergy Asthma Immunol.* 1999 83:471–475

Cimmino MA. Epidemiology of psoriasis and psoriatic arthritis. *Reumatismo.* 2007;59 Suppl 1:19-24

Ciocon DH, & Kimball AB. 2007. Psoriasis and psoriatic arthritis: separate or one and the same? *Br J Dermatol* 2007 157: 850–860.

Coates LC, & Helliwell PS. 2008. Classification and categorization of psoriatic arthritis. Clin Rheumatol 2008. 27:1211-1216.

Coates LC, & Helliwell PS. 2010. Disease measurement--enthesitis, skin, nails, spine and dactylitis. Best Pract Res Clin Rheumatol. 2010 Oct 24 (5):659-670.

Cohen AD, Weitzman D, & Dreiher J. 2010. Psoriasis and hypertension: a case-control study. *Acta Derm Venereol.* 2010 90(1):23-6.

Das RP, Jain AK, & Ramesh V. 2009. Current concepts in the pathogenesis of psoriasis. *Indian J Dermatol.* 2009 54:7–12

Davidovici BB, Sattar N, Prinz JC, Puig L, Emery P, Barker JN, van de Kerkhof P, Ståhle M, Nestle FO, Girolomoni G, &

de Felice C, Ardigo M, Berardesca E. Biologic therapies for psoriasis. *J Rheumatol* Suppl. 2009 Aug;83:62-4.

Di Cesare A, Di Meglio P, & Nestle FO. 2009. The IL-23/Th17 axis in the immunopathogenesis of psoriasis. *J Invest Dermatol.* 2009 Jun 129(6):1339-1350. Epub 2009 Mar 26.

Elder JT. 2009. Genome-wide association scan yields new insights into the immunopathogenesis of psoriasis. *Genes Immun.* 2009;10:201–209

Elder JT, Bruce AT, Gudjonsson JE, Johnston A, Stuart PE, Tejasvi T, Voorhees JJ, Abecasis GR, & Nair RP. 2010.Molecular dissection of psoriasis: integrating genetics and biology. J Invest Dermatol. 2010 May 130(5):1213-26. Epub 2009 Oct 8.

El-Nour H, Santos A, Nordin M, Jonsson P, Svensson M, Nordlind K, & Berg M. 2009. Neuronal changes in psoriasis exacerbation. *J Eur Acad Dermatol Venereol.* 2009 Nov 23(11):1240-1245. Epub 2009 May 6.

Epub 2007 Aug 13.

Fantini F, Magnoni C, Bracci-Laudiero L, & Pincelli C. 1995. Nerve growth factor is increased in psoriatic skin. *J Invest Dermatol* 1995; 105:854-855.

Farber EM, & Nall ML (1974). The natural history of psoriasis in 5,600 patients. *Dermatologica* 148:1–18

Farley E, Masrour S, McKey J, & Menter A. 2009. Palmoplantar psoriasis: a phenotypical and clinical review with introduction of a new quality-of-life assessment tool. *J Am Acad Dermatol.* 2009 Jun;60(6):1024-31

Federman DG, Shelling M, Prodanovich S, Gunderson CG, & Kirsner RS. Psoriasis: an opportunity to identify cardiovascular risk. *Br J Dermatol.* 2009 Jan;160(1):1-7. Epub 2008 Oct 25.

Fernandez-Guerrero ML, Aguado JM, Barros C, Montalban C, Martin T, & Bouza E. 1987. Visceral leishmaniasis in immunocompromised hosts. *Am J Med.* 1987 83:1098–1102.

Fortune DG, Richards HL, & Griffiths CE. Psychologic factors in psoriasis: consequences, mechanisms, and interventions, *Dermatol. Clin.* 2005 23:681–694.

Fruth U, Solioz N, & Louis JA. 1993. Leishmania major interferes with antigen presentation by infected macrophages. *J Immunol* 1993. 150:1857–1864.

García-Kutzbach A, Montenegro A, Iraheta I, Bará C, & Saénz R. 2011. Epidemiology of spondyloarthropathies in Central America. *Am J Med Sci.* 2011 Apr 341(4):295-297.

Garg A, & Gladman D. 2010. Recognizing psoriatic arthritis in the dermatology clinic *J Am Acad Dermatol* 2010 63:733-748

Gelfand JM, Mehta NN, & Langan SM. 2011. Psoriasis and Cardiovascular Risk: Strength in Numbers, Part II. *J Invest Dermatol.* 2011 May 131(5):1007-1010.

Ghazizadeh R, Shimizu H, Tosa M, & Ghazizadeh M. 2010. Pathogenic mechanisms shared between psoriasis and cardiovascular disease. *Int J Med Sci.* 2010 Aug 19;7(5):284-9.

Gilliver SC, Emmerson E, Bernhagen J, & Hardman MJ. 2011 MIF: a key player in cutaneous biology and wound healing. *Exp Dermatol.* 2011 Jan;20(1):1-6. doi: 10.1111/j.1600-0625.2010.01194.x.

Gisondi P, Del Giglio M, Cozzi A. & Girolomoni G. 2010. Psoriasis, the liver, and the gastrointestinal tract. *Dermatol Ther* 23: 155–159

Gladman DD, Shuckett R, Russell ML, Thorne JC, & Schachter RK.1987. Psoriatic arthritis (PSA)—an analysis of 220 patients. *Q J Med* 1987. 62:127–141.

Gottlieb A, Korman NJ, Gordon KB, Feldman SR, Lebwohl M, Koo JY, Van Voorhees AS, Elmets CA, Leonardi CL, Beutner KR, Bhushan R, & Menter A. 2008. Guidelines of care for the management of psoriasis and psoriatic arthritis. Section 2. Psoriatic arthritis: Overview and guidelines of care for treatment with an emphasis on the biologics. *J Am Acad Dermatol.* 2008. 58(5):851-864.

Guenther L, & Gulliver W. 2009. Psoriasis comorbidities. *J Cutan Med Surg.* 2009 Sep-Oct;13 Suppl 2:S77-8

Handman E. 2001. Leishmaniasis: Current status of vaccine development. *Clin.Microbiol Rev.* 2001. 14:229–243.

Hanova P, Pavelka K, Holcatova I, & Pikhart H. 2010. Incidence and prevalence of psoriatic arthritis, ankylosing spondylitis, and reactive arthritis in the first descriptive population-based study in the Czech Republic. *Scand J Rheumatol.* 2010 Aug 39(4):310-7.

Harper EG, Guo C, Rizzo H, Lillis JV, Kurtz SE, Skorcheva I, Purdy D, Fitch E, Iordanov M, & Blauvelt A. 2009. Th17 cytokines stimulate CCL20 expression in keratinocytes in vitro and in vivo: implications for psoriasis pathogenesis. *J Invest Dermatol.* 2009 Sep 129(9):2175-83. Epub 2009 Mar 19;doi:10.1038/jid.2009.65;

Harvima IT, Nilsson G, Suttle MM, & Naukkarinen A. 2008. Is there a role for mast cells in psoriasis? *Arch. Dermatol. Res.* 2008 300:461–476.

Harvima IT, Viinamäki H, Naukkarinen A, Paukkonen K, Neittaanmäki, & Horsmanheimo M, 1993. Association of cutaneous mast cells and sensory nerves with psychic stress in psoriasis, *Psychother. Psychosom.* 1993 60:168–176.

Harvima RJ, Viinamäki H, Harvima IT, Naukkarinen A, Savolainen A, Aalto AML, M. & Horsmanheimo M. 1996. Association of psychic stress with clinical severity and symptoms of psoriatic patients, *Acta Derm.-Venereol. (Stockh.)* 1996. 76:467–471

Helliwell PS. 2009. Established Psoriatic Arthritis: Clinical Aspects J Rheumatol 2009. 83:21-23

Herron MD, Hinckley M, Hoffman MS, Papenfuss J, Hansen CB, Callis KP, & Krueger GG. 2005. Impact of obesity and smoking on psoriasis presentation and management. *Arch Dermatol.* 2005. 141:1527-1534.

Husted JA, Tom BD, Farewell VT, & Gladman DD. 2010. Longitudinal analysis of fatigue in psoriatic arthritis. J Rheumatol. 37:1878-1884.

Husted JA, Tom BD, Farewell VT, Schentag CT, & Gladman DD. 2007. A longitudinal study of the effect of disease activity and clinical damage on physical function over the course of psoriatic arthritis: Does the effect change over time? *Arthritis Rheum.* 2007. 56:840-849.

Ibrahim G, Waxman R, & Helliwell PS. 2009. The prevalence of psoriatic arthritis in people with psoriasis. *Arthritis Rheum.* 2009 Oct 15 61(10):1373-1378.

Iikura M, Suto H, Kajiwara N, Oboki K, Ohno T, Okayama Y, Saito H, Galli SJ, & Nakae S. 2007. IL-33 can promote survival, adhesion and cytokine production in human mast cells, *Lab. Invest.* 2007 Oct. 87(10):971–978.

Ilkovitch D. 2011. Role of immune-regulatory cells in skin pathology. *J Leukoc Biol.* 2011 Jan 89(1):41-49. Epub 2010 Jul 13.

Jamnitski A, Visman IM, Peters MJ, Boers M, Dijkmans BA, & Nurmohamed MT. 2010. Prevalence of cardiovascular diseases in psoriatic arthritis resembles that of rheumatoid arthritis. Ann Rheum Dis. doi: 10.1136/ard.2010.136499

Janković S, Raznatović M, Marinković J, Maksimović N, Janković J, & Djikanović B. 2009. Relevance of psychosomatic factors in psoriasis: a case-control study. *Acta Derm Venereol.* 2009;89(4):364-8.

Jerner B, Skogh M, & Vahlquist A. 1997. A controlled trial of acupuncture in psoriasis: noconvincing effect. *Acta Derm Venereol* 1997 77:154–156.

Kandere-Grzybowska K, Gheorghe D, Priller J, Esposito P, Huang M, Gerard N, & Theoharides TC. 2003. Stress-induced dura vascular permeability does not develop in mast cell-deficient and neurokinin-1 receptor knockout mice, *Brain Res.* 2003 980:213–220.)

Katsarou-Katsari A, Filippou A, Theoharides TC. 1999. Effect of stress and other psychological factors on the pathophysiology and treatment of dermatoses, *Int. J. Immunopathol. Pharmacol.* 1999. 12: 7–11.

Kawana S, Liang Z, Nagano M, & Suzuki H. 2006. Role of substance P in stress-derived degranulation of dermal mast cells in mice, *J. Dermatol. Sci.* 2006 42:47–54.

Keeren K, Friedrich M, Gebuhr I, Philipp S, Sabat R, Sterry W, Brandt C, Meisel C, Grütz G, Volk HD, & Sawitzki B. 2009. Expression of tolerance associated gene-1, a mitochondrial protein inhibiting T cell activation, can be used to predict response to immune modulating therapies. *J Immunol.* 2009 Sep 15 183(6):4077-4087. Epub 2009 Aug 14

Kemp M, Hansen MB, & Theander TG. 1992. Recognition of leishmania antigens by T lymphocytes from nonexposed individuals. *Infect Immun.* 1992 60: 2246–2251

Kilarski WW, & Gerwins P. 2009A new mechanism of blood vessel growth - hope for new treatment strategies. *Discov Med.* 2009 Jun;8(40):23-7.

Kim N, Thrash B, & Menter A. 2010. Comorbidities in psoriasis patients. *Semin Cutan Med Surg.* 2010. 29(1):10-15.

Kima PE, Soong L, Chicharro C, Ruddle NH, & McMahon-Pratt D. 1996. Leishmania-infected macrophages sequester endogenously synthesized parasite antigens from presentation to CD4+ T cell. *Eur J Immunol* 1996. 26:3163–3169.

Körner H, McMorran B, Schlüter D, & Fromm P. 2010. The role of TNF in parasitic diseases: still more questions than answers. *Int J Parasitol.* 2010 40:879–888.

Krathen MS, Gottlieb AB, & Mease PJ. 2010. Pharmacologic immunomodulation and cutaneous malignancy in rheumatoid arthritis, psoriasis, and psoriatic arthritis. J Rheumatol. 2010. 37:2205-2215.

Krueger JG Psoriasis and systemic inflammatory diseases: potential mechanistic links between skin disease and co-morbid conditions. J Invest Dermatol. 2010 Jul;130(7):1785-96. Epub 2010 May 6.

Kunz M. 2009. Current treatment of psoriasis with biologics. *Curr Drug Discov Technol.* 2009 Dec 6(4):231-40.

Langner MD, & Maibach HI. 2009. Pruritus measurement and treatment. *Clin Exp Dermatol.* 2009 Apr 34(3):285-288.

Leeman SE, & Ferguson SL. 2000. Substance P: an historical perspective, Neuropeptides 34 (2000) 249–254.

Lin HW, Wang KH, Lin HC, & Lin HC. 2011. Increased risk of acute myocardial infarction in patients with psoriasis: a 5-year population-based study in Taiwan. *J Am Acad Dermatol.* 2011 Mar 64(3):495-501. Epub 2011 Jan 8.

Lonsdorf AS, Hwang ST, & Enk AH. 2009. Chemokine receptors in T-cell-mediated diseases of the skin. *J Invest Dermatol.* 2009 Nov; 129(11):2552-2566. Epub 2009 May 28. doi:10.1038/jid.2009.122;

Lotti T, Hercogova J, & Prignano F. 2010. The concept of psoriatic disease: can cutaneous psoriasis any longer be separated by the systemic comorbidities? *Dermatol Ther.* 2010. 23(2):119-122.

Maejima H, Taniguchi T, Watarai A, & Katsuoka K. 2010. Evaluation of nail disease in psoriatic arthritis by using a modified nail psoriasis severity score index. Int J Dermatol. 2010 49:901-906.

Major, E. (2010). "Progressive multifocal leukoencephalopathy in patients on immunomodulatory therapies". *Annual review of medicine* 2010. 61 (1): 35–47. doi:10.1146/annurev.med.080708.082655. PMID 19719397

Marji JS, Marcus R, Moennich J, & Mackay-Wiggan J. 2010. Use of biologic agents in pediatric psoriasis. J Drugs Dermatol. 2010. 9:975-986.

Mazzoccoli G, Notarsanto I, de Pinto GD, Dagostino MP, De Cata A, D'Alessandro G, Tarquini R, & Vendemiale G. 2010. Anti-tumor necrosis factor-α therapy and changes of flow-mediated vasodilatation in psoriatic and rheumatoid arthritis patients. Intern Eme

McFadden JP, Baker BS, Powles AV, & Fry L. 2009. Psoriasis and streptococci: the natural selection of psoriasis revisited. *Br J Dermatol.* 2009 May 160(5):929-37.

McGonagle D, Palmou Fontana N, Tan AL, & Benjamin M. 2010. Nailing down the genetic and immunological basis for psoriatic disease. Dermatology 2010. 221 (Suppl. 1):15-22 (DOI: 10.1159/000316171)

McHugh NJ. 2009. Traditional schemes for treatment of psoriatic arthritis. J Rheumatol 2009. 83:49-51.

McInnes IB, Illei GG, Danning CL, Yarboro CH, Crane M, Kuroiwa T, Schlimgen R, Lee E, Foster B, Flemming D, Prussin C, Fleisher TA, & Boumpas DT. 2001. IL-10 improves skin disease and modulates endothelial activation and leukocyte effector function in pat

Mease P. 2006. Psoriatic Arthritis Update. Bull NYU Hosp Jt Dis 2006. 64, Numbers 1 & 2,

Mease PJ. 2008. Assessment tools in psoriatic arthritis. *J Rheumatol.* 2008 35:1426-1430.

Mease PJ. 2009. Psoriatic arthritis assessment and treatment update. Curr Opin Rheumatol. 2009. 21:348-55.

Mease PJ. 2010a. Psoriatic arthritis - update on pathophysiology, assessment, and management. *Bull NYU Hosp Jt Dis.* 2010 68(3):191-8.

Mease PJ. 2010b. Psoriatic Arthritis: Pharmacotherapy Update Curr Rheumatol Rep 2010 12:272-280)

Migliore A, Bizzi E, Laganà B, Altomonte L, Zaccari G, Granata M, Canzoni M, Marasini B, Massarotti M, Massafra U, Ranieri M, Pilla R, Martin LS, Pezza M, Vacca F, & Galluccio A. 2009. The safety of anti-TNF agents in the elderly. Int J Immunopathol Pharm

Mok C, Ko G, Ho L, Yu K, Chan P, & To C. 2010. Prevalence of atherosclerotic risk factors and the metabolic syndrome in patients with chronic inflammatory arthritis. *Arthritis Care Res (Hoboken).* DOI 10.1002/acr.20363)

Moll JM, & Wright V. 1973. Psoriatic arthritis. *Semin Arthritis Rheum* 1973. 3(1):55–78.

Monteleone G, Pallone F, MacDonald TT, Chimenti S, & Costanzo A. 2011. Psoriasis: from pathogenesis to novel therapeutic approaches. *Clin Sci (Lond).* 2011 Jan;120(1):1-11.

Moulin D, Donze O, Talabot-Ayer D, Mezin F, Palmer G, & Gabay C, Interleukin (IL)-33 induces the release of pro-inflammatory mediators by mast cells, *Cytokine* 2007 40:216–225.

Mrowietz U, & Reich K. 2009. Psoriasis—new insights into pathogenesis and treatment.*Dtsch Arztebl Int.* 2009;106:11–19.

Mrowietz, U, Elder JT, & Barker J. 2007. The importance of disease associations and concomitant therapy for the long term management of psoriasis patients. *Arch Dermatol Res.* 2007;298:309–319

Murray HW, Lu CM, Mauze S, Freeman S, Moreira AL, Kaplan G, & Coffman RL. 2002. Interleukin 10 (IL-10) in experimental visceral leishmaniasis and IL-10 receptor blockade as immunotherapy. *Infect Immun.* 2002 70:6284–6293.

Nakai K, Yoneda K, Maeda R, Munehiro A, Fujita N, Yokoi I, Moriue J, Moriue T, Kosaka H, & Kubota Y. 2009. Urinary biomarker of oxidative stress in patients with psoriasis vulgaris and atopic dermatitis. *J Eur Acad Dermatol Venereol.* 2009 Dec 23(12):1405-1408.

Naldi L, & Mercuri SR. 2010 Epidemiology of comorbidities in psoriasis. *Dermatologic Ther.* 2010;23:114–118.)

Naldi L, & Rzany B. 2009. Psoriasis (chronic plaque). *Clin Evid (Online).* 2009 Jan 9 2009. pii: 1706.

Naukkarinen A, Jarvikallio A, Lakkakorpi J, Harvima IT, Harvima RJ, & Horsmanheimo M. 1996. Quantitative histochemical analysis of mast cells and sensory nerves in psoriatic skin, *J. Pathol.* 1996 180:200–205.

Nestle FO, Kaplan DH, & Barker J. 2009 Psoriasis, *N. Engl. J. Med.* 361 (2009) 361:496–509.

Nijsten T, & Wakkee M. 2009. Complexity of the association between psoriasis and comorbidities. *J Invest Dermatol.* 2009 Jul 129(7):1601-1603.

Nofal A, Al-Makhzangy I, Attwa E, Nassar A, & Abdalmoati A. 2009. Vascular endothelial growth factor in psoriasis: an indicator of disease severity and control. *J Eur Acad Dermatol Venereol.* 2009 Jul;23(7):803-6. Epub 2009 Mar 6.

O'Daly JA, & Gleason J. 2010c. Antigens from Leishmania amastigotes inducing clinical remission of psoriasis: Relationship between leishmaniasis and psoriasis. Journal of Clinical Dermatology DERMA 2010 1:47-57

O'Daly JA, Gleason J, Lezama R, Rodriguez PJ, Silva E, & Indriago NR. 2011. Antigens from Leishmania amastigotes inducing clinical remission of psoriatic arthritis. Arch Dermatol Res. 10.1007/s00403-011-1133-0

O'Daly JA, Gleason JP, Peña G, & Colorado I. 2010a. Purified proteins from leishmania amastigotes-induced delayed type hypersensitivity reactions and remission of collagen-induced arthritis in animal models. Arch Dermatol Res 2010. 302:567-581.

O'Daly JA, Lezama R, & Gleason J. 2009b. Isolation of Leishmania amastigote protein fractions which induced lymphocyte stimulation and remission of psoriasis. *Arch Dermatol Res* 2009b. 301:411-427.

O'Daly JA, Lezama R, Rodriguez PJ Silva E, Indriago NR, Peña G, Colorado I, Gleason J, Rodríguez B, Acuña L, & Ovalles T. 2009a. Antigens from Leishmania amastigotes induced clinical remission of psoriasis. Arch Dermatol Res 2009. 301:1-13.

O'Daly JA, Rodriguez B, Ovalles T, & Pelaez C. 2010b. Lymphocyte subsets in peripheral blood of patients with psoriasis before and after treatment with leishmania antigens. Arch Dermatol Res 2010. 302:95-104.

O'Daly JA, Spinetti H, Rodríguez MB, Acuña L, Garcia P. Castillo LM, Ovalles T, Zambrano L, Yanes A, Iannello JG, Garcia R, Papapietro A, Zamora C & Salinas O.1995a. Proteínas de amastigotes de varias cepas de leishmanias protegen a seres humanos contra la Leishmaniasis en el área de Guatire, Edo. Miranda, Venezuela. *Gac Méd Caracas.* 1995 103:133–177.

O'Daly JA, Spinetti H, Rodríguez MB, Acuña L, Garcia P, Castillo LM, Zambrano L, Ovalles T, & Zamora C. 1995b Comparación de los efectos terapéuticos de la mezcla de promastigotes + BCG, antígenos purificados de amastigotes y el Glucantime en un área hiperendémica de Leishmaniasis cutánea, en Guatire, Edo, Miranda, Venezuela. *Gac Méd Caracas* 103:327-357.

O'Neill T, & Silman AJ. 1994. Psoriatic arthritis. Historical background and epidemiology [review]. *Baillieres Clin Rheumatol* 1994. 8:245-261

O'Rielly DD, & Rahman P. 2010. Where Do We Stand With the Genetics of Psoriatic Arthritis? Curr Rheumatol Rep 2010. 12:300–308.

O'Connor TM, O'Connell J, O'Brien DI, Goode T, Bredin CP, & Shanahan F. 2004. The role of substance P in inflammatory disease, J. Cell. Physiol. 2004 201:167–180.

Okwor I, & Uzonna J. 2009. Vaccines and vaccination strategies against human cutaneous leishmaniasis. *Hum Vaccin.* 2009. 5:291–301.

Olivieri I, D'Angelo S, Palazzi C, Lubrano E, & Leccese P. 2010. Emerging drugs for psoriatic arthritis. Expert Opin Emerg Drugs. 2010. 15:399-414.

Olivieri I, Padula A, D'Angelo S, & Cutro MS. 2009. Psoriatic arthritis sine psoriasis. J Rheumatol 2009. 83:28-29.

Ortega C, Fernandez S, Carrillo JM, Romero P, Molina IJ, Moreno JC, & Santamarıa M. 2009. IL-17-producing CD8+ T lymphocytes from psoriasis skin plaques are cytotoxic effector cells that secrete Th17-related cytokines *J. Leukoc. Biol.* 2009 86: 435–443

Özdamar SO, Seckin D, Kandemir B, & Turanlt AY. 1996. Mast cells in psoriasis, Dermatology 192 (1996) 190.

Papo D, Hein R, & Ring J. 2010. Psoriasis as an independent risk factor for development of coronary artery disease. *Dtsch Med Wochenschr.* 135:1749-54.

Parafianowicz K, Sicińska J, Moran A, Szumański J, Staniszewski K, Rudnicka L, & Kokoszka A. 2010. [Psychiatric comorbidities of psoriasis: pilot study]. *Psychiatr Pol.* 2010 Jan-Feb 44(1):119-126.

Pastore S, & Korkina L. 2010. Redox imbalance in T cell-mediated skin diseases. *Mediators Inflamm.* Volume 2010, Article ID 861949, 9 pages doi:10.1155/2010/861949 Epub 2010 Aug

Paus R, Theoharides TC, & Arck PC. 2006. Neuroimmunoendocrine circuitry of the'brain-skin connection', *Trends Immunol.* 2006 27: 32–39.

Peternel S, & Kastelan M. 2009. Immunopathogenesis of psoriasis: focus on natural killer T cells. *J Eur Acad Dermatol Venereol.* 2009 Oct; 23(10):1123-1127. Epub 2009 Apr 30.

Pincelli C. 2000. Nerve growth factor and keratinocytes: a role in psoriasis. *Eur J Dermatol* 2000; 10:85-90.

Piruzian E, Bruskin S, Ishkin A, Abdeev R, Moshkovskii S, Melnik S, Nikolsky Y, & Nikolskaya T. Integrated network analysis of transcriptomic and proteomic data in psoriasis. *BMC Syst Biol.* 2010 Apr 8 4:41-53.

Prignano F, Ricceri F, Pescitelli L, & Lotti T. 2009. Itch in psoriasis: epidemiology, clinical aspects and treatment options. *Clin Cosmet Investig Dermatol.* 2009 Feb 19;2:9-13.

Prodanovich S, Kirsner RS, Kravetz JD, Ma F, Martinez L, & Federman DG. Association of psoriasis with coronary artery, cerebrovascular, and peripheral vascular diseases and mortality. *Arch Dermatol.* 2009 Jun 145(6):7

Pushparaj PN, Tay HK, H'ng SC, Pitman N, Xu D, McKenzie A, Liew FY, & Melendez AJ. 2009. The cytokine interleukin-33 mediates anaphylactic shock, *Proc. Natl Acad. Sci. USA* 2009 106:9773–9778.

Radtke MA, Reich K, Blome C, Rustenbach S, & Augustin M 2009. Prevalence and clinical features of psoriatic arthritis and joint complaints in 2009 patients with psoriasis:

results of a German national survey. *J Eur Acad Dermatol Venereol.* 2009 Jun 23(6):683-691. Epub 2009 Mar 6.

Rambukkana A, Das PK, Witkamp L Rambukkana A, Das PK, Witkamp L, Yong S, Meinardi MM, & Bos JD.1993. Antibodies to mycobacterial 65-kDa heat shock protein and other immunodominant antigens in patients with psoriasis. *J Invest Dermatol* 100:87–92.

Rashmi R, Rao KS, & Basavaraj KH. A comprehensive review of biomarkers in psoriasis. *Clin Exp Dermatol.* 2009 Aug;34(6):658-63. Epub 2009 Jun 25

Raychaudhuri SK, & Raychaudhuri SP. 2009 NGF and its receptor system: a new dimension in the pathogenesis of psoriasis and psoriatic arthritis. Ann N Y Acad Sci. 2009. 1173:470-477.

Raychaudhuri SP, Jiang WY, & Farber EM. 1998. Psoriatic keratinocytes express high levels of nerve growth factor. *Acta Derm Venereol* 1998; 78:84-86.

Rehal B, Modjtahedi BS, Morse LS, Schwab IR, Maibach HI. 2011. Ocular psoriasis. *J Am Acad Dermatol.* 2011 May 5. [Epub ahead of print]

Reich K, Krüger K, Mössner R, & Augustin M. 2009. Epidemiology and clinical pattern of psoriatic arthritis in Germany: a prospective interdisciplinary epidemiological study of 1511 patients with plaque-type psoriasis. *Br J Dermatol* 160:1040–1047

Reiner NE, Ng W, & McMaster WR. 1987. Parasite-accessory cell-interactions in murine leishmaniasis. Leishmania donovani suppresses macrophage expression of Class-I and class-II major histocompatibility complex geneproducts. *J. Immunol.* 1987. 138:1926–1932.

Reiner NE, Ng W, & McMaster WR. 1988. Kinetics of gamma interferon binding and induction of major histocompatibility complex class II mRNA in leishmania infected macrophages. *Proc Natl Acad Sci USA* 1988. 85: 4330–4334.

Remröd C, Lonne-Rahm L, & Nordliond K. 2007. Study of substance P and its receptor neurokinin-1 in psoriasis and their relation to chronic stress and pruritus, *Arch. Dermatol. Res.* 2007 299:85–91

Reveille JD. 2011. Epidemiology of spondyloarthritis in North America. *Am J Med Sci.* 2011 Apr. 341(4):284-6.

Rico T, Marchione R, & Kirsner RS. 2009. Vascular disease in psoriasis. *J Invest Dermatol.* 2009 Oct 129(10):2327.

Rodriguez Coura J, Galvao-Castro B, & Grimaldi G 1987. Disseminated American cutaneous leishmaniasis in a patient with AIDS. *Memorias do Instituto Oswaldo Cruz.* 1987 82:581–582.

Rohekar S, Tom BDM, Hassa A, Schentag CT, Farewell VT, & Gladman DD. 2008. Prevalence of Malignancy in Psoriatic arthritis. Arthritis & Rheumatism 2008. 58:82–87.

Rosamond W, Flegal K, Furie K, Go A, Greenlund K, Haase N, Hailpern SM, Ho M, Howard V, Kissela B, Kittner S, Lloyd-Jones D, McDermott M, Meigs J, Moy C, Nichol G, O'Donnell C, Roger V, Sorlie P, Steinberger J, Thom T, Wilson M, & Hong Y. 2008. American Heart Association Statistics Committee and Stroke Statistics SubcommitteeHeart disease and stroke statistics--2008 update: a report from the American Heart Association Statistics Committee and Stroke Statistics Subcommittee. *Circulation.* 2008 Jan 29 117(4):e25-146. Epub 2007 Dec 17.

Rosenthal PJ, Chaisson RE, Hadley WK, & Leech JH. 1988. Rectal leishmaniasis in a patient with acquired immunodeficiency syndrome. *Am J Med.* 1988 84:307–309.

Rudwaleit M, & Taylor WJ. 2010. Classification criteria for psoriatic arthritis and ankylosing spondylitis/axial spondyloarthritis. Best Pract Res Clin Rheumatol. 2010 Oct 24(5):589-604

Saber TP, Ng CT, Renard G, Lynch BM, Pontifex E, Walsh CA, Grier A, Molloy M, Bresnihan B, Fitzgerald O, Fearon U, & Veale DJ. 2010. Remission in psoriatic arthritis: is it possible and how can it be predicted? Arthritis Res Ther. 2010. 12:R94.

Sampaio-Barros PD. 2011. Epidemiology of spondyloarthritis in Brazil. *Am J Med Sci.* 2011 Apr 341(4):287-288.

Santamaria Babi LF, Maser R, Perez Soler MT, Picker LJ, Blaser K, & Hauser C. 1995. Migration of skin homing T cell across cytokine activated human endothelial cell layers involves interaction of the cutaneous lymphocyte-associated antigen (CLA) the very late antigen 4 (VLA-4) and the lymphocyte function-associated antigen-1 (LFA-1) *J Immunol.* 1995;154:1543–1550.

Saraceno R, Kleyn CE, Terenghi G, & Griffiths CE. 2006. The role of neuropeptides in psoriasis, *Br. J. Dermatol.* 2006 155:876–882.

Saraceno R, Mannheimer R, & Chimenti S. 2008. Regional distribution of psoriasis in Italy. *J Eur Acad Dermatol Venereol.* 2008 Mar, 22(3):324-9.

Scaglia M, Villa M, Gatti S, & Fabio F. 1989. Cutaneous leishmaniasis in acquired immunodeficiency syndrome. *Trans Roy Soc TropMed Hyg* 1989 83:338–339.

Scarpa R, Altomare G, Marchesoni A, Balato N, Matucci Cerinic M, Lotti T, Olivieri I, Vena GA, Salvarani C, Valesini G, & Giannetti A. 2010. Psoriatic disease: concepts and implications. J Eur Acad Dermatol Venereol. 2010 Jun;24(6):627-30. Epub 2010 Feb 25.

Scarpa R, Atteno M, Costa L, Peluso R, Iervolino S, Caso F, & Del Puente A. 2009. Early psoriatic arthritis. *J Rheumatol* 83 26-27

Schäfer I, Rustenbach SJ, Radtke M, Augustin J, Glaeske G, & Augustin M. 2011 [Epidemiology of Psoriasis in Germany - Analysis of Secondary Health Insurance Data.] *Gesundheitswesen.* 2010 Jun 11. 2010, 73(5):308-313.

Seifert M, Sterry W, Effenberger E, Rexin A, Friedrich M, Haeussler-Quade A, Volk HD, Asadullah K. 2000. The antipsoriatic activity of IL-10 is rather caused by effects on peripheral blood cells than by a direct effect on human keratinocytes. *Arch Dermatol Res.* 2000 292:164–172.

Sfikakis PP. 2010. The first decade of biologic TNF antagonists in clinical practice: lessons learned, unresolved issues and future directions. Curr Dir Autoimmun. 2010. 11:180-210.

Shbeeb M, Uramoto KM, Gibson LE, O'Fallon WM, & Gabriel SE. 2000. The epidemiology of psoriatic arthritis in Olmsted County, Minnesota, USA, 1982-1991. *J Rheumatol.* 2000. 27(5):1247-1250.

Shelling ML, Federman DG, Prodanovich S, Kirsner RS.Psoriasis and vascular disease: an unsolved mystery. Am J Med. 2008 May;121(5):360-5.

Singh S, Singh U, Singh S. 2010. Prevalence of autoantibodies in patients of psoriasis. *J Clin Lab Anal.* 2010;24(1):44-8.

Soriano ER, & Rosa J. 2009. Update on the treatment of peripheral arthritis in psoriatic arthritis. Curr Rheumatol Rep. 11:270-277.

Stager S, Joshi T, & Bankoti R. Immune evasive mechanisms contributing to persistent Leishmania donovani infection. *Immunol Res.* 2010 47:14–24.

Tagen M, Stiles L, Kalogeromitros D, Gregoriou DS, Kempuraj D, Makris, Donelan J, Vasiadi M, Staurianeas NG, & Theoharides TC, Skin corticotropinreleasing hormone receptor expression in psoriasis, *J. Invest. Dermatol.* 2007 127:1789–1791)

Tam LS, Leung YY, & Li EK. 2009. Psoriatic arthritis in Asia. *Rheumatology (Oxford).* 2009 Dec 48(12):1473-7. Epub 2009 Aug 27.

Taylor W, Gladman D, Helliwell P, Marchesoni A, Mease P, & Mielants H. 2006. Classification criteria for psoriatic arthritis: development of new criteria from a large international study. Arthritis Rheum 2006 54:2665–2673

Theoharides TC, Alysandratos KD, Angelidou A, Delivanis DA, Sismanopoulos N, Zhang B, Asadi S, Vasiadi M, Weng Z, Miniati A, & Kalogeromitros D. 2010. Mast cells and inflammation. *Biochim Biophys Acta.* Dec 23, 2010 doi:10.1016/j.bbadis.2010.12.014

Theoharides TC, Donelan JM, Papadopoulou N, Cao J, Kempuraj D, & Conti P. 2004. Mast cells as targets of corticotropin-releasing factor and related peptides, *Trends Pharmacol. Sci.* 25 (2004) 563–568.

Theoharides TC, Zhang B, Kempuraj D, Tagen M, Vasiadi M, Angelidou A, Alysandratos KD, Kalogeromitros D, Asadi S, Stavrianeas N, Peterson E, Leeman S, & Conti P. 2010. IL-33 augments substance P-induced VEGF secretion from human mast cells and is increased in psoriatic skin. *Proc. Natl Acad. Sci. USA* 2010 107:4448–4453.

Tobin AM, Veale DJ, Fitsgerald O, Rogers S, Collins P, O'Shea D, & Kirby B. 2010. Cardiovascular Disease and Risk Factors in Patients with Psoriasis and Psoriatic Arthritis. *J Rheumatol* 2010. 37:1386-1394.

Truzzi F, Marconi A, & Pincelli C. 2011. Neurotrophins in healthy and diseased skin *Dermato-Endocrinology* 3:1, 32-36; January/February/March 2011

Tsai TF, Wang TS, Hung ST, Tsai PI, Schenkel B, Zhang M, & Tang CH. 2011. Epidemiology and comorbidities of psoriasis patients in a national database in Taiwan. *J Dermatol Sci.* 2011 Mar 16. [Epub ahead of print])

Van Voorhees AS, & Fried R. 2009. Depression and quality of life in psoriasis. *Postgrad Med.* 2009 July 121:154–161.

Vaz A, Lisse J, Rizzo W, & Albani S. 2009. Discussion: DMARDs and biologic therapies in the management of inflammatory joint diseases. Expert Rev Clin Immunol. 2009. 5:291-299.

Vena GA, Vestita M, & Cassano N. 2010. Can early treatment with biologicals modify the natural history of comorbidities? Dermatol Ther 23:181–193.

Vilanova X, & Pinol J. 1951. Psoriasis arthropathica. *Rheumatism* 1951. 7:197-208.

Virkki LM, Sumathikutty BC, Aarnio M, Valleala H, Heikkilä R, Kauppi M, Karstila K, Pirilä L, Ekman P, Salomaa S, Romu M, Seppälä J, Niinisalo H, Konttinen YT, & Nordström DC. 2010. Biological therapy for psoriatic arthritis in clinical practice: outcomes

Vojdani A, & Lambert J. 2009. The Role of Th17 in Neuroimmune Disorders: Target for CAM Therapy. Part I. *Evid Based Complement Alternat Med.* 2009 Jul 21. eCAM 2009;Page 1-8 doi:10.1093/ecam/nep062

von Bubnoff D, Andrès E, Hentges F, Bieber T, Michel T, & Zimmer J. 2010. Natural killer cells in atopic and autoimmune diseases of the skin. *J Allergy Clin Immunol.* 2010 Jan 125(1):60-68.

Wang D, Eiz-Vesper B, Zeitvogel J, Dressel R, Werfel T, Wittmann M. *Experimental Dermatology* DOI: 10.1111/j.1600-0625.2011.01287.x

Weger W. 2010. Current status and new developments in the treatment of psoriasis and psoriatic arthritis with biological agents. *Br J Pharmacol.* 160:810-820.

Weiss E, Mamelak AJ, La Morgia S, Wang B, Feliciani C, Tulli A, Sauder DN. 2004. The role of interleukin 10 in the pathogenesis and potential treatment of skin diseases. *J Am Acad Dermatol.* 2004 50:657–675.

Wilson FC, Icen M, Crowson CS, McEvoy MT, Gabriel SE, & Kremers HM. 2009. Time trends in epidemiology and characteristics of psoriatic arthritis over 3 decades: a population based study. *J Rheumatol.* 2009. 36(2):361-367.

Wolkenstein P, Revuz J, Roujeau JC, Bonnelye G, Grob JJ, & Bastuji-Garin S. 2009 Psoriasis in France and associated risk factors: results of a case-control study based on a large community survey. *Dermatology* 2008 Dec 6, 218(2):103-109.

Wollina U, Unger L, Heinig B, & Kittner T. 2010. Psoriatic arthritis. Dermatol Ther 23:123–136.

World Health Organization, Leishmaniasis Control home page: http://www.who.int/ctd/html/leis.html.

Wright V. 1956. Psoriasis and arthritis. *Ann Rheum Dis* 1956. 15:348-356.

Wright V. 1959a. Rheumatism and psoriasis: a re-evaluation. *Am J Med* 1959. 27:454-462.

Wright V. 1959b. Psoriatic arthritis: a comparative study of rheumatoid arthritis, psoriasis and arthritis associated with psoriasis. *Arch Dermatol* 1959 80:27-35.

Wu Y, Mills D, & Bala M. 2009. Impact of psoriasis on patients' work and productivity: a retrospective, matched case-control analysis. *Am J Clin Dermatol.* 2009;10:407–410.

Xu D, Jiang H, Kewin P, Li Y, Mu R, Fraser AR, Pitman N, Kurowska-Stolarska M, McKenzie ANJ, Mclinnes IB, & Liew FY. 2008. IL-33 exacerbates antigeninduced arthritis by activating mast cells, *Proc. Natl. Acad. Sci.* 2008 105:10913–10918.

Zeljko-Penavi´c J, Situm M, Simi´c D, & Vurnek-Zivkovi M. 2010. Quality of life in psoriatic patients and the relationship between type I and type II psoriasis. Coll Antropol. 2010 Mar, 34:195–198. 14.

Zhou Q, Mrowietz U, & Rostami-Yazdi M. 2009. Oxidative stress in the pathogenesis of psoriasis. *Free Radic Biol Med.* 2009 Oct 1;47(7):891-905. Epub 2009 Jul 3.

Zügel U, & Kaufmann SHE. 1999. Role of heat shock proteins in protection from and pathogenesis of infectious diseases. *Clin Microbiol Rev* 12:19–39

Zumiani G, Zanoni M, & Agostini G. 2000. Evaluation of the efficacy of Comano thermal baths water versus tap water in the treatment of psoriasis. *G Ital Dermatol Venereol* 2000 135:259–263.

2

History of Psoriasis

Ines Brajac and Franjo Gruber
Department of Dermatovenerology, University Hospital Centre Rijeka
Croatia

"It is not a disease on which to build a medical reputation"
E. Wilson

1. Introduction

Psoriasis is probably as old as mankind. Today, it is a well defined skin disease, in which genetic, environmental and immunologic factors participate in etiopathogenesis. However, despite its frequency, chronicity and visibility, it is quite hard to find a description of psoriasis in the works of the ancient physicians.

Dermatology developed slowly, first with appearance of the protodermatologists at the end of the 18th century, and continued with the arrival of the first dermatologists. From those times psoriasis became a distinct entity.

However, until the last century, the descriptions of disease considered «morbi in pulchredine», were rather vague, the denomination not standardized and the translation from one language to others discrepant. Different authors called the disease with various names, while diverse diseases had the same names. The confusion in terminology and description of psoriasis lasted for centuries.

2. Psoriasis through history: Description and definition

2.1 Psoriasis in the old age

The medicine developed in Mesopotamia, peopled by Sumers, Assirs, and Babylons. The oldest written witness regarding their medicine is clay tablets 3000-5000 year old (Radbill, 1975). Skin diseases have been known to Mesopotamian physicians, called asu, but was cured usually by seers and priests. Definitely there is not notice of psoriasis.

According to Herodotus in the pharaonic Egypt there were physicians for every organ. Numerous medicaments were used, along with magical ceremonies and enchantments (Herodotus, 1989). Hovewer, nothing relate to psoriasis in their medical papyruses. In the largest writing, the Ebers papyrus written about the 15th century BC, found in 1873 in Luxor, numerous skin diseases were described (paragraph 90-95 and 104-118). The term šuf. t for scale was find, but it was impossible to recognize psoriasis (Ebbel, 1937).

Data about medicine among ancient Hebrews were scarce, mostly preventive in nature, and can be found only in their religious books the Old Testament and the Talmud. In the Leviticus, a short description of a cutaneous disease called zaraath (translated in Greek as lepra) was found, which some believed to be leprosy, psoriasis, vitiligo, fungal diseases, or even some other skin condition (Goldman et al., 1966).

The Ayurvedic, religious medicine, developed in India during antiquity. It was based on magic-religious rites, with using of certain plants. Among the medical books from that period the great importance had the Charaka Samitha. In this book and in the Bower manuscript, the disease named Khusta was described briefly. The disease was probably leprosy, although Paul Richter supposed it was psoriasis (Menon & Haberman, 1969; Richter, 1928).

In the golden age of Greek science, the father of western medicine - Hippocrates (ca. 460- 377 BC), separated diseases from divine influences and religious procedures. He used the word *psora* that meant itch for itchy lesions on the eyelids and genitals. This condition was not psoriasis undoubtedly, though he used tars and climate to treat that disease (Hippocrate, 1839). He also grouped various skin conditions under the term of lopoi, that in Greek mean scale and introduced the word alphos and leukos for some skin diseases with maculae but doubtless not for psoriasis (G. Sticker, 1931).

The first description of psoriasis appear during the Roman Empire in the 1st century AD in the books of A. Cornelius Celsus » De re medica libri octo». The disease was described as impetigo that can appear on the skin of the extremities and nails (the second, the 4th or third type according to different authors). The disease was treated with medicaments containing pitch and sulphur. Interestingly, Celsus did not use the words psoriasis, psora, lepra (Bechet, 1936).

The word psora had been mentioned in the books «Naturalis historia» of the other Roman encyclopedist Pliny, but he did not describe better the disease, for which he recommended the root of cucumber. It is possible that the term alphos also described psoriasis (Celsus, 1989).

Galen (131-201 AD) of Pergamon, physician of some Roman imperators, was the first who used the term psoriasis, but only for an itchy, scaly eruption of the eyelids and scrotum, that was probably seborrheic dermatitis (Galenus, 1830; Plinius, 1969).

In the manuscripts of the greatest physicians of antiquity we found little about psoriasis, probably because they gave little importance to the skin, believing the organ merely a web to hold together the other parts of the body. Recently Karl Holubar wrote minutely about the semantic aspects of the word psoriasis, and stated that no clear clinical description of psoriasis can be found in the works of the ancient writers (Holubar, 1990).

In the pre-Columbian period in America the Maya, the Aztecs, the Incas, and the Nahuas had a kind of medicine in which magic and religious elements were interwoven, but also treated skin diseases with plants. A disease, probably psoriasis, they treated topically and internally with herbs and resins (Obermeyer, 1974).

2.2 Psoriasis in the middle age

After the extinction of the Roman Empire by the Goths take place the darkness of the Middle Age, a period of stagnation which negatively affected the development of science (Porter, 1999). The literate men were confined to monastic cloisters and medicine was full of superstition, ignorance and mysticism and gave little attention to skin diseases. Writers according to Hebra spent their time in frivolous commentaries of the ancient classic writers, physicians or no, while the cause of the diseases remained unknown (Bechet, 1936). The majority of the people was cured by quacks and barbers often illiterate.

The Arabian physicians perhaps first distinguished psoriasis from other skin diseases already in the VIII century A.D., and it seem they used a kind of psychotherapy in treatment (Shafii & Shafii, 1979).

In Western the first medical School was founded in Salerno, where Constantine the African translated old medical manuscripts from Greek and Arabic to Latin. By the 13th century most manuscripts had been translated into Latin that became the dominant language of the educated people.

2.3 Psoriasis in the renaissance

The Renaissance was a cultural movement that spanned roughly the 14th to the 17th century, beginning in Florence in the Late Middle Ages and later spreading to the rest of Europe. During this time some authors mentioned the diseases psora and lepra in their books. Among these was Johannes Manardi (1462-1536) from Ferrara, who mentioned the disease "psora" in his "Epistolae medicinales", but wrote nothing more about (Manardi,1542).

The most important work on skin disease was written by Hieronymus Mercurialis (1530-1606), professor of medicine at the universities of Padua, and Bologna. The book was entitled »De morbis cutaneis et omnibus corporis humani excrementis» and based on his lectures transcribed by his student Acardius. For this book Garrison said «the first systematic text book on diseases of the skin". Mercurialis divided the skin diseases, similarly to Galen "a capite ad pedes" in those of the scalp and then of the entire body, both subdividing in change of the color, change in structure and bulks. He described psoriasis under the name of "lepra grecorum" and for other condition used the term "psora" (Mercurialis, 1572).

In 1700, B. Ramazzini (1633-1714) published his original work "De morbis artificum diatriba" in which the diseases caused by the work in certain professions was described, among them also skin conditions. Ramazzini pointed out a lot of new causes of diseases different from the Hippocrates's theory of a dyscrasia of humors (Ramazzini, 1700).

2.4 Psoriasis in 18th century

During the 18th century a few surgeons and physicians tried to devote oneself to the study of the skin and its diseases. Among them was Daniel Turner (1667-1740), who firstly started to work as a surgeon, then obtained in America at Yale a honorary degree of doctor medicine. In 1714 he published the book entitled «De morbis cutaneis a treatment of diseases incident to the skin», that went through a few editions and was soon translated in other languages (Turner, 1726). He gave not an accurate description of psoriasis that he called "leprosy of the Greek", while "leprosy of the Arabian" was our leprosy. He was aware that the local application of ointments and drugs transfer them internally.

In the second part of the 18th century the great Swedish naturalist and physician Carl Linnaeus (1707-1787) introduced the binomial terminology and first classified the plants in a comprehensible manner. In 1735 he published this in his book »Systema naturae» and later even proposed to classify the human diseases in his «Genera morborum» (Linnaeus, 1763). The same topic, in the same year, one can find in Francois Boissier de Sauvages who in his work »Nosologia methodica" classified diseases in ten classes with about 2400 species (Grmek, 1996). These types of classifications were soon used in the classification of skin diseases.

In 1777 Charles Anne Lorry (1726-1783), who became the physician of Louis XVI and can be considered the first French dermatologist, published in Paris his «Tractatus de morbis cutaneis». The book contained more than 700 pages, in which one can find the first attempt of an etiologic classification of skin diseases as well the interaction between internal organs, especially the gastrointestinal, nerve system and the "skin organ" (organum constitutit). Perhaps he was the first who described the Auspitz sign (Lorry, 1777).

Joseph Jacob von Plenck (1738-1807) a Hungarian excellent surgeon and obstetrician in Vienna and expert in botany compiling a list of about 800 medicinal plants, in 1776 published the little book entitled «Doctrina de morbis cutaneis». In his book the diseases was classified on morphological basis i.e. the elementary lesions of 120 skin diseases in 14 classes, even the entities were often unidentifiable (Plenck, 1776). He gave only marginally attention to psoriasis (seated in the class of squames) and its therapy, and used the old term impetigo for it (from Latin impetus - to attack).

For long time the surgeon treated skin diseases and therefore D. Turner, C. Lorry, and J. Plenck can be considered the protodermatologist (Holubar & Ferenčić, 2002). Their effort opened the way to the first dermatologist like R.Willan and JL. Alibert.

Two decades after Plenck, the English physician Robert Willan (1757-1812), working at the London Public Dispensary published the Book «On cutaneous disease» in which he developed a simpler, better and usable classification of the skin diseases on the basis of eight elementary lesions (Willan, 1798). He used the term psoriasis for the papulosquamous disease, in the order squamae, together with lepra, pityriasis and ichthyosis and partly differentiated psoriasis from leprosy (psora leprosa and lepra grecorum). He described different forms of psoriasis: guttata, diffusa, gyrata, palmaria, unguium, inveterata. He also noticed that the disease begin on the knees and elbows, attack the scalp and also the finger and toe-nails. During his life he published the skin diseases of the first four orders (Willan, 1809). After his premature death, his work was continued and completed by his disciple and successor Thomas Bateman (1778-1821), who also published some books on the subject paying attention on the treatment.

At the beginning of the XIX century the great French physician Jean Louis Alibert (1768-1837) worked and taught at the Hospital of St. Louis in Paris, dedicated to skin diseases. He opposed to Willan classification and also attempt to make order and systematize the skin diseases. He followed the ideas to classify diseases in agreement with another botanist B. de Jussieu based on the analogy and divided the skin diseases in 12 classes or groups. He also later (1829) proposed an « arbre des dermatoses» (in English-tree of skin diseases), a rather naive scheme, which made only a greater confusion. Psoriasis classified in the group of dartrous dermatoses together with leprosy (Alibert, 1832).

In this century hospitals or dispensaries were opened only for treatment of skin or venereal diseases giving to the physicians the opportunity to study more cases of skin diseases and psoriasis as well.

It was Ferdinand von Hebra (1806-1880) who in 1841, working in Vienna at the Allgemeines Krankenhaus definitely divided psoriasis from leprosy (improving the terminology and classification of R. Willan). He was a popular teacher and became the first professor of dermatology of German languages, and more importantly he classified the skin diseases in 12 groups not only on the basis of gross anatomy, but after Karl Rokitansky (1804-1878) used also the microscopic criteria for their classification (Hebra, 1856), introducing general pathology to describe skin diseases. Regard psoriasis treatment he believed in pilulae asiaticae (arsenic) (Bechet, 1936). His successor Moritz Kaposi also continued on this way.

2.5 Psoriasis in 19th century

During the 19th century the dermatologists continued to dispute about the classification of skin diseases. Dermatology and also psoriasis grew and develop with the introduction of pathohistological classifications (F. Hebra, Auspitz). Regard psoriasis it is to underline that Alibert noted in 1822 the association of the disease with joint deformities (Alibert, 1818), for which Besnier coined the name arthritis psoriatica. The association was later detailed by Charles BOURDILLON (Bourdillon,1888), while Erasmus Wilson described the association of psoriasis with gout and rheumatic diseases.

The description of the varieties of psoriasis followed: psoriasis pustulosa generalisata in 1910 by Leo von Zumbusch (1884-1940) (von Zumbusch,1910), and later the of psoriasis palmo-plantaris by Barber-Königsbeck.

Some authors described signs that helped the diagnosis of this disease. Heinrich Köbner (1838-1904), professor of dermatology in Breslau, described the isomorphous effect of irritation or Köbner phenomenon in 1872, i.e. appearence of a psoriatic lesion at the site of a physical or other injury (Köbner,1877). Later this phenomenon was used experimentally to study the early changes that appear in the disease.

Heinrich Auspitz (1835-1886), a Hebra pupil, described the appearance of papillary bleeding after the removal of the scales from a psoriatic lesion (Auspitz sign or bloody dew phenomenon), even this sign had been before noted by D.Turner, R.Willan and F.Hebra. Auspitz was interested in dermatopathology, and introduced a few pathohistological terms such parakeratosis and acanthoma typical for psoriasis (Pusey, 1933). In 1879 Duncan and Bulckley described the "pellicole decolable". Hard debates followed about the possibility of psoriatic manifestation on mucous membranes particularly on the oral cavity.

At the end of the 19th century psoriatic micro morphology was described by Hebra, Unna, and William Munro who described the microabscess (micropustule), i.e. the accumulation of neutrophils in the stratum corneum.

2.6 Psoriasis in 20th century

During the first part of the 20th century the Woronoff ring was described around the psoriatic plaque (1926) especially after treatment with antrarobin (Woronoff , 1926; Kogoj , 1927)

The spongiform pustule in pustular psoriasis was described 1927. by Franjo Kogoj (1894-1981) who working in Zagreb and later better defined by Mladen Rupec through a ultramicroscopic study (Kogoj,1927; Rupec, 1970).

In the second part of the 20th century it was demonstrated that the psoriatic epidermis contains 25 times more mitoses per unit than the epidermis from healthy persons. van Scott and Ekel demonstrated that the keratinocytes of psoriatic patients have a significant shortening of their cell cycle from about 311 h in normal person to 36 h; (van Scott, 1963) and the turnover time of the epidermis is markedly shortened, from 27 days to 4 days (Weinstein, 1968).

In 20th century many authors studied the genetic alteration and today there is undisputed evidence that the disease is multifactorial i.e. caused by multiple genes. Many of these " susceptible " genes are mapped on different chromosomes (PSOR1-PSOR 10). The disease is triggered also by different environmental factors (Sanchez, 2007; Bowcock & Barker, 2003).

The association with the HLA molecules was described especially for type 1 of psoriasis, that is frequently inherited, has a more severe course and develops early, while in type 2 the disease develop later and is rarely inherited (Henseler & Christopher, 1985).

Last decades numerous immunological researches accumulate evidence of presence of alteration of the innate and adaptive immune response in psoriatic patients. Investigations evidentiated an accumulation of activated lymphocytes, mostly CD4 in the dermis and CD8 in the epidermis. This imply a primary disregulation in of the immune system and permitted a better understanding and new insight in the pathogenesis as well new possibilities in the management of psoriasis (Krueger, 2002). Psychological stress also can influence the course of the disease.

3. The treatment of psoriasis through history

D. Turner describe very realistically in his book cases of psoriasis treated with inunctions of a ointment containing ammoniated mercury (Hydrargyri amidochlorati) or with a broth of boiled vipers (Turner, 1726). Although very interesting, such details of the treatment are beyond the scope of our article. As the diagnosis of psoriasis before the 19th century was rather debatable, and the treatment usually problematic and ingenuous, we will expose the treatment of psoriasis from the beginning of the XIX century. The treatment of course was topical and/or internal, but for a long period of time the physicians gave more attention to the internal, believing that the external application of drugs on the skin can drive inward the lesions and so cause « metastases» to the internal organs. It was Hebra who asserted this is only speculation.

3.1 The treatment of psoriasis in 19th century

One of the first used internally medicaments for psoriasis treatment was arsenic. In 1806 Thomas Girdlestone was the first who used potassium arsenite as solutio Fowleri, following a moderate use, usually 6 drops 3 times a day (Girdlestone, 1806). This solution was introduced into medicine in 1780 by the English physician and pharmacist Fowler (Fowler, 1786). The drug was easily absorbed and then deposited in various organs, especially in the skin and hair, actihg through inhibiting some enzymes. Years after, F. Hebra, M.Kaposi and E. Wilson also recommended solutio Fowleri (before a meal in water or a bland tea) and pilulae asiaticae (consisting of arsenic, black pepper, acacia and water) in the treatment of psoriasis (Bechet, 1936). It seems that arsenic compounds improved mostly psoriasis guttata, sometimes other forms of the disease.

In 1869 Lipp introduced the subcutaneous injections of arsenous acid (Piffard, 1881).

The protracted use of arsenic in a chronic disease like psoriasis with time led to its accumulation and toxicity. On the skin, liver, and other organs pigmentations, keratoses and malignant tumors appeared. In spite of this horrible adverse reactions arsenic remained in use to the middle of the XX century and the introduction of corticosteroids in the therapy of psoriasis (Gruber et al., 2004).

Mercury was used for centuries in the treatment of syphilis and skin diseases. Mercury ointments was used also by Bateman and by other physicians during the XIX century. According to Henry Pfiffard (1842-1910) the internal use of calomel was also extolled by Biett, Rayer and other physicians (Piffard, 1881) Brault in 1895 used organic mercury compound injections in the treatment of arthritis psoriatica (Brault, 1895). Still in 1972 W. Jadassohn and F. Kogoj recommended a mercury ointment for psoriasis capillitii (Jadassohn & Kogoj, 1972).

Many disease as well as psoriasis were considered infectious diseases and an antibacterial treatment introduced (iodine, phenol, acetic acid). Among other drugs used internally for psoriasis treatmen were diuretics (petroselinum apium, foliae uvae ursi, digitalis, tinctura cantharides), with little benefit.

The local or internal (intramuscular) use of sulphur and salicylic acid in treatment of skin disease in general is very old. Hebra and Kaposi used sulphur and salicylic acid in various ointments, obtaining the removal of the scales (Hebra, 1845).

For centuries in India Chrysarobin was used in the treatment of dermatomycoses and perhaps psoriasis i.e. long before the English physician Balmanno Squire in 1876 wrote about its use for psoriasis (Squire, 1878). The drug was present in the Goa (or Bahia) powder, obtained from the center of the trunk of the tree Andira Araroba (*Vataireopis araroba*), which grows in some parts of Brasil (Swanbeck, 1992). Chrysarobin is an antranone that easily oxidizes and its concentration in the powder was very variable. This drug was used in the form of 1-5% ointment and when applied on skin it cause itching and colored the skin and linen. These effects prevented a larger use of this drug at home. The drug was effective, but expensive and toxic.

3.2 The treatment of psoriasis in the 20th century

Around the change of the century the development of chemistry and technology especially in Germany and England favored the synthesis of new drugs for disease treatment. The chemist Galewsky synthesized dithranol (cignolin) in 1916., which permitted easier to cure psoriasis. The first to use it were the Galewsky brother and PC Unna (Galewsky, 1916). It was applied as ointment or paste (0.1%) or later as a stick for short contact therapy of psoriasis.

Already Hippocrates used tars in the treatment of skin disease (mostly pine tar). Tars were often used during the last two centuries. Little improvement in psoriasis was obtained with wood tars (of pine, birch, juniper, pix betulina) containing acetic acid, phenol, carbonic acid. They were incorporated in ointments, paste, oils and applied directly on the skin, or used for baths (Leigheb, 1958). Because of their acidic character tars were irritative and also stained brown or purple the skin and clothes. Bituminous tars such as ichthyol were also used.

After the introduction of coal tar obtained from distillation of coal in the manufacture of illuminating gas, greater improvement in psoriasis treatment was observed. This substance had an antiproliferative and antimflammatory action but also had an unpleasant odor and irritating potential. It was also phototoxic under UVA and visible rays.

In 1925 Goeckerman (1884-1954) used coal tar in conjunction with ultraviolet light irradiation (Goeckerman, 1925). Because of possible carcinogenic action this method is today only used in the treatment of psoriasis palmoplantaris. Ingram developed a treatment of psoriasis based on coal tar and UVB irradiation.

For centuries diet was used in the treatment of different diseases. Naturally there were also numerous attempts to treat psoriasis with diets like low fat(Grütz and Bürger), high fat, vegetarian (Brocq, Buckley), low or high contains of kalium (Weirich, 1960). Probably some effect, if it was, can be linked to a diminished intake of calories that can lower the epidermal proliferation as the cells for this need energy.

The benefical effect of sun on skin diseases was known among the old civilizations, and heliomarinotherapy is used also in our time. Artificial ultraviolet radiation was introduced in medicine by Finsen at the beginning of XX century. Alderson, in the twenties, reported an improvement with UVR in psoriasis (Alderson, 1923). In the last decennia lamps were developed with wavebands between 300 and 320 nm, with narrow spectrum around 311 nm and PUVA therapy. In 1973 Tronnier and Schule first found a good improvement of psoriasis after the topical use of psoralens and UVA (Tronnier / Schule, 1973). The next year JA Parish at Harvard used oral 8-methoxy- psoralens and UVA irradiation, and soon later H. Hönigsmannn (Parrish et al., 1974; Wolff et al., 1975) Few years later, 5- methoxypsoralen in photochemotherapy was introduced in Vienna (1979). This treatment was highly effective and gave long lasting remissions.

At the middle of the 20th century corticosteroids were introduced into medicine. The first treatment of psoriasis with topical corticosteroids made M.B. Sulzberger and V.Witten in 1952., but the local application of cortisone and hydrocortisone was without effects on psoriasis (Sulzberger, 1952).

Changing the steroid molecule with fluoridation permitted to obtain more potent steroids like fluocinolone acetonide, betamethasone valerate and clobetasol propionate. These drugs were effective in clearing most cases of psoriasis. Their efficacy can be enhanced with occlusive dressing or using combination with salicylic acid, tars and other. The drawbacks of this therapy are atrophy of the skin, telangiectasias, suppression of the hypothalamus-pituitary-adrenal axis and tachyphylaxis.

Among other drugs employed in the treatment of psoriasis are the cytostatics and antimetabolits. Particular mention deserve folate inhibitors like aminopterin and methotrexate, introduced in the 1950s, which in disabling cases of psoriasis and psoriatic arthritis can give a satisfactory response (Gubner, 1951; Edmundson & Guy, 1958). In recent years the internal use of Cyclosporine, an immunosuppressive drug, inhibiting T cell activation, showed favorable results in the treatment of the disease, but a problem represents its nephrotoxicity (Mueller & Herrmann, 1979).

In the '70s the Retinoids, analogs of Vitamin A, were introduced in treatment of psoriasis, especially of erythrodermic and pustular form. The introduction of systemic retinoids represented a great step forward for the patients. First was synthesized isotretinoin and used for psoriasis in 1972, later were introduced etretinate and acitretin that showed a better efficacy and lower toxicity. (Orfanos & Runne, 1976; Kingston et al., 1987). They act through the nuclear receptors RAR and RXR and on the expression of genes important for the proliferation and differentiation of keratinocytes. Retinoids can be used in combination with PUVA. It is important to avoid their use during pregnancy being teratogenic (Lammer et al., 1985).

Last decades analogs of vitamin D3 (calcipotriol, tocalcitol) showed to slowing the epidermopoiesis and stimulate the differentiation of keratinocytes in cultures and were introduced in the topical treatment of psoriasis (Smith et al., 1986).

3.3 The future: The 21th century

Decades of research evidenced he importance of the immune mechanisms in the insurgence of psoriasis. The introduction of biological agents in he therapy of psoriasis and further elucidation in the pathogenesis of the disease (Tutrone et al., 2004) permitted us to believe to bolster in the future use of drugs that act on specific receptors (IL-2), cytokines, chemokines or on some other molecules of the lymphocytes (Mrowietz, 2003). Monoclonal antibody humanized or recombinant and fusion proteins will find employment in the treatment of psoriasis as they can act on molecules on the surface of lymphocytes such CD4, CD2, or on molecules present on the surface of antigen presenting cells. Other may block some of the proimflammatory cytokines like tumor necrosis factor α or perhaps interleukins that deviate the TH1 to TH2 immune response. Monitoring for infections, autoimmune reactions are necessary.

Also, the discovery done by O'Daly opens a new door for understanding and treatment of psoriasis. While injecting volunteers with vaccine for prevention of leishmaniasis, clinical remission of psoriasis was observed. The results confirmed in a controlled study demonstrated favorable benefit/risk profile and merits further development for the treatment of psoriasis (O'Daly et al.,2008). There are factors in Leishmania species which induce remission of psoriasis by stimulating lymphocytes (O'Daly et al; 2010). Furthermore, Antigens from Leishmania amastigotes inducing clinical remission of psoriatic arthritis (O'Daly et al.,2011).

The new local, systemic, photochemotherapy and psychological treatments can be a substantial aid in the management of the disease, and will permit to improve the quality of life in psoriatic patients. Psoriasis vulgaris and other forms burden are not only related to alteration of the skin, but frequently can involve also to the joints, cardiovascular problems, and a metabolic syndrome. This historical review of psoriasis and its treatment from the Ancient times until today, alike the study of the skin and its diseases, illustrate efficiently the complexity of its etiology, the dilemmas of language barriers, chaos of the confounding nomenclature that endurated in this fields, and this is well illustrated by the innumerable books and articles written in the last centuries about this enigmatic disease.

Psoriasis as a common disease has a significant socio-economic impact on the individual and on the society.Today dermatology and so fairly psoriasis need the support of other scientific disciplines like molecular medicine, genetics, immunology, and pharmacogenetics.

4. References

Alibert, JL. (1818). *Precis theorique et pratique sur les maladies de la peau.Vol 2, Caille et Ravier,* Paris.

Alibert, JL. (1832). Monographie des dermatoses. *Precis theorique et pratique des maladies de la peau.* Daynac, Paris.

Alderson, HE. (1923). Heliotherapy for psoriasis. *Arch Dermatol,* 8, , pp 79-80.

Bechet, PE. (1936). Psoriasis. A brief historical review, *Arch Derm Syph* 33,No2, pp327-334.

Bowcock, AM., & Barker, JN. (2003). Genetics of psoriasis: the potential impact on new therapies, *J Am Acad Dermatol* 49 (suppl 2):s51-56.

Bourdillon,C. (1888). *Psoriasis et arthropathies.* These, Paris.

Brault, J. (1895). Deux cas de psoriasis traite par les injections mercurielles. *Bull Soc Franc Dermatol,* pp 332.

Celsus, CA. (1989) De Medicina, Transl by Spencer WG, Book V, 17. Harward University Press, Cambrige, pp168-173.

Ebbel, B. (1937).*The papirus Ebers,* Levinn-Munksgaard, Copenhagen.

Edmundson, WF., & Guy BW. (1958) Treatment of psoriasis with folic acid antagonists. *Arch Dermatol* ,78 , No2,pp 200-203.

Fowler, T.(1786) Medical reports on the effects of arsenic in the cure of agues remitting fevers and periodical head aches. *London Med J*,7, pp192-205.

Galewsky, E. (1916). Űber Cignolin, ein Ersatzpräparat des Chrysarobins. *Derm Wschr*,62, pp 113-115.

Galenus, C. (1830). *Opera omnia.* C. Kuhn ed, Cnobloch, Lipsia, pp 449.

Girdlestone, T. (1806). Observation the effect of dr. Fowler's mineral solution in lepra et either disease. *Med Phys J*,15 pp 297.

Goldman, L., Moraites, RS., & Kitzmiller, K. (1966) White spots in Biblical times. *Arch Dermatol;* 93, No 6, pp748-753.

Goeckerman, WH.(1925) Treatment of psoriasis. *Northwest Med* ,24, pp229.

Gubner, R.(1951) Effect of Aminopterin on epithelial tissue. *Arch Derm Syph,* 64, No6, pp 688-699.

Grmek, M.(1996). Il concetto di malattia. In :M. Grmek,ed, *Storia del pensiero medico occidentale. 2 Dal rinascimento all' inizio dell' Ottocento,* Laterza, Bari, pp279.

Gruber, F., Kaštelan, M.,& Brajac, I.(2004). Psoriasis treatment - Yesterday, today, and tomorrow. *Acta Dermatovenerol Croat*,12, No2, pp30-34.

Hebra, F. (1856-1876) *Atlas der Hautkrankheiten.* Vol I-X , Wien.

Hebra, F. (1845) Versuch einer auf pathologische Anatomie gegründeten Einteilung der Hautkrankheiten. *Zeitschr der K uK Gesellschaft der Aertze in Wien*:2, pp211-231.

Henseler, T.,& Christopher, E. (1985) Psoriasis of early and late onset: characterization of two types of psoriasis vulgaris . *J Am Acad Dermatol* ,13,No3, pp450- 456.

Herodotus.(1989) *Le storie* Vol 1-2.(Greek-Ital. transl.)p84, Garzanti, Milano.

Hippocrate.(1839-1861). Ouvres completes. Transl. et ed. E. Littre, Bailliere et fils, Paris vol I-X.

Holubar, K., & Ferenčić –Fatović, S. (2002).*The roots of international dermatology: seven useful tables on the first dermatological personalities and achievements.* European Society for history of dermatology and venereology, Paris,pp 1-7.

Holubar, K. (1990).Psoriasis 100 years ago. *Dermatologica*,180,No1, pp1-4.

Jadassohn, W.,& Kogoj, F.(1972). Bemerkungen zur psoriasistherapie. Proceeding VII Congres dermatovenerologists Jugoslavije, Opatija - Rijeka, 1972, pp 65.
Kogoj, F.(1927).Un cas de maladie de Hallopeau. *Acta Dermatovenereol*,8, No1,pp1
Köbner, H.(1877) Zur Aetiologie der Psoriasis. *Wschr Derm*, 4,pp203-20.
Krueger, JG. (2002)The immunologic basisfor the treatment of psoiasis with new biologic agents. *J Am Acad Dermatol*,46, No1, pp1-23.
Kingston,T., Matt, L.,& Lowe, N.(1987). Etretin therapy for severe psoriasis. Arch Dermatol, 123,No1 pp55-58.
Lammer, EJ, Chen, DT,Hoar, RM ret al.(1985). Retinoic acid embriopathy *N E J M*, 313,No14, pp 837-841.
Lorry, C. (1777).*Tractatus de morbis cutaneis*. G. Cavelier, Paris.
Leigheb, V.(1958). Il valore pratico attuale della terapia esterna medicamentosa delle malattie cutanee. *Minerva Dermatol* ,vol 33(suppl 1), pp81-82.
Linnaeus, C. (1763). *Genera morborum*. Uppsala.
Menon, IA., & Haberman, HF.(1969) Dermatological writings of Ancient India. *Med Hist*,13, pp387- 392.
Manardi, J.(1542) *Epistolae medicinales*, Schaeffer, Venetii.
Mercurialis, H.(1572). De morbis cutaneis et omnibus corporis humani excrementis. P.A. Meietos, Venetiis
Mueller, W.,& Herrmann, B. (1979) Ciclosporin A for psoriasis. *N Engl J Med* 301, No10,pp 555.
Mrowietz, U.(2003). Therapie der Psoriasis mit Biologicals. *Hautarzt*, 54, No3, pp 224-229.
O'Daly, JA., Lezama, R., & Rodriguez, PJ. et al. (2008). Antigens from Leishmania amastigotes induced clinical remission of psoriasis. *Arch Dermatol Res*,No 301, pp 1-13 .
O'Daly, JA., Lezama, R., & Gleason, J. (2009) Isolation of Leishmania amastigote protein fractions which induced lymphocyte stimulation and remission of psoriasis. *Arch Dermatol Res*,No 301, pp 411-27 .
O'Daly, JA., Gleason, J., Lezama, R., et al. (2011). Antigens from Leishmania amastigotes inducing clinical remission of psoriatic arthritis. *Arch Dermatol Res*,No 303, pp 399-415.
Obermeyer, ME.(1974) Mexican dermatology of the Pre- Columbian period. *Intern J. Dermatol* 3, pp293-299
Orfanos, CE, & Runne, U. (1976) Systemic use of a new retinoid with and without local dithranol treatment in generalized psoriasis. *Br J Dermatol*, 95, No1, pp101-103.
Parrish, JA., Fitzpatrick,TB., Tannenbaum, L.,& Pathak MA.(1974). Photochemotherapyof psoriasis with oral methoxsalen and long wave ultraviolet light. *N Engl J Med*, 291,No23,pp1207-211.
Piffard, HG.(1881). A treatise on the materia medica and therapeutics of the skin. W. Wood, New York.
Plinius, C. (1969).*Naturalis historia*. Harward University Press, Cambrige, XXIII,3.
Plenck, J J. (1776). *Doctrina de morbis cutaneis*, R. Graeffer, Wien.
Porter, R. (1999).*The greatest benefit to mankind*. Harper Collins, . UK, pp106
Pusey, WA. (1933). *History of dermatology*. CC Thomas, Springfield, pp33.
Radbill, SX.(1975) Pediatric dermatology in Antiquity (part1). *Intern J Dermatol* ,14, No 5, pp 363-368.

Richter, P.(1928) Geschichte der Dermatologie. In J Jadassohn ed: *Handbuch der Haut u. GeschlechtsKrankheiten*,Vol XIV/2, J Springer, Berlin pp1-240.

Ramazzini, B.(1700). *De morbis artificium diatriba.* Modena 1700

Rupec, M.(1970) Zur Ultrastruktur der spongiform Pustel. *Arch Klin Exp Derm*, 239,pp30

van Scott, EJ.,& Ekel, TM.(1973) Kinetics of hyperplasia in psoriasis. *Arch Dermatol* ,88, No4,pp 373- 381.

Sanchez, F. (2007).The genetic of psoriasis susceptibility. *G It Dermat Venereol*,142, No5, pp 489-501.

Shafii, M., & Shafii, SL. (1979) Exploratory psychotherapy in the treatment of psoriasis twelve hundred years ago. *Arch Gen Psychiatry*, 36,pp1242-1245.

Smith, EL.,Walworth, ND., & Holick, HK.(1986). Effect of 1 alpha -25 dihydroxy vitamin D3 on the morphology and biochemical differentiation of cultured human epidermal keratinocytes grown in serum free. *J Invest Dermatol* , 86, No6, pp709-714.

Squire, B.(1878). On *the treatment of psoriasis by an ointment of chrysophanic acid.* Churchill, London, pp8.

Sticker, G.(1931) Entwurf einer Geschichte der ansteckenden Geschlechtskrankheiten. In J. Jadassohn ed: *Handbuch der Haut u. GeschlechtsKrankheiten*,Vol XXIII, J Springer, Berlin.264- 603

Sulzberger, M.B., & Witten, VH.(1952) The effect of topically applied compound F in selected dermatoses. J Invest Dermatol, 19, No2,pp101-102.

Swanbeck, G.(1992). Der Baum, aus welchem Chrysarobin gewonnen wurde. *Hautarzt*, 43, No 6, pp 388-389.

Tronnier, H., & Schule, N. (1973).Zur dermatologischen Therapie von Dermatosen mit Langwelligen UV nach Photosensibilisirung der Haut mit Methoxsalen, erste Ergebnisse bei Psoriasis vulgaris. *Zeitschr Haut Geschlkr*, 48,pp385-393.

Smith, EL.,Walworth, ND., & Holick, HK.(1986). Effect of 1 alpha -25 dihydroxy vitamin D3 on the morphology and biochemical differentiation of cultured human epidermal keratinocytes grown in serum free. *J Invest Dermatol* , 86, No6, pp709-714.

Tutrone, WD., Saini, R., & Weinberg, JM.(2004) Biological therapy for psoriasis: An overview of infliximab, etanercept, efalizumab and alefacept. Drugs, 7, pp 45-49.

Turner, D. (1726). *Disease incident to the skin.* III ed. Bonurike, London, pp45.

Willan, R.(1798). *On cutaneous diseases*: Johnsen, London.

Willan, R.(1809). *On cutaneous diseases.*Vol 1, Johnson St. Pauls Church Yard, London.

von Zumbusch, L.(1910). Psoriasis und pustuloses Exanthem. *Arch Dermatol syphilol* 1910:99:335.

Weinstein, GD. et al,(1968) Abnormal cell proliferation in psoriasis. *J Invest Dermatol*, 50,No 3, pp254.

Weirich, E G.(1960) Die systemisce Therapie der Psoriasis. *Hautarzt*, 11, No5,pp193-201.

Wolff, K., Königsmann, H., Gschnait, F et al.(1975). Photochemotherapie bei Psoriasis Klinische Erfahrungen bei 153 Patienten. *Dtsch Med Wschr*, 100, pp 2471-2477.

Woronoff, DL.(1926).Die peripherenVeranderungen der Haut um die Effloreszenzen der Psoriasis vulgaris und Syphilis corymbosa. *Derm Wschr*, 82, pp249-258.

3

Psoriasis: Epidemiology, Clinical and Histological Features, Triggering Factors, Assessment of Severity and Psychosocial Aspects

Susana Coimbra[1,2], Hugo Oliveira[3], Américo Figueiredo[3], Petronila Rocha-Pereira[1,4] and Alice Santos-Silva[1,5]
[1]*Instituto de Biologia Molecular e Celular (IBMC), Universidade do Porto, Porto*
[2]*Centro de Investigação das Tecnologias da Saúde (CITS) – Instituto Politécnico da Saúde Norte, CESPU, Gandra-Paredes,*
[3]*Serviço de Dermatologia, Hospitais da Universidade de Coimbra, Coimbra*
[4]*Centro de Investigação em Ciências da Saúde (CICS), Universidade da Beira Interior, Covilhã*
[5]*Departamento de Ciências Biológicas, Laboratório de Bioquímica, Faculdade de Farmácia, Universidade do Porto, Porto*
Portugal

1. Introduction

Psoriasis, a chronic erythematosquamous dermatitis that affects about 2-3% of the population, is characterized by abnormal keratinocyte hyperproliferation, resulting in thickening of the epidermis and of the stratum corneum. Psoriasis *vulgaris* accounts for 90% of the psoriasis cases and is characterized by well delineated reddish and scaly papules and plaques, typically on the elbows, knees and scalp or in other cutaneous surfaces.

Psoriatic skin changes have been described since biblical times. The first documented description is found in the Old Testament in the third book of Moses. It was confused with leprosy for hundred of years, and, therefore, many people with psoriasis was ostracised in the Middle Age. At the beginning of the 19th century, Robert Willan, an English physician, was the first to clinically describe psoriasis (Crissey and Parish 1998). Humankind suffered and studied this disease for at least 3000 years, and, naturally, several possible causes for the disease have been hypothesized.

Nowadays it is accepted that psoriasis is a chronic, recurrent, immune-mediated inflammatory disease, with a recognised genetic predisposition. The primary immune defect appears to be an increase in cell signalling via chemokines and cytokines that act up-regulating gene expression, causing keratinocyte hyperproliferation. T lymphocytes and their cytokines and chemokines appear to be the driver of lesion development and persistence, although other cells, such as endothelial cells, dendritic cells, neutrophils and keratinocytes play also an important role, along with other cytokines and growth factors (Chen, de Groot et al.; Wollenberg, Wagner et al. 2002; Sano, Chan et al. 2005). Currently, it is proposed that psoriasis development depends on skin infiltration of T helper (Th)1/Th17 cells that stimulate macrophages and dermal dendritic cells to release mediators that sustain inflammation and cause abnormal keratinocyte proliferation. Interleukin (IL)-23 has the potential to activate Th17 cells, stimulating their survival and proliferation and serving as a key master cytokine regulator in psoriasis (Blauvelt 2008). Th17 cells secrete IL-17, IL-21 and IL-22, with the latter mediating IL-23 induced acanthosis and dermal inflammation (Zheng, Danilenko et al. 2007; Kunz 2009).Therefore, the IL-23/Th17 axis seem to play an important role in psoriasis and explains the hyperplasia of psoriatic keratinocytes (by IL-22), and why neutrophils appear in a chronic inflammatory disease, such as psoriasis (IL-8 production induced by IL-17) (Di Cesare, Di Meglio et al. 2009). More recently, functional interactions between IL-33 and mast cells were also found to contribute to inflammatory conditions, such as psoriasis (Xu, Jiang et al. 2008; Castellani, Kempuraj et al. 2009; Theoharides, Zhang et al. 2010). Nonetheless, the immunologic target molecule that would allow to classify psoriasis as an autoimmune disease, as well as, the events that trigger the inflammatory process, remain to be determined.

Patients with psoriasis require an individual management and long-term planning of therapeutic strategies. The ratio risk *versus* benefit, and the cost-effectiveness of the different treatments should be carefully evaluated. The therapy is chosen in accordance with skin type, clinical history, patient's age, severity of psoriasis and the response to previous treatments. Topical agents are, usually, chosen for milder forms and limited psoriasis; phototherapy, photochemotherapy and systemic agents for moderate and severe psoriasis. Biological therapies, the more recent therapies for psoriasis, are particularly used for severe psoriasis.

2. Epidemiology

Psoriasis affects about 125 million of people worldwide (National Psoriasis Foundation), is common in Caucasians and affects equally men and women. The prevalence of psoriasis in the population of Northern Europe and Scandinavia is 1.5-3%. While relatively common in Japanese, it is less common in Chinese, Eskimos, West Africans and North American blacks, and very uncommon in North American and South American natives and aboriginal Australians (Langley, Krueger et al. 2005). The causes for these variations are likely to be genetical and environmental; actually, population-based and twin studies indicate psoriasis as an heritable disease with a polygenic mode of inheritance, with variable penetrance (Elder, Nair et al. 1994). The prevalence of psoriasis seems to be affected by latitude (Vazquez, Carrera et al. 2006).

The onset of psoriasis can be at any time of life and, afterwards, it usually persists for life. The mean age of onset of psoriasis *vulgaris* is at 33 years, and 75% of the patients develop psoriasis before 46 years of age (Nevitt and Hutchinson 1996). It has been also suggested that psoriasis onset is bimodal, with a peak at 16- 22 and the other peak at 57-60 years of age. The age of onset is slightly earlier in women than in men.

Psoriasis is a relapsing disease, although natural remission occurs in about one-third of the psoriatic patients (Farber and Nall 1974).

According to Henseler and Christophers (Henseler and Christophers 1985) there are two types of psoriasis, defined by the age of psoriasis onset: type I, when it occurs at or before 40 years of age, and type II, when it occurs after the age of 40 years. Type I disease accounts for more than 75% of the cases. These patients are much more likely to express susceptibility alleles at the human leukocyte antigen (HLA) *loci*, to have affected first-degree relatives and to experience a more severe and recurrent disease than patients with type II psoriasis.

The course and progress of psoriasis is apparently unpredictable.

3. Clinical features

Psoriasis *vulgaris* or chronic plaque psoriasis, is the classic and the most common form of psoriasis presentation. The other forms of psoriasis include guttate, erythrodermic and pustular psoriasis. It is characterized by papulosquamous plaques well-defined from surrounding normal skin (Figure 1A). These plaques are red or salmon pink, covered by white or silvery scales, and the plaques may be thick, thin, large or small. They are more active at the edge and are, usually, symmetrically distributed, occurring commonly on elbows, knees, scalp, lumbosacral region and umbilicus.

Psoriasis *vulgaris* may have a variable course, presenting chronic stable lesions or plaques with a rapid onset and widespread involvement. It is, usually, symptomatic, with patients complaining of intense pruritus or burning; about 30% of the patients suffer from itch and pain, mostly due to the dryness and cracking of the psoriatic area.

Early lesions frequently start as small pinpoint papules, which, soon in their evolution, show scaling. The amount of scaling varies among patients, and at different body areas on a given patient, and its removal may reveal tiny bleeding points (Auspitz sign) (Murphy, Kerr et al. 2007). A white blanching ring, known as Woronoff`s ring may be observed in the skin surrounding a psoriatic plaque.

In inactive disease, the few existing plaques remain with the same size, and new ones do not appear.

Worsening of the disease is associated with enlargement of existing lesions and appearance of new, small lesions. With gradual peripheral extension, the plaques may develop different configurations: in psoriasis gyrata, a curved linear pattern predominates; in annular psoriasis, ring-like lesions develop secondary to central clearing; and in psoriasis follicularis, minute scaly papules are present at the opening of the pilosebaceous follicles (Langley, Krueger et al. 2005). The terms rupioid and ostraceous are related to distinct morphological subtypes of plaque psoriasis. Rupioid plaques are small and highly hyperkeratotic, resembling limpet shells. Ostraceous psoriasis refers to hyperkeratotic plaques, with concave centres, similar in shape to oyster shells (Langley, Krueger et al. 2005).

Site-specific variants of psoriasis *vulgaris* exist. Flexural or inverse psoriasis occurs in intertriginous sites. Seborrhoeic psoriasis occurs in eyebrows, nasolabial folds, postauricular and presternal sites. Psoriatic nail disease is most commonly found in patients with psoriatic arthritis. Fingernails are more commonly affected than toenails, and the clinical manifestations range from pitting, yellowish discoloration, and paronychia, to subungual hyperkeratosis, onycholysis, and severe onychodystrophy (Salomon, Szepietowski et al. 2003).

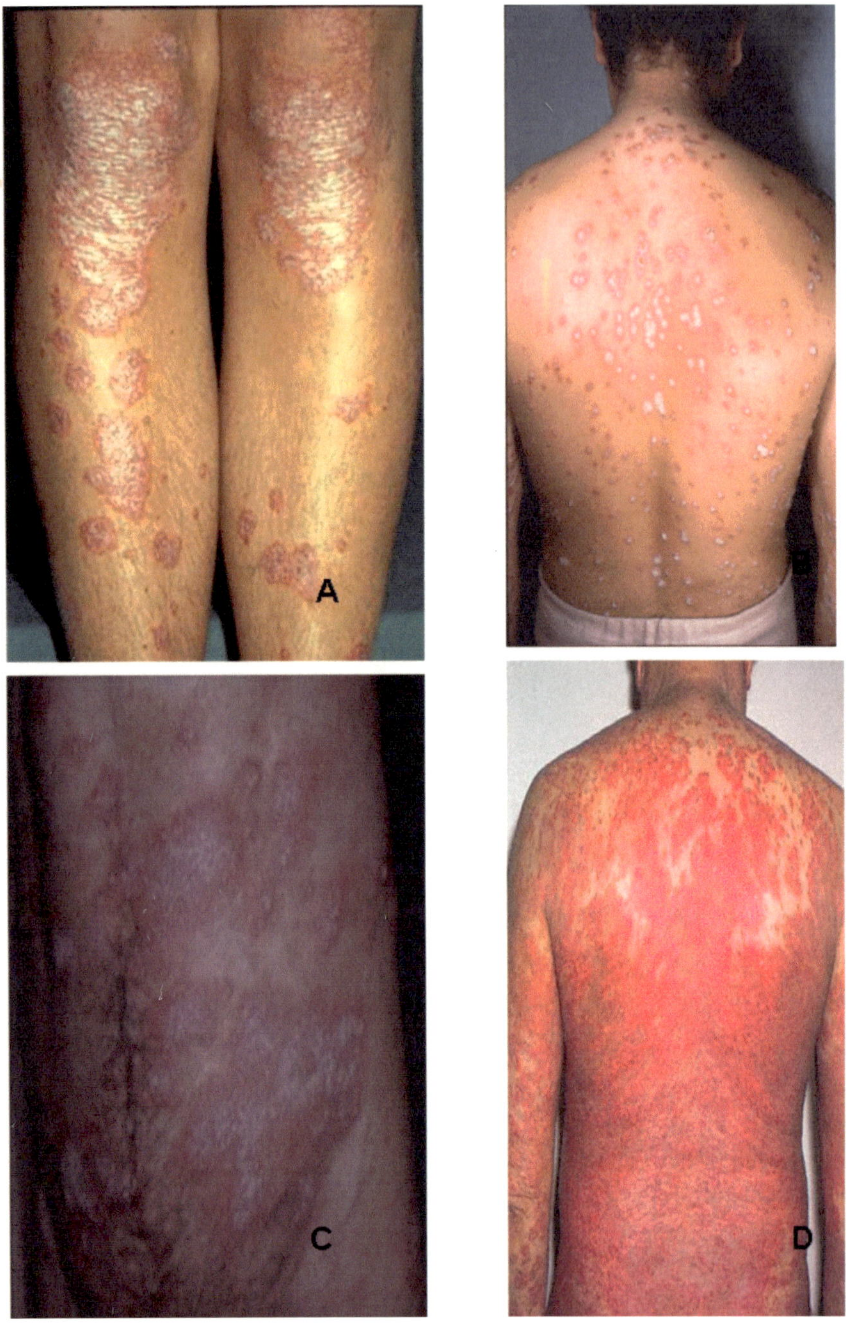

Fig. 1. Psoriasis clinical manifestations: A - chronic plaque psoriasis, B - guttate psoriasis, C - pustular psoriasis, D - erythrodermic psoriasis (With permission of Américo Figueiredo, PhDMD, and of Hugo Oliveira, MD).

Psoriatic arthritis is a seronegative inflammatory arthritis that occurs in the presence of psoriasis *vulgaris*. Five types of this psoriasis have been proposed: distal interphalangeal joint only, asymmetrical oligoarthritis, polyarthritis, spondylitis and arthritis mutilans (Wright 1956; Wright 1959a; Wright 1959b). Gladman expanded the five sub-groups to seven: distal disease, oligoarthritis (<4 joints), polyarthritis, spondylitis only, distal disease plus spondylitis, oligoarthritis plus spondylitis and polyarthritis plus spondylitis (Gladman, Shuckett et al. 1987). About 10-30% of patients with psoriasis *vulgaris* develop psoriatic arthritis. It is controversial whether or not the skin condition and arthritis represent a different manifestation of the same disease. Immunological studies, genetic evidence and different responses to treatment, suggest that they might be different conditions with a similar underlying inflammatory process (Pitzalis, Cauli et al. 1996; Ho, Bruce et al. 2005).

Psoriasis *vulgaris* can be classified in accordance with the configuration of the lesions and their localization. It is also classified, according to the severity of clinical presentation, in mild, moderate and severe (see Assessing psoriasis severity).

Guttate psoriasis (Figure 1B), an acute form of psoriasis that develops especially in children, adolescents and young adults, is characterized by papules with less than 1 cm in diameter that erupt in the trunk and extremities, about 2 weeks after a β-haemolytic streptococcal or a viral infection, and/or after acute stressful life events. Usually, it is self-limited, resolving in 3-4 months, however its long-term prognosis is unknown. Some affected individuals may progress to a chronic form of plaque psoriasis and sparkles of guttate lesions may appear during the course of chronic plaque psoriasis (Martin, Chalmers et al. 1996).

Pustular psoriasis (Figure 1C) is an acute form of psoriasis, in which small, monomorphic, sterile pustules develop in painful inflamed skin. It can be generalized and potentially life-threatening or it can be localized, presenting as palmoplantar pustulosis or acrodermatitis continua of Hallopeau. Acrodermatitis continua is a rare, chronic, pustular eruption of the fingers and toes. Palmoplantar pustulosis is characterized by hyperkeratosis and clusters of pustules over the hands and/or feet; some authors claim, however, that this form is not really a psoriasis form (Asumalahti, Ameen et al. 2003). Patients with generalized pustular psoriasis may have pre-existing plaque psoriasis or develop it after pustular episodes. An intercurrent infection, or the abrupt withdrawal of systemic and, occasionally, of ultrapotent topical corticosteroids may also trigger this form of psoriasis.

In erythrodermic psoriasis (Figure 1D), more than 90% of the skin surface area is affected, which may lead to hypothermia, due to an impairment in the thermoregulation of the skin, high output cardiac failure, infection and metabolic changes. These changes include hypoalbuminaemia and anaemia due to loss of iron, vitamin B_{12} and folate. This form of psoriasis can be a life-threatening condition. It may present as chronic plaque psoriasis that gradually worsens, as plaques become confluent and extensive. Erythroderma may also be precipated by infection, tar, drugs, or withdrawal of corticosteroids (Langley, Krueger et al. 2005).

4. Genetic predisposition

A genetic predisposition to develop the disease appears to exist. Indeed, psoriasis develops in bone marrow transplant recipients from donors with psoriasis, and clears in recipients from donors without psoriasis (Wahie, Alexandroff et al. 2006).

About 30% of psoriatic patients present a family history of the disease in a first or second-degree relative. In fact, the probability to develop psoriasis is raised when first-grade relatives suffer from the disease. The risk to develop psoriasis appears to be about 20% if one parent has psoriasis and about 75% if both parents are affected (Watson, Cann et al. 1972).

Psoriasis has been associated with certain HLA-types (HLA-Cw6, HLA-B13, HLA-B17, HLABw57, HLA-DR4), and those with HLA-Cw6 seem to have a 10-fold higher risk to develop the disease. A collaborative genome-wide association study of psoriasis involving thousands of cases and controls revealed association between psoriasis and seven genetic loci: HLA-C, IL12B, IL23R, IL23A, IL4/IL13, TNFAIP3, and TNIP1 (Elder, Bruce et al. 2010). Moreover, a family history of psoriasis, an early-onset of the disease and the presence of HLA-Cw*0602 (the major determinant of phenotypic expression), have been associated to a more unstable and severe clinical course, as compared to those patients with late onset psoriasis and negative for HLA-Cw*0602 (Henseler and Christophers 1985; Gudjonsson, Karason et al. 2006).

The molecular genetic basis of psoriasis is complex, with evidence that multiple genes are involved. At least nine chromosomal susceptibility *loci* have been revealed (PSORS1-9). The PSORS1 gene, in the major histocompatibility complex region on chromosome 6 (6p21), appears to be associated with most cases of psoriasis. However, the exact location of PSORS1 gene remains controversial. Furthermore, the penetrance of PSORS1 *locus* is estimated to be less than 15%, implying that other genetic and/or environmental factors may also contribute to the liability of the disease. Moreover, an association of PSORS with functional polymorphisms in modifier genes that mediate inflammation (e.g., tumour necrosis factor (TNF)-α) and vascular growth (e.g., vascular endothelial growth factor), has been found (Capon, Munro et al. 2002).

Thus, whereas the existence of a genetic component in psoriasis is certain, the exact location of the genes involved remains to be determined.

Psoriatic patients present a substantial genetic heterogeneity and it is likely that this genetic heterogeneity could lead to subtle differences in disease pathogenesis, explaining the different responses to treatment observed in the patients.

5. Triggering factors

Psoriasis has a complex genetic predisposition, with a complex inheritance pattern, plus an environmental component. The development and exacerbation of psoriasis appears to involve an interaction between multiple genetic and environmental risk factors. Usually, psoriasis is triggered by infection, inflammation, stress, skin injury and drugs.

Several microbial infections are associated with the development and/or worsening of psoriasis. A strong association is the induction of guttate psoriasis by a preceding tonsilar *Streptococcus pyogenes* infection. Disease exacerbation has been associated with skin and/or gut colonization by *Staphylococcus aureus, Malassezia* and *Candida albicans* (Noah 1990; Waldman, Gilhar et al. 2001). Streptococcal infections precede the development or worsening of psoriasis in more than 90% of patients with type I psoriasis (Weisenseel, Laumbacher et al. 2002). The role, if any, of viruses (papilomaviruses, retroviruses, endogenous retroviruses) present in lesional skin is unknown.

In about 30% of patients, the lesions appear at sites of skin injury - the Koebner phenomenon (Holzmann, Werner et al. 1992). This phenomenon is an indicator of disease activity and may have a prognostic value, as it is, usually, associated with early onset of psoriasis. Interestingly, light-induced psoriasis, resulting from an excessive sun exposure (that may improve psoriasis if used appropriately), is also a form of Koebner phenomenon.

There is a growing list of drugs that may aggravate existing psoriasis or induce it for the first time. The frequency of this adverse event varies between drugs. The most commonly proposed causative agents are β-blockers, lithium, synthetic anti-malarial drugs, non-steroidal anti-inflammatory drugs, angiotensin-converting enzyme inhibitors and tetracycline antibiotics (Wolf, Lo Schiavo et al. 1997; O'Brien and Koo 2006).

Evidences confirm that the onset of plaque psoriasis is highly associated with a preceding stressful life event (Mallbris, Larsson et al. 2005); indeed, chronic psychological stress may influence the development of psoriasis and affect its clinical expression (Naldi, Chatenoud et al. 2005).

Diet is sometimes referred as a possible triggering factor for psoriasis, but no consistent data exist. Apparently, fish oil diet or a diet consisting predominantly of glucose and unsaturated fatty acids has beneficial effects on psoriasis (Lithell, Bruce et al. 1983; Caspary, Elliott et al. 2005).

Alcoholism, cigarette smoking, obesity, type 2 diabetes *mellitus*, and metabolic syndrome increase the risk for developing psoriasis (Naldi, Chatenoud et al. 2005; Neimann, Shin et al. 2006). These factors may influence clinical severity and prognosis of psoriasis and, as risk factors for cardiovascular diseases (CVD), may underlie the increased morbidity and mortality for CVD events observed in psoriatic patients.

Some authors stated (Mallbris, Larsson et al. 2005; Naldi, Chatenoud et al. 2005) that obesity precedes and may represent a risk factor to develop psoriasis. Moreover, after the onset of psoriasis, obesity seems to contribute to its exacerbation (Sterry, Strober et al. 2007). We found (Coimbra, Oliveira et al. 2010a) that the prevalence of overweight/obesity in psoriatic patients is high, with overweight/obese patients presenting higher leptin, resistin, TNF-α and IL-6 levels, and lower adiponectin values, as compared to patients with a normal body mass index. Obesity itself, by increasing friction and trauma in the waistline and intertriginous areas, may worsen psoriasis by the Koebner phenomenon (Higa-Sansone, Szomstein et al. 2004). Furthermore, obesity may favour the onset of the disease, by providing a chronic level of low-grade inflammation that may contribute to trigger the development of psoriasis and may account for its severity (Hamminga, van der Lely et al. 2006).

Indeed, inflammation seems to be a central key in psoriasis onset and exacerbation. Studies in our lab (Coimbra, Oliveira et al. 2010b; Coimbra, Oliveira et al. 2010c) showed that worsening of psoriasis is linked to an enhanced inflammatory response with neutrophil activation and in which the cytokine network is disturbed. We also found that after a successful treatment the inflammatory markers levels decreased. Nonetheless, at clearing of the disease, a residual inflammatory response still persists, what may be important for the relapse episodes that are characteristic of psoriasis.

6. Psoriasis *vulgaris* histological features

Psoriasis presents three main histological features: epidermal hyperplasia (acanthosis), dilated and prominent blood vessels in the dermis, and an inflammatory infiltrate of leukocytes, predominantly in the dermis (Gonzalez, Rajadhyaksha et al. 1999; Werner,

Bresch et al. 2008). The histopathological findings in psoriasis lesions, however, may vary as a consequence of the recurrent courses of exacerbation of the disease. The increase in epidermal proliferation and in inflammation are not uniform, even within the same lesion of chronic plaque type psoriasis. Typically, they are higher at the centre of the pinpoint of early lesions, whereas in more developed plaque lesions these changes are found at the border.

A sparse superficial perivascular T-lymphocytic infiltrate of the dermis is, usually, the earliest alteration observed in the lesions. This is followed by the development of dilated and tortuous blood vessels within dermal papillae, by mild dermal oedema, and by minimal spongiosis, with rare T-lymphocyte and/or neutrophil exocytosis. Subsequently, a slight epidermal hyperplasia, with higher neutrophil exocytosis and small mounds of parakeratosis (retention of nuclei in cells of the stratum corneum) containing neutrophils are observed. The infiltrate in the dermis at this early plaque stage is, usually, composed of lymphocytes, histiocytes and neutrophils, in addition to red blood cells.

The developed plaques show marked epidermal hyperplasia, with regular elongation of epidermal rete ridges with characteristic bulbous enlargement of their tips; elongation of intervening dermal papillae containing dilated and tortuous capillaries; fine fibrillary collagen and thinning of epidermis that lies immediately above the dermal papillae. Additionally, there is pallor of the superficial layers of the epidermis and spongiosois is minimal or absent. There is marked hyperkeratosis, as well as, hypogranulosis subjacent to areas of parakeratosis. In most cases, neutrophils within the parakeratosis are present (Munro's microabscesses). Spongiform pustules of Kojog may be formed, due to the migration of neutrophils from the papillary capillaries that aggregate beneath the stratum corneum and in the upper Malpighian layer between degenerating and thinned keratinocytes (Mehta, Singal et al. 2009). Subsequently, the keratynocytes at the centre of the pustule degenerate, with formation of a large single cavity surrounded by thinned keratinocytes.

Both T cell subsets, CD4+ and CD8+ T cells, are present in early stage and developed lesions, but, whereas CD8+ T cells are preferentially present within the epidermis (Bos, Hagenaars et al. 1989), CD4+ T cells are mainly in the dermis. Currently, it is also believed that a separate population of T-helper (Th) cells beside the Th1 cells, namely, the Th17 cells, are present at psoriatic lesions (Lowes, Kikuchi et al. 2008).

The characteristic massive scaling is a consequence of a thickened, irregular stratum corneum with parakeratosis and epidermal thickening with acanthosis, papillomatosis, and absence of granular layer. Epidermal thickening is caused by increased keratinocyte proliferation, reflecting the increased mitotic activity within the basal and suprabasal layers. In normal skin, the maturation of keratinocytes from the basal layer to the cornified layer takes about 28 days, whereas in the psoriatic lesion, it is shortened to 5 days. This shortened maturation is associated with massively disrupted terminal differentiation of keratinocytes and is mainly reflected by parakeratosis.

As referred, the psoriatic plaque is characterized by profound histological disturbances and by the presence of different and unusual cell types. There is a marked infiltration of mononuclear leukocytes, the development of elongated/hyperplastic blood vessels in the papillary dermal region that accounts for the visible redness of psoriatic skin lesions. At the early stage of the plaque, infiltration of T cells, dendritic cells and monocytes/macrophages occurs. Later, the cellular density of these infiltrates increases, and infiltrates of CD8+ T cells and neutrophilic granulocytes occur, particularly in the epidermis. Many lymphocytes, monocytes, and neutrophils are clearly adherent to endothelial cells.

Leukocytes can gain skin parenchyma by transmigration through reactive blood vessels, and resident skin leukocytes might increase creating the dense infiltrates, observed in psoriatic lesions. Although Langerhans cells and dermal dendritic cells have long been recognized as the main types of dendritic cells in skin, only more recently the types of dendritic cells in psoriatic lesions were identified, such as, CD11c+ (myeloid) and plasmocytoid dendritic cells. CD11c+ dendritic cells correspond to interstitial dendritic cells in other tissues and are the most abundant dendritic cell type in the dermis (Lowes, Chamian et al. 2005; Nestle, Conrad et al. 2005).

Polymorphonuclear neutrophils seem to play a pivotal role in the acute inflammatory changes of psoriatic lesions. Areas of parakeratosis appear to contain abundant neutrophils (Cox and Watson 1972). In addition, it is known that pronounced parakeratosis is associated with the presence of neutrophils and that Munro's microabscesses are located exclusively within areas of parakeratosis (van de Kerkhof and Lammers 1987). Coexistence of neutrophils and parakeratosis is in part explained by the tissue destructive properties of active oxygen intermediates and proteolytic enzymes that are released by activated neutrophils attached to the stratum corneum (Terui, Ozawa et al. 2000).

It is of interest, the fact that resolving or treated plaques of psoriasis show initially a progressive reduction of neutrophils within the stratum corneum and of the parakeratosis, with regeneration of the granular zone. The epidermal changes resolve later. The histopathologic clue of the disease that may remain is a residual mild superficial dermal fibrosis with persistence of papillary dermal capillary dilatation and tortuosity (Murphy, Kerr et al. 2007).

In summary, histologically, in psoriasis, there is marked acanthosis, accompanied by parakeratosis and a mixed dermal infiltrate, including CD4+ T cells, dendritic cells, macrophages, and mast cells. Indeed, by immunostaining for IL-17A and IL-22, it has been shown numerous cells present in the psoriasis lesions which are able to produce these cytokines (Harper, Guo et al. 2009). In the epidermis, neutrophilic exudates and CD8+ T cells are often seen. Dermal papillary blood vessels are dilated and tortuous.

7. Assessing psoriasis severity

In clinical practice, broad global assessments of psoriasis activity and its effect on patient's quality of life are used to define the severity of patient's disease and to define the more appropriate treatment. Furthermore, in clinical trials, the quantification of the disease severity is critical to measure the efficacy of the treatment under study, by comparing the severity of disease before and after the treatment.

The severity of psoriasis can be defined by the percentage of body surface area involved. In mild cases, the lesions cover less than 10% of the body surface, in moderate cases 10-20% and in the severe cases the lesions affect more than 20% of skin surface (Naldi and Gambini 2007).

There are several other approaches to measure the severity of psoriasis, which consider not only the affected skin surface, but also the degree of scaling and the type of infiltration.

The Psoriasis Area and Severity Index (PASI) is the prototype for such measures, and is the most widely used tool to assess psoriasis severity in clinical trials and in clinical practice. It was developed as an outcome measure in clinical trials on oral retinoids in 1978 (Frederiksson T 1978).

The PASI score ranges from 0 to 72. It combines the assessment of four body areas: head and neck, upper limbs, trunk and lower limbs. To assess affected body surface area, the proportion of skin affected in each area is given by a numerical score, representing the proportion involved. Within each area the severity of the lesions is assessed by three signs, erythema, thickness/induration, and desquamation/scaling; each of the three signs is assessed on a five-point scale. Finally, the PASI score is calculated according to an appropriate formula (Figure 2).

Score	0	1	2	3	4	5	6
Erythema Induration Desquamation	none	mild	moderate	severe	very severe	—	—
True Area (%)	0	1-9	10-29	30-49	50-69	70-89	90-100

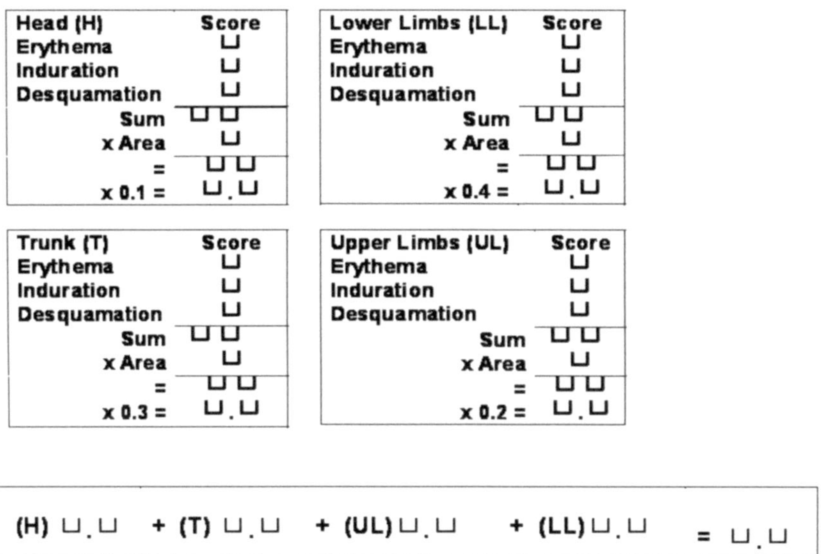

Fig. 2. Psoriasis Area and Severity Index (PASI) score assessment (H, head; LL, lower limbs; T, trunk; UL, upper limbs).

A PASI score below 10 defines psoriasis as mild, between 10 and 20 as moderate, and above 20 as severe (Naldi and Gambini 2007). The evaluation of PASI presents some subjectivity, which is reduced when patients are evaluated always by the same dermatologist.

The PASI system has two major advantages: it is sensitive to changes in the area of the affected skin and in the severity of the lesions; therefore, the changes in PASI score reflect improvement or worsening of the disease. Its widespread use in the research setting means that it is possible to compare information from different studies. When conducting a clinical trial for treatment of psoriasis, a predetermined endpoint is required, on which the efficacy of the drug will be assessed. It is established that a 75% improvement in PASI, defined as PASI 75, is a clinically meaningful endpoint for clinical trials, and there is strong evidence demonstrating that 50% improvement in PASI (PASI 50) could also be a clinically meaningful endpoint (Carlin, Feldman et al. 2004). A major limitation of the PASI is that it is not routinely used by clinicians and, therefore, is poorly understood by both clinicians and patients. It also presents poor sensitivity to changes in small areas of involvement. Therefore, PASI is not the best tool to be used in patients with mild disease.

Another traditional assessment tool to evaluate psoriasis severity is the Physician's Global Assessment (PGA), a simple instrument that provides a subjective global evaluation. There are several variants for PGA. Typically, the patient is asked to rate the disease, using a scale of seven categories, "clear", "almost clear", "mild", "mild to moderate", "moderate", "moderate to severe" and "severe". It is less objective than PASI, but the result is more easily understood by the patient (Berth-Jones, Grotzinger et al. 2006).

The Lattice System Physician's Global Assessment (LS-PGA), formerly known as Lattice System Global Psoriasis Scale, applies a more objective approach to global assessment of disease severity than PGA, because it considers the body surface area involved and the morphological characteristics of the plaques (Berth-Jones, Grotzinger et al. 2006). Total body surface area involved is estimated using a scale of seven categories (0, 1-3, 4-9, 10-20, 21-29, 30-50, ≥ 51%). Then, using a matrix system, the average of plaque characteristics (elevation, erythema and scaling) will be evaluated. The categories, on an eight-point scale, are: "clear", "almost clear", "mild", "mild to moderate", "moderate", "moderate to severe", "severe", and "very severe".

Despite the importance of the evaluation of psoriasis severity, there is a lack of consensus on the most appropriate measures (van de Kerkhof 1997; Chalmers and Griffiths 2003; Langley and Ellis 2004), though PASI, PGA, and LS-PGA appear to be highly correlated with each other (Langley and Ellis 2004). Despite the referred limitations, the PASI score is the most accepted and widely used measure in clinical trials and in clinical practice (Ashcroft, Wan Po et al. 1999).

Other important psoriasis measurement tools are under development, especially those that also measure the patient's perception of well-being. The National Psoriasis Foundation has developed the National Psoriasis Foundation Psoriasis Score, a responder index, that include six subdomains: induration at two target sites, current and baseline body surface area, physician global assessment, patient global assessment, and patient assessment of itch (Gottlieb, Chaudhari et al. 2003).

Two other quantitative ways of measuring psoriasis are biopsies and photographs. Biopsies are attractive because they are objective, however, their major limitation is that psoriasis does not resolve in a uniform way, and, therefore, biopsies may not provide a representative sampling of lesions. In theory, photographs could be used to confirm real time assessments of disease severity. It is not clear, however, if thickness/induration or even scaliness of lesions can be accurately assessed using the photographs. Nevertheless, photographs do make a strong impact in educating physicians and, therefore, they are commonly incorporated into clinical trials.

Most of these tools do not include a measure about the quality-of-life or considers the patient's perception of well-being. Thus, any direct information about psychological and/or social disease consequences is not provided. Indeed, a major component in the assessment of psoriasis should be the measurement of the quality of life, because the improvement in patients' lives is the primary goal of therapy. The term quality of life, or health related quality of life (HRQOL), refers to a quantitative estimation of the global impact of a disease on physical, social, and psychological well-being of a patient. It appears that there is not always a strong correlation between the HRQOL and the severity of the disease, as defined by PASI. For instance, the visibility of psoriatic lesions or the impairment of daily activities may incapacitate a patient to work; itch and pain may cause severe impairment of HRQOL.

The estimation of quality of life is obtained through standardized questionnaires exploring the relevant dimensions of the patient's life that may be affected by the disease. Non-specific queries, such as the Medical Outcome Survey Short Form 36 (SF-36) and the Euro QOL, are used to assess patients' overall quality of life (Ware and Sherbourne 1992; Brazier, Jones et al. 1993).

There are more specific instruments, focusing on aspects of quality of life that are affected by skin disease. These, include the Dermatology Life Quality Index (DLQI) and the Skindex (Finlay and Khan 1994; Chren, Lasek et al. 1997). There are even more specific measures for psoriasis. For instance, scores that include psychological impact along with the severity of the skin lesions are the Salford Psoriasis Index and the Psoriasis Disability Index (Kirby, Fortune et al. 2000). A psoriasis-specific study of QOL, the PSORIQOL, is a recently introduced 25-item instrument (McKenna, Cook et al. 2003).

The DLQI and the SF-36 have been previously used to evaluate the HRQOL on psoriatic patients (Feldman, Gottlieb et al. 2008; Reich and Griffiths 2008). The generic queries, such as the SF-36, are useful to show the impact of psoriasis. The SF-36 has showed that the impact of psoriasis was similar or higher than that imposed by many other serious medical conditions.

The DLQI has been most widely used in psoriasis trials as a measure to assess the quality of life related to skin disease. Indeed, it has been used in more than 35 psoriasis studies, and it has been used very extensively over the last years in the study of the new generation of systemic therapies for psoriasis. Furthermore, it has been shown that the value of clinical research in psoriasis is improved in the DLQI, as the DLQI score banding proposes: 0-1 means "no effect on QOL"; 2-5, "small effect"; 6-10, "moderate effect"; 11-20, "very large effect"; 21-30, "extremely large effect". Apparently, a total DLQI higher than 10 represents a skin disease having a very large effect on patient's life, needing intervention, and, from the individual point of view, a DLQI of 5 or less is associated with improved QOL.

Quality of life clarified the multidimensional nature of disease assessment and outcome, which should include the evaluation of disease associated discomfort, level of disability, and social disruption. It is important to define the severity of psoriasis, but it is also important to identify psoriasis that severely affects the quality of life.

8. Psoriasis psychosocial aspects

A number of psychiatric/psychological comorbidities have been observed in psoriatic patients. Psoriasis deeply affects the well-being of the patient and has emotional and social consequences (Jobling and Naldi 2006). Thus, to define psoriasis as only a skin problem is a very restrictive approach.

Psoriatic patients present a variety of psychological problems, including poor self esteem, sexual dysfunction, anxiety and depression. Indeed, about 35% of psoriatic patients report symptoms of depression (Friedewald, Cather et al. 2008); about 80% of patients refer that the disease has a negative impact on their lives for a variety of reasons, including the physical symptoms, upsetting physical appearance (particularly because its onset is before 30 years of age in 60% of the cases), frustration, anger, anxiety, depression, and increased use of alcohol (Mease and Menter 2006). Since psoriasis is a persistent, disfiguring and stigmatizing disease, clinicians need to be aware of the emotional and psychological impact of psoriasis in the patient.

Major depression seems to be a significant predictor of CVD events. It may be an independent risk factor for death, after suffering an acute myocardial infarction (Carney, Blumenthal et al. 2003), and it may increase the risk for coronary artery disease (Barth, Schumacher et al. 2004). An association between depressive symptoms and the levels of serum inflammatory markers was also reported (Stewart, Janicki-Deverts et al. 2008). Acute or chronic psychological stress, may induce a chronic inflammatory process that may culminate in atherosclerosis (Black and Garbutt 2002).

It is known that in psoriatic patients, psychological stress, by itself, can play a role in exacerbation of psoriasis, and that higher stress reactivity has been associated with the onset of psoriasis at an earlier age (Naldi, Chatenoud et al. 2005). Indeed, 31% of the patients reported the onset of psoriasis in periods of increased everyday life stress, and in 71% of patients, psoriasis symptomatology worsened during stressful life episodes (Griffiths and Richards 2001; Zachariae, Zachariae et al. 2004). The importance of stress in psoriasis has been further highlighted, since psychological distress affects treatment outcome in psoriatic patients. For instance, the level of stress may prolong the time taken for psoralen plus UVA (PUVA) to clear the symptoms of psoriasis (Fortune, Richards et al. 2003). Accordingly, stress reduction by stress management, relaxation or cognitive techniques shortened the time to clear psoriasis symptoms by PUVA, and, moreover, improved the clinical severity of psoriasis (Kabat-Zinn, Wheeler et al. 1998; Fortune, Richards et al. 2002). An interesting finding is the increase in the catecholamine levels after stress exposure in psoriatic patients (Buske-Kirschbaum, Ebrecht et al. 2006), pointing to a hyper responsive sympatho-adrenomedullary system in psoriasis.

The relevance of stress in psoriasis is broadly accepted, however, the underlying mechanisms, of how psychological distress exacerbates or triggers psoriasis, are poorly understood. It is known that psychological stress has the potential to regulate the immune response, and there is emerging evidence that abnormal neuroendocrine response to stress may contribute to the pathogenesis of chronic autoimmune diseases (Jorgensen, Bressot et al. 1995).

Psoriatic patients often manifest not only a profound psychosocial disability, but also a significant impairment of health related quality of life (Reich and Griffiths 2008). The lack of understanding by the family members may increase the level of anxiety in the patient; the QOL of relatives and partners of patients with psoriasis can also be significantly affected (Eghlileb, Davies et al. 2007).

Some authors believe that HRQOL is more determined by how an individual mentally copes with the disease than by the amount of skin affected (Stern, Nijsten et al. 2004;

Friedewald, Cather et al. 2008). Others, refer that the impact of the disease in HRQOL seem to be greater in patients with more extensive skin involvement (Gelfand, Feldman et al. 2004). Thus, clinicians need to try to perceive the severity of psoriasis from the patient's point of view. From the patient's perspective, psoriasis is usually considered as severe, if it causes embarrassment or anxiety, pruritus or soreness; if it affects relationships, everyday activities, working, studying or sport activities, or if there is joint involvement. In a survey of patients with severe forms of psoriasis, 79% reported that psoriasis had a negative impact on their lives, 40% felt frustration with recurrent treatments, and 32% did not perceive their treatment to be sufficiently aggressive (Krueger, Koo et al. 2001). The impact of psoriasis seems to be more severe for young adults (18-24 years old), particularly, for women, singles, patients with visible psoriasis, patients who developed psoriasis in early childhood, patients who have a negative state of mind as a result of psoriasis, or patients who have experienced additional problems due to psoriasis (Young 2005).

It is known that the stress caused by living with psoriasis can be manifested as avoidance behaviours. Active psoriasis seems to lead to a marked loss of productivity (Fowler, Duh et al. 2008). In fact, the two main contributors to stress in patients with psoriasis are engaging in avoidance behaviour and the belief that they are being evaluated on the basis of their skin disease, which may lead to low grade persistent stress. It has been reported that psoriatic patients present a reduction in physical and mental functioning comparable to that observed in patients with cancer, arthritis, hypertension, heart disease and depression (Rapp, Feldman et al. 1999). Furthermore, the general health status of the patient may be affected by all the diseases that associate with psoriasis, creating a substantial impact on HRQOL.

Psychological sequelae of the disease can impair the response to treatment, since patients with pathological levels of anxiety are less likely to respond to therapy (Fortune, Richards et al. 2003). Thus, stress in the form of pathological worry has a deleterious effect on response to therapy. In consequence, psychological intervention may play an important role in the management of psoriasis patients.

9. Acknowledgements

We are greatful to Fundação para a Ciência e Tecnologia (FCT: POCI/SAU - OBS/58600/2004) and Fundo Europeu de Desenvolvimento Regional (FEDER).

10. References

Ashcroft, D. M., A. L. Wan Po, et al. (1999). "Clinical measures of disease severity and outcome in psoriasis: a critical appraisal of their quality." Br J Dermatol 141(2): 185-91.

Asumalahti, K., M. Ameen, et al. (2003). "Genetic analysis of PSORS1 distinguishes guttate psoriasis and palmoplantar pustulosis." J Invest Dermatol 120(4): 627-32.

Barth, J., M. Schumacher, et al. (2004). "Depression as a risk factor for mortality in patients with coronary heart disease: a meta-analysis." Psychosom Med 66(6): 802-13.

Berth-Jones, J., K. Grotzinger, et al. (2006). "A study examining inter- and intrarater reliability of three scales for measuring severity of psoriasis: Psoriasis Area and

Severity Index, Physician's Global Assessment and Lattice System Physician's Global Assessment." Br J Dermatol 155(4): 707-13.

Black, P. H. and L. D. Garbutt (2002). "Stress, inflammation and cardiovascular disease." J Psychosom Res 52(1): 1-23.

Blauvelt, A. (2008). "T-helper 17 cells in psoriatic plaques and additional genetic links between IL-23 and psoriasis." J Invest Dermatol 128(5): 1064-7.

Bos, J. D., C. Hagenaars, et al. (1989). "Predominance of "memory" T cells (CD4+, CDw29+) over "naive" T cells (CD4+, CD45R+) in both normal and diseased human skin." Arch Dermatol Res 281(1): 24-30.

Brazier, J., N. Jones, et al. (1993). "Testing the validity of the Euroqol and comparing it with the SF-36 health survey questionnaire." Qual Life Res 2(3): 169-80.

Buske-Kirschbaum, A., M. Ebrecht, et al. (2006). "Endocrine stress responses in TH1-mediated chronic inflammatory skin disease (psoriasis vulgaris)--do they parallel stress-induced endocrine changes in TH2-mediated inflammatory dermatoses (atopic dermatitis)?" Psychoneuroendocrinology 31(4): 439-46.

Capon, F., M. Munro, et al. (2002). "Searching for the major histocompatibility complex psoriasis susceptibility gene." J Invest Dermatol 118(5): 745-51.

Carlin, C. S., S. R. Feldman, et al. (2004). "A 50% reduction in the Psoriasis Area and Severity Index (PASI 50) is a clinically significant endpoint in the assessment of psoriasis." J Am Acad Dermatol 50(6): 859-66.

Carney, R. M., J. A. Blumenthal, et al. (2003). "Depression as a risk factor for mortality after acute myocardial infarction." Am J Cardiol 92(11): 1277-81.

Caspary, F., G. Elliott, et al. (2005). "A new therapeutic approach to treat psoriasis by inhibition of fatty acid oxidation by Etomoxir." Br J Dermatol 153(5): 937-44.

Castellani, M. L., D. Kempuraj, et al. (2009). "The latest interleukin: IL-33 the novel IL-1-family member is a potent mast cell activator." J Biol Regul Homeost Agents 23(1): 11-4.

Chalmers, R. J. and C. E. Griffiths (2003). "Resetting the research agenda for psoriasis." J Invest Dermatol 120(5): ix-x.

Chen, S. C., M. de Groot, et al. "Expression of chemokine receptor CXCR3 by lymphocytes and plasmacytoid dendritic cells in human psoriatic lesions." Arch Dermatol Res 302(2): 113-23.

Chren, M. M., R. J. Lasek, et al. (1997). "Improved discriminative and evaluative capability of a refined version of Skindex, a quality-of-life instrument for patients with skin diseases." Arch Dermatol 133(11): 1433-40.

Coimbra, S., H. Oliveira, et al. (2010a). "C-reactive protein and leucocyte activation in psoriasis vulgaris according to severity and therapy." J Eur Acad Dermatol Venereol 24(7): 789-96.

Coimbra, S., H. Oliveira, et al. (2010b). "Circulating adipokine levels in Portuguese patients with psoriasis vulgaris according to body mass index, severity and therapy." J Eur Acad Dermatol Venereol 24(12): 1386-94.

Coimbra, S., H. Oliveira, et al. (2010c). "Interleukin (IL)-22, IL-17, IL-23, IL-8, vascular endothelial growth factor and tumour necrosis factor-alpha levels in patients with

psoriasis before, during and after psoralen-ultraviolet A and narrowband ultraviolet B therapy." Br J Dermatol 163(6):1282-90.
Cox, A. J. and W. Watson (1972). "Histological variations in lesions of psoriasis." Arch Dermatol 106(4): 503-6.
Crissey, J. T. and L. C. Parish (1998). "Two hundred years of dermatology." J Am Acad Dermatol 39(6): 1002-6.
Di Cesare, A., P. Di Meglio, et al. (2009). "The IL-23/Th17 axis in the immunopathogenesis of psoriasis." J Invest Dermatol 129(6): 1339-50.
Eghlileb, A. M., E. E. Davies, et al. (2007). "Psoriasis has a major secondary impact on the lives of family members and partners." Br J Dermatol 156(6): 1245-50.
Elder, J. T., A. T. Bruce, et al. (2010). "Molecular dissection of psoriasis: integrating genetics and biology." J Invest Dermatol 130(5): 1213-26.
Elder, J. T., R. P. Nair, et al. (1994). "The genetics of psoriasis." Arch Dermatol 130(2): 216-24.
Farber, E. M. and M. L. Nall (1974). "The natural history of psoriasis in 5,600 patients." Dermatologica 148(1): 1-18.
Feldman, S. R., A. B. Gottlieb, et al. (2008). "Infliximab improves health-related quality of life in the presence of comorbidities among patients with moderate-to-severe psoriasis." Br J Dermatol 159(3): 704-10.
Finlay, A. Y. and G. K. Khan (1994). "Dermatology Life Quality Index (DLQI)--a simple practical measure for routine clinical use." Clin Exp Dermatol 19(3): 210-6.
Fortune, D. G., H. L. Richards, et al. (2002). "A cognitive-behavioural symptom management programme as an adjunct in psoriasis therapy." Br J Dermatol 146(3): 458-65.
Fortune, D. G., H. L. Richards, et al. (2003). "Psychological distress impairs clearance of psoriasis in patients treated with photochemotherapy." Arch Dermatol 139(6): 752-6.
Fowler, J. F., M. S. Duh, et al. (2008). "The impact of psoriasis on health care costs and patient work loss." J Am Acad Dermatol 59(5): 772-80.
Frederiksson T, P. U. (1978). "Severe psoriasis - oral therapy with a new retinoid." Dermatologica 157: 238-44.
Friedewald, V. E., Jr., J. C. Cather, et al. (2008). "The editor's roundtable: psoriasis, inflammation, and coronary artery disease." Am J Cardiol 101(8): 1119-26.
Gelfand, J. M., S. R. Feldman, et al. (2004). "Determinants of quality of life in patients with psoriasis: a study from the US population." J Am Acad Dermatol 51(5): 704-8.
Gladman, D. D., R. Shuckett, et al. (1987). "Psoriatic arthritis (PSA)--an analysis of 220 patients." Q J Med 62(238): 127-41.
Gonzalez, S., M. Rajadhyaksha, et al. (1999). "Characterization of psoriasis in vivo by reflectance confocal microscopy." J Med 30(5-6): 337-56.
Gottlieb, A. B., U. Chaudhari, et al. (2003). "The National Psoriasis Foundation Psoriasis Score (NPF-PS) system versus the Psoriasis Area Severity Index (PASI) and Physician's Global Assessment (PGA): a comparison." J Drugs Dermatol 2(3): 260-6.
Griffiths, C. E. and H. L. Richards (2001). "Psychological influences in psoriasis." Clin Exp Dermatol 26(4): 338-42.

Gudjonsson, J. E., A. Karason, et al. (2006). "Distinct clinical differences between HLA Cw*0602 positive and negative psoriasis patients-an analysis of 1019 HLA-C- and HLA-B-typed patients." J Invest Dermatol 126(4): 740-5.

Hamminga, E. A., A. J. van der Lely, et al. (2006). "Chronic inflammation in psoriasis and obesity: implications for therapy." Med Hypotheses 67(4): 768-73.

Harper, E. G., C. Guo, et al. (2009). "Th17 cytokines stimulate CCL20 expression in keratinocytes in vitro and in vivo: implications for psoriasis pathogenesis." J Invest Dermatol 129(9): 2175-83.

Henseler, T. and E. Christophers (1985). "Psoriasis of early and late onset: characterization of two types of psoriasis vulgaris." J Am Acad Dermatol 13(3): 450-6.

Higa-Sansone, G., S. Szomstein, et al. (2004). "Psoriasis remission after laparoscopic Roux-en-Y gastric bypass for morbid obesity." Obes Surg 14(8): 1132-4.

Ho, P., I. N. Bruce, et al. (2005). "Evidence for common genetic control in pathways of inflammation for Crohn's disease and psoriatic arthritis." Arthritis Rheum 52(11): 3596-602.

Holzmann, H., R. J. Werner, et al. (1992). "[Detection of the Kobner phenomenon of the skeleton of patients with psoriasis]." Hautarzt 43(10): 645-51.

Jobling, R. and L. Naldi (2006). "Assessing the impact of psoriasis and the relevance of qualitative research." J Invest Dermatol 126(7): 1438-40.

Jorgensen, C., N. Bressot, et al. (1995). "Dysregulation of the hypothalamo-pituitary axis in rheumatoid arthritis." J Rheumatol 22(10): 1829-33.

Kabat-Zinn, J., E. Wheeler, et al. (1998). "Influence of a mindfulness meditation-based stress reduction intervention on rates of skin clearing in patients with moderate to severe psoriasis undergoing phototherapy (UVB) and photochemotherapy (PUVA)." Psychosom Med 60(5): 625-32.

Kirby, B., D. G. Fortune, et al. (2000). "The Salford Psoriasis Index: an holistic measure of psoriasis severity." Br J Dermatol 142(4): 728-32.

Krueger, G., J. Koo, et al. (2001). "The impact of psoriasis on quality of life: results of a 1998 National Psoriasis Foundation patient-membership survey." Arch Dermatol 137(3): 280-4.

Kunz, M. (2009). "Current treatment of psoriasis with biologics." Curr Drug Discov Technol 6(4): 231-40.

Langley, R. G. and C. N. Ellis (2004). "Evaluating psoriasis with Psoriasis Area and Severity Index, Psoriasis Global Assessment, and Lattice System Physician's Global Assessment." J Am Acad Dermatol 51(4): 563-9.

Langley, R. G., G. G. Krueger, et al. (2005). "Psoriasis: epidemiology, clinical features, and quality of life." Ann Rheum Dis 64 Suppl 2: ii18-23; discussion ii24-5.

Lithell, H., A. Bruce, et al. (1983). "A fasting and vegetarian diet treatment trial on chronic inflammatory disorders." Acta Derm Venereol 63(5): 397-403.

Lowes, M. A., F. Chamian, et al. (2005). "Increase in TNF-alpha and inducible nitric oxide synthase-expressing dendritic cells in psoriasis and reduction with efalizumab (anti-CD11a)." Proc Natl Acad Sci U S A 102(52): 19057-62.

Lowes, M. A., T. Kikuchi, et al. (2008). "Psoriasis vulgaris lesions contain discrete populations of Th1 and Th17 T cells." J Invest Dermatol 128(5): 1207-11.

Mallbris, L., P. Larsson, et al. (2005). "Psoriasis phenotype at disease onset: clinical characterization of 400 adult cases." J Invest Dermatol 124(3): 499-504.

Martin, B. A., R. J. Chalmers, et al. (1996). "How great is the risk of further psoriasis following a single episode of acute guttate psoriasis?" Arch Dermatol 132(6): 717-8.

McKenna, S. P., S. A. Cook, et al. (2003). "Development of the PSORIQoL, a psoriasis-specific measure of quality of life designed for use in clinical practice and trials." Br J Dermatol 149(2): 323-31.

Mease, P. J. and M. A. Menter (2006). "Quality-of-life issues in psoriasis and psoriatic arthritis: outcome measures and therapies from a dermatological perspective." J Am Acad Dermatol 54(4): 685-704.

Mehta, S., A. Singal, et al. (2009). "A study of clinicohistopathological correlation in patients of psoriasis and psoriasiform dermatitis." Indian J Dermatol Venereol Leprol 75(1): 100.

Murphy, M., P. Kerr, et al. (2007). "The histopathologic spectrum of psoriasis." Clin Dermatol 25(6): 524-8.

Naldi, L., L. Chatenoud, et al. (2005). "Cigarette smoking, body mass index, and stressful life events as risk factors for psoriasis: results from an Italian case-control study." J Invest Dermatol 125(1): 61-7.

Naldi, L. and D. Gambini (2007). "The clinical spectrum of psoriasis." Clin Dermatol 25(6): 510-8.

National Psoriasis Foundation. "Psoriasis Statistics." Retrieved 27th of May of 2011, from http://www.psoriais.org/about//stats.

Neimann, A. L., D. B. Shin, et al. (2006). "Prevalence of cardiovascular risk factors in patients with psoriasis." J Am Acad Dermatol 55(5): 829-35.

Nestle, F. O., C. Conrad, et al. (2005). "Plasmacytoid predendritic cells initiate psoriasis through interferon-alpha production." J Exp Med 202(1): 135-43.

Nevitt, G. J. and P. E. Hutchinson (1996). "Psoriasis in the community: prevalence, severity and patients' beliefs and attitudes towards the disease." Br J Dermatol 135(4): 533-7.

Noah, P. W. (1990). "The role of microorganisms in psoriasis." Semin Dermatol 9(4): 269-76.

O'Brien, M. and J. Koo (2006). "The mechanism of lithium and beta-blocking agents in inducing and exacerbating psoriasis." J Drugs Dermatol 5(5): 426-32.

Pitzalis, C., A. Cauli, et al. (1996). "Cutaneous lymphocyte antigen-positive T lymphocytes preferentially migrate to the skin but not to the joint in psoriatic arthritis." Arthritis Rheum 39(1): 137-45.

Rapp, S. R., S. R. Feldman, et al. (1999). "Psoriasis causes as much disability as other major medical diseases." J Am Acad Dermatol 41(3 Pt 1): 401-7.

Reich, K. and C. E. Griffiths (2008). "The relationship between quality of life and skin clearance in moderate-to-severe psoriasis: lessons learnt from clinical trials with infliximab." Arch Dermatol Res 300(10): 537-44.

Salomon, J., J. C. Szepietowski, et al. (2003). "Psoriatic nails: a prospective clinical study." J Cutan Med Surg 7(4): 317-21.

Sano, S., K. S. Chan, et al. (2005). "Stat3 links activated keratinocytes and immunocytes required for development of psoriasis in a novel transgenic mouse model." Nat Med 11(1): 43-9.

Stern, R. S., T. Nijsten, et al. (2004). "Psoriasis is common, carries a substantial burden even when not extensive, and is associated with widespread treatment dissatisfaction." J Investig Dermatol Symp Proc 9(2): 136-9.

Sterry, W., B. E. Strober, et al. (2007). "Obesity in psoriasis: the metabolic, clinical and therapeutic implications. Report of an interdisciplinary conference and review." Br J Dermatol 157(4): 649-55.

Stewart, J. C., D. Janicki-Deverts, et al. (2008). "Depressive symptoms moderate the influence of hostility on serum interleukin-6 and C-reactive protein." Psychosom Med 70(2): 197-204.

Terui, T., M. Ozawa, et al. (2000). "Role of neutrophils in induction of acute inflammation in T-cell-mediated immune dermatosis, psoriasis: a neutrophil-associated inflammation-boosting loop." Exp Dermatol 9(1): 1-10.

Theoharides, T. C., B. Zhang, et al. (2010). "IL-33 augments substance P-induced VEGF secretion from human mast cells and is increased in psoriatic skin." Proc Natl Acad Sci U S A 107(9): 4448-53.

van de Kerkhof, P. C. (1997). "The Psoriasis Area and Severity Index and alternative approaches for the assessment of severity: persisting areas of confusion." Br J Dermatol 137(4): 661-2.

van de Kerkhof, P. C. and A. M. Lammers (1987). "Intraepidermal accumulation of polymorphonuclear leukocytes in chronic stable plaque psoriasis." Dermatologica 174(5): 224-7.

Vazquez, R., O. Carrera, et al. (2006). "Exploring the association between anorexia nervosa and geographical latitude." Eat Weight Disord 11(1): e1-8.

Wahie, S., A. Alexandroff, et al. (2006). "Psoriasis occurring after myeloablative therapy and autologous stem cell transplantation." Br J Dermatol 154(1): 194-5.

Waldman, A., A. Gilhar, et al. (2001). "Incidence of Candida in psoriasis--a study on the fungal flora of psoriatic patients." Mycoses 44(3-4): 77-81.

Ware, J. E., Jr. and C. D. Sherbourne (1992). "The MOS 36-item short-form health survey (SF-36). I. Conceptual framework and item selection." Med Care 30(6): 473-83.

Watson, W., H. M. Cann, et al. (1972). "The genetics of psoriasis." Arch Dermatol 105(2): 197-207.

Weisenseel, P., B. Laumbacher, et al. (2002). "Streptococcal infection distinguishes different types of psoriasis." J Med Genet 39(10): 767-8.

Werner, B., M. Bresch, et al. (2008). "Comparative study of histopathological and immunohistochemical findings in skin biopsies from patients with psoriasis before and after treatment with acitretin." J Cutan Pathol 35(3): 302-10.

Wolf, R., A. Lo Schiavo, et al. (1997). "The in vitro effect of hydroxychloroquine on skin morphology and transglutaminase." Int J Dermatol 36(9): 704-7.

Wollenberg, A., M. Wagner, et al. (2002). "Plasmacytoid dendritic cells: a new cutaneous dendritic cell subset with distinct role in inflammatory skin diseases." J Invest Dermatol 119(5): 1096-102.

Wright, V. (1956). "Psoriasis and arthritis." Ann Rheum Dis 15(4): 348-56.

Wright, V. (1959a). "Psoriatic arthritis; a comparative study of rheumatoid arthritis, psoriasis, and arthritis associated with psoriasis." AMA Arch Derm 80(1): 27-35.

Wright, V. (1959b). "Rheumatism and psoriasis: a re-evaluation." Am J Med 27: 454-62.
Xu, D., H. R. Jiang, et al. (2008). "IL-33 exacerbates antigen-induced arthritis by activating mast cells." Proc Natl Acad Sci U S A 105(31): 10913-8.
Young, M. (2005). "The psychological and social burdens of psoriasis." Dermatol Nurs 17(1): 15-9.
Zachariae, R., H. Zachariae, et al. (2004). "Self-reported stress reactivity and psoriasis-related stress of Nordic psoriasis sufferers." J Eur Acad Dermatol Venereol 18(1): 27-36.
Zheng, Y., D. M. Danilenko, et al. (2007). "Interleukin-22, a T(H)17 cytokine, mediates IL-23-induced dermal inflammation and acanthosis." Nature 445(7128): 648-51.

4

Psoriasis and *Malassezia* Yeasts

Asja Prohić
Department of Dermatovenerology,
University Clinical Center of Sarajevo
Bosnia and Herzegovina

1. Introduction

There is evidence that psoriasis is principally a T cell-mediated skin disease. The interaction between T cells and keratinocytes via cytokines probably plays a very important role in the pathogenic process (Lee & Cooper, 2006). However, little is known about the initial stimulus that leads to the abnormal T-cell activation.

Yeasts of the genus *Malassezia* are now considered synonymous with those previously named *Pityrosporum,* which are members of the normal cutaneous microbiota from humans and other warm-blooded animals. They have also been associated with several skin diseases such as pityriasis versicolor, seborrheic dermatitis and atopic dermatitis (Gupta et al., 2004; Ashbee 2007).

Although streptococcal infection is the commonest and best delineated infective trigger for psoriasis, fungal infections have been noted on occasion to cause an exacerbation of psoriasis or psoriatic arthritis (Fry & Baker, 2007).

The role of *Malassezia* species in psoriasis is still undetermined, but several reports have associated these lipophilic yeasts with the development of skin lesions in psoriasis. Mostly of these studied are treatment studies, showing the efficacy of antifungal drugs, both topical and systemic, in the treatment of the disease (Rosenberg & Belew, 1982; Alford et al., 1986).

Currently, the genus *Malassezia* includes 14 species, which have been identified traditionally based on their morphology and biochemical features (Cafarchia et al., 2011). Since the description of new species a number of studies have evolved to elucidate the role of the different species in the ecology and pathogenicity in a range of dermatoses, in which variable results have been reported from different geographical regions.

2. Malassezia yeasts

2.1 Description and natural habitats

The genus *Malassezia* (former *Pityrosporum*) belongs to basidiomycetous yeasts and is classified in the *Malasseziales (Ustilaginomycetes, Basidiomycota)* (Boekhout & Gueho, 2003).

Malassezia yeasts are part of the normal cutaneous commensal flora. However, under the influence of predisposing factors these yeasts are able to cause a number of cutaneous and systemic diseases in humans and different animal species. Unlike many other microorganisms, *Malassezia* yeasts are rarely found in the environment. Their natural habitat is primarily the skin of most warm-blooded vertebrates (Midgley, 2000).

Malassezia yeasts have an affinity for lipids as substrates and the term 'lipophilic yeasts' is frequently used to identify the genus. Due to their dependence on lipids for survival, they are most often found in sebum rich areas of the skin such as scalp, face and the trunk. Less frequently, they may be also found on other areas of the body including arms, legs and genitalia.

Colonization with *Malassezia* may occur as early as neonatal period and increases after puberty, which is related to the increase in skin surface lipids that results from higher sebaceous gland activity during this period. Their density varies depending on age, body site, geographic area, and the presence of normal or diseased skin (Ashbee, 2006).

2.2 Historical review and taxonomy

The taxonomy of *Malassezia* has been confused because yeasts are dimorphic, existing in both yeast and mycelial (hyphal) forms, depending on culture conditions.

For many years two taxonomy systems existed. The yeast phase was originally described as *Pityrosporum* and the mycelial phase as *Malassezia,* with two species *M. furfur* and *M. pachydermatis,* before they were unified in 1986 with both phases included in *Malassezia* (Cannon, 1986).

On the basis of genome differences, in 1990, the third species *M. sympodialis* was described (Simmons & Gueho, 1990), and some years later, with the use of new molecular techniques, the genus was taxonomically revised and enlarged with four new species: *M. slooffiae, M. globosa, M. obtusa* and *M. restricta* (Gueho et al., 1996). *M. pachydermatis* is the only non lipid-depended species confirmed to be associated with animals, while remaining species are obligatory lipophilic and found primarily in humans (Guillot & Bond, 1999).

Furthermore, in last few years some new species have been isolated from human (*M. dermatis, M. japonica* and *M. yamotensis*) and animal skin (*M. nana, M. caprae and M. equina, M. cuniculi*) (Sugita et al., 2002; Sugita et al, 2003; Sugita et al, 2004; Hirai et al., 2004; Cabañes et al., 2007; Cabañes et al., 2011). At present, 14 species of *Malassezia* have been identified.

The different species of *Malassezia* yeasts that are known so far are shown in Table 1. No doubt that additional new species will be identified from both humans and animals in close future.

2.3 Biological, cultural and immunological characteristics

The different *Malassezia* species are distinguished based on their morphology, growth characteristics, enzyme activities, as well as by molecular characteristics.

Malassezia specijes	First description	Isolation from humans	Isolation from animals
M. furfur	Baillon 1889	Healthy skin Skin diseases: mainly pityriasis versicolor, systemic infections	Healthy skin
M. pachydermatis	(Weidman) Dodge 1925	Systemic infections	Healthy skin: mainly dogs and cats Skin diseases: seborrheic dermatitis and otitis in dogs
M. sympodialis	Simmons & Guého 1990	Healthy skin Skin diseases: atopic dermatitis	Healthy skin Skin diseases: otitis in cats
M. slooffiae	Guillot, Midgley & Guého 1996	Healthy skin: external ear canal Skin diseases: pityriasis versicolor	Healthy skin: pigs Skin diseases: dermatitis in goats
M. globosa	Midgley, Guého & Guillot 1996	Healthy skin Skin disease: mainly pityriasis versicolor	Healthy skin Skin lesions: otitis in cats
M. obtusa	Midgley, Guillot & Guého 1996	Healthy skin Skin diseases: mainly pityriasis versicolor	
M. restricta	Guého, Guillot & Midgley 1996	Healthy skin Skin diseases: mainly seborrheic dermatitis and scalp psoriasis	
M. dermatis	Sugita, Takashima, Nishikawa & Shinoda 2002	Healthy skin Skin diseases: atopic dermatitis	
M. japonica	Sugita, Takashima, Kodama, Tsuboi & Nishikawa 2003	Healthy skin Skin diseases: atopic dermatitis	
M. yamatoensis	Sugita, Takashima, Tajima, Tsuboi & Nishikawa 2004	Healthy skin Skin diseases: seborrheic dermatitis	
M. nana	Hirai, Kano, Makimura, Yamaguchi & Hasegawa 2004		Skin diseases: cats and cows
M. caprae	Cabanes & Boekhout 2007		Healthy skin: goats
M. equina	Cabanes & Boekhout 2007		Healthy skin: horses
M. cuniculi	*Cabanes, Vega & Castella 2011*		Healthy skin: rabits

Table 1. *Malassezia* species isolated from humans and animals

The fungus is dimorphic, existing in both saprophytic yeast and a parasitic mycelial form. The yeast form is most commonly associated with normal skin and predominates in culture, although hyphae may be seen with some species (Saadatzadeh et al., 2001).

For direct demonstration of the yeasts, the specimen is collected from the clinical lesions by scraping or tape stripping and a potassium hydroxide mount is prepared. The cells are morphologically variable, occurring in round, oval or cylindrical forms. They show the production of blastoconidia by a process of repetitive monopolar or sympodial budding. Direct microscopy of the pityriasis versicolor scales reveals predominantly hyphae with clusters of yeast cells (spaghetti and meatball appearance), due to the phase transition from yeast to mycelium seen in this disease (Figure 1).

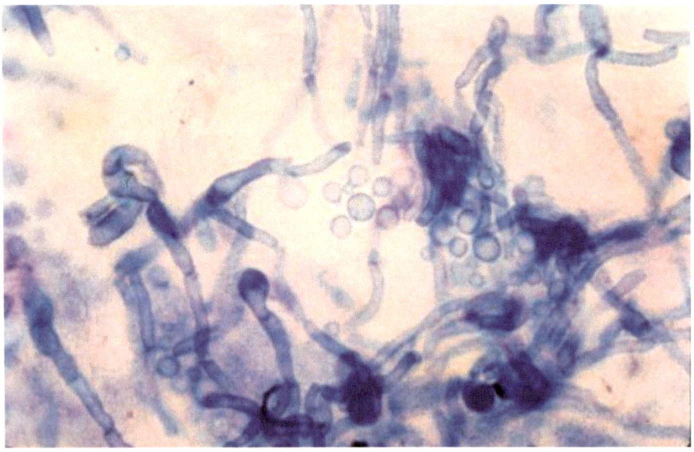

Fig. 1. The typical appearance of the hyphae and spores of *Malassezia* in the scales of pityriasis versicolor

The colonies of *Malassezia* spp. are raised, dull, creamy yellow and have a characteristic brittle texture (Figure 2). The characteristic morphological features of *Malassezia* yeasts include thick, multi-layered cell wall which is surrounded by a lamellar layer which contains lipids (Gueho et al., 1996).

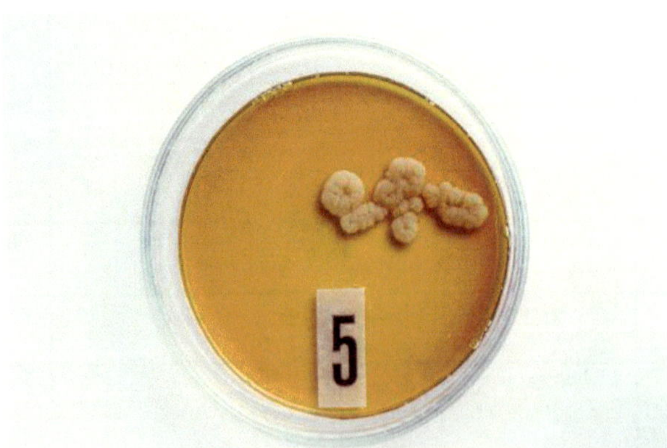

Fig. 2. The colonies of *M. globosa* on modified Dixon agar

Malasezia species produce a wide range of enzymes, including lipases, phospholipases and hydrolase. The lipases are essential in providing the lipids required for growth in vitro and in vivo. All species of *Malassezia* with the exception of *M. pachydermatis,* are lipid-dependent due to an inability to synthesize long-chain saturated fatty acids (Nazzaro Porro et al., 1986; Juntachai et al., 2009).

To differentiate among the *Malassezia* species, cultures should be done in special media (Leeming and Notman agar or modified Dixon agar), except for *M. pachydermatis,* the only one that is able to grow in Sabouraud agar (Guillot et al., 1996).

However, difficulties in cultivating *Malassezia* organisms may limit the analyses and bias the observations (Batra et al., 2005). Thus, molecular approaches, particularly analyses of ribosomal genes and internal transcribed regions, have been used for detection, identification, and characterization of *Malassezia* species (Cafarchia et al., 2011).

Malassezia has the ability to stimulate the immune system via classical and alternative complement pathways, acting as an adjuvant and elicits both humoral and cellular immune response. In contrast, it is able to resist phagocytic killing by neutrophils and downregulate cytokine responses when co-cultured with peripheral blood mononuclear cells. With the interaction of yeasts with keratinocytes they induce the production of different cytokines, especially IL-6, IL-8 and IL-10 (Asbbee 2006; Blanco & Garcia 2008).

2.4 Human diseased associated with *Malassezia* yeasts

In recent years, the genus *Malassezia* has come to be considered important in the etiology of various skin and systemic diseases. Both immunocompetent and immunosuppressed patients may be affected by this type of infection. In immunologically competent hosts, *Malassezia* species are implicated in the pathogenesis of variety of skin infections such as pityriasis versicolor, *Malassezia* folliculitis, seborrheic dermatitis, and, rarely, in a range of other dermatological disorders (Midgley 2000; Gupta et al., 2004). In contrast, in immunocompromised patients, including patients with AIDS, immune-haematological, oncological, and solid organ and bone marrow transplant recipients, these yeasts have been associated with catheter-related fungemia, sepsis and a variety of deeply invasive infections (Tragiannidis et al., 2010).

The etiological role of *Malassezia* yeasts in pityriasis versicolor is unquestioned; the organism found in the lesions is predominantly in its mycelial phase (Crespo et al., 1999; Gupta et al., 2001; Prohic & Ozegovic, 2007; Trabelsi et al., 2010).

In the case of the other skin diseases such as seborrheic dermatitis, *Malassezia* folliculitis, confluent and reticulate papillomatosis, atopic dermatitis, and psoriasis, the pathogenic role of *Malassezia* yeasts remains less clear; transition of the yeast cells to their pathogenic hyphal form cannot be clearly demonstrated (Gupta et al., 2004; Ashbee 2007).

With the revision of the taxonomy of *Malassezia,* new questions have been raised about their significance and relative prevalence in various dermatologic disorders.

The diseases where *Malassezia* species have been implicated and the most frequent species isolated are summarized in Table 2.

Pityriasis versicolor	*M. globosa, M. furfur*
Seborrheic dermatitis	*M. restricta, M. globosa, M. sympodialis*
Malassezia folliculitis	*M. globosa, M. restricta*
Atopic dermatitis	*M. sympodialis, M. globosa, M. furfur*
Confluent and reticulate papillomatosis	*M. furfur, M. sympodialis*
Psoriasis	*M. globosa, M. restricta*
Onychomycosis	*Malassezia* spp.
Acne	*Malassezia* spp.
Otitis	*M. sympodialis*
Neonatal pustulosis	*M. globosa, M. sympodialis*
Oportunitic systemic infections	*M. furfur, M. pachydermatis*

Table 2. Human diseases associated with *Malassezia* yeasts and the most frequent species isolated

3. Psoriasis

3.1 Superantigens

The pathogenesis of psoriasis is quite complex, but there is compelling evidence that T-cell activation and resultant overproduction of proinflammatory cytokines are critical for the development and maintenance of psoriatic lesion (Lee & Cooper, 2006; Tokura et al., 2010).

A variety of different environmental factors are accepted as of importance in provoking new episodes of psoriasis or in modifying preexisting diseases. They include trauma, infections, drugs and psychological stress (Fry & Baker, 2007). However, definite proof that particular autoantigens, antigens or both contribute to the immunopathology of psoriasis is still lacking.

Nevertheless, a number of keratins microbial proteins have been postulated as putative candidates (Jones et al., 2004). Keratin (K) 13 has significant homology with K17, which was previously identified as candidate autoantigen based on the presence of both antibodies and T cells that cross-react with a streptococcus M protein (Gudmundsdottir et al, 1999). Furthermore, K13 is not present in adult skin normally, but is present in fetal skin (van Muijen et al, 1987), and is up-regulated during trauma or inflammation. (Kallioinen et al, 1995). This could potentially provide an explanation for the Koebner phenomenon, where new psoriasis plaques can flare up at or old lesions spread to a site of injury.

Superantigens may exacerbate psoriasis by stimulating T cells to initiate the pathogenic events of psoriasis. Microorganisms such as β-haemolytic streptococci, *Staphylococcus aureus* and *Candida albicans* have been suggested as external triggers that activate large number of T cells and release proinflammatory cytokines, particularly tumour necrosis factor (TNF)-a (Macias et al., 2011). Massive cytokine production could lead to reduced vascular tone, resulting in widespread organ hypoperfusion, acidosis and multiorgan failure.

3.1.1 Bacterial superantigens

Streptococcal superantigens appear to play a direct role in the pathogenesis of guttate psoriasis. It is well documented that streptococcal infection can trigger guttate psoriasis or exacerbate chronic plaque psoriasis, possibly through the release of bacterial superantigenic toxins, now known as streptococcal pyrogenic exotoxins (Gudjonsson et al., 2003).

The high level of streptococcal throat cultures and sore throats in chronic plaque psoriasis implies that patients with chronic plaque psoriasis are extremely efficient at streptococcal throat carriage. It was purposed that part of the psoriatic genotype protects against death during epidemics of invasive streptococcal infections, but at the expense of increased streptococcal carriage and predisposition to the development of psoriasis (McFadden et al., 2009).

Furthermore, T lymphocytes specific for group A streptococci have been isolated and cloned from the skin of guttate psoriatic patients suggesting a role of these cells in the disease process (Baker et al., 1993; Valdimarsson et al., 1995).

These observations indicate that streptococcal infections are major etiological factors for psoriasis in genetically predisposed individuals. However, this does not exclude a role for other microorganisms in the disease.

3.1.2 Fungal superantigens

Fungal organisms have also been suggested as external triggers that release factors which serve as superantigens and stimulate T cells to initiate the pathogenic events of psoriasis (Waldman et al., 2001)

Regarding the prevalence of *Candida albicans* infections in psoriasis, data are controversial. Some authors found no increase in the prevalence of Candida in intertriginous area of psoriatic patients as compared with healthy individuals (Flytstrom et al., 2003; Leibovici et al., 2008). As ketoconazole appeared to be helpful in the treatment of some inverse psoriasis patients, the authors suggested an anti-inflammatory effect, which may explain some of its beneficial effects irrespective of *Candida* infection. However, Rebora reported the presence of *Candida* in the intertriginous areas of psoriatic patients and commented that *Candida* present in the intertriginous areas disappears when replaced by Gram negative bacteria, but leaves a kobnerising effect (Rebora, 2004).

4. *Malassezia* and psoriasis

4.1 Historical review

Rivolta made the first association of the lipophilic yeasts and psoriasis in 1873 (Rivolta, 1873). He reported on round double-contoured budding cells in the epidermis of a patient with psoriasis and named them *Cryptococcus psoriasis.*

The role of *Malassezia* yeasts in psoriasis is still undetermined, but there are several reports indicating that these microorganisms are able to elicit psoriasiform lesions in both human and animals. Rosenberg reported that, after heavy dense suspensions of *Malassezia* were applied to the shaved rabbits skin, lesions both grossly and microscopically similar to psoriasis developed. The lesions persisted as long as *Malassezia* continued to be applied but otherwise resolved within 3 to 4 days (Rosenberg et al., 1980).

The same group claimed to be able to induce lesions that developed following patch testing with sonicates of heat killed *Malassezia* cells on nonlesional skin of patients with psoriasis and biopsy specimens showed features consistent with psoriasis (Lober et al., 1982).

Although a Koebner phenomenon could not be excluded, their hypothesis was that psoriasis was produced by *Malassezia* yeasts through activation of the alternative pathway of complement, and also activated by other microorganisms and endotoxins.

Elewski reported of a patient developing guttate psoriasis in sites of *Malassezia* folliculitis. In this case, pustules transformed into guttate lesions prior and during erythromycin therapy but resolved when ketoconazole was applied (Elewski, 1990). Although this transformation could also be Koebner phenomenon, this case report supported the proposal that psoriasis may be included in *Malassezia*-associated diseases.

The beneficial effect of both oral and topical ketoconazole, followed by reduction of yeasts, indicates that *Malassezia* yeasts may represent another antigenic stimulus in psoriasis (Rosenberg & Belew, 1982). Although this antimycotic drug may act through a direct mode of action, it has also been shown that it can suppress *Malassezia*-induced proliferation of lymphocytes in psoriatic patients and thus reduce the response to the antigenic stimulation in skin lesions (Alford et al., 1986).

More recent studies have indicated that *Malassezia* yeasts cause exacerbation of psoriasis by triggering the release of cytokines, in particular IL-8 through a Toll-like receptor 2-mediated pathway (Baroni et al., 2006). However, convincing evidence of their importance in the pathogenesis of the disease is still lacking.

4.2 Isolation to the species level

Since the description of the new species some studies have focused on their distribution in various diseases, and also in psoriasis.

The identification of *Malassezia* yeasts to a species level is of no diagnostic value in skin diseases, as the same species form an integral part of normal cutaneous microflora in humans. However, it is of great importance to determine which species are implicated in certain skin disease and whether there is variation in the distribution of the yeasts with clinical data, body site, origin of the population, etc.

The results of the *in vitro* susceptibility studies have shown variations in susceptibility of the seven *Malassezia* species to ketoconazole, variconazole, itraconazole, and terbinafine. Strains of *M.furfur, M.globosa, and M.obtusa* were more tolerant to terbinafine than other species, while *M.sympodialis* was found to be highly susceptible (Gupta et al., 2000). Therefore, correct identification of *Malassezia* species is required for the selection of appropriate antifungal therapy.

Some authors have stated that *M. globosa* predominate (Prohic, 2003; Zomorodian et al., 2008) whilst others have found *M. restricta* (Amaya et al., 2007) or *M. sympodialis* (Hernandez et al., 2003) to be the most common species in scalp lesions of psoriasis.

The higher detection rate of *Malassezia* species was observed using molecular determination method than by conventional culture methods. These variations may be attributed to the different sampling technique and inadequate determination of the relative proportion of species on the skin, or the consent ability of the fungus to grow in each specified medium that have impact on the range of species recovered. Geographical and racial factors were also suspected as playing a part in the results yielded by conventional culture systems (Sandstrom Falk et al., 2005).

4.3 Immune response to *Malassezia* yeasts

Psoriasis is also known to have a strong genetic component. Therefore, several studies have examined the immune responses of psoriasis patients to *Malassezia*.

It has been shown that these individuals have immunologic responses to both *Malassezia* yeasts and to proteins derived from them. T cells reactive to the various morphological variants of yeasts have been isolated from lesional skin, but they were not specific for the disease (Baker et al., 1997). Furthermore, antibodies to proteins from *Malassezia* have been reported in patients with psoriasis, but not healthy subjects (Squiquera et al., 1994; Liang et al., 2003). These antibodies were subsequently shown to recognize the *N*-acetylglucosamine terminals of glycoproteins present in *Malassezia* (Mathow et al., 1996). However, both of these proteins are recognized by sera from patients with atopic dermatitis (Lintu et al., 1997; Nissen et al., 1998), and so they are not specific markers for psoriasis.

Kanda et al. found that *Malassezia* yeasts induce Th-1 and Th2-related cytokine, chemokine and prostaglandin E2 production in peripheral blood mononuclear cells from patients with psoriasis vulgaris (Kanda et al., 2002).

Furtermore, *Malassezia* can invade cultured human keratinocytes, modulate proinflammatory and immunomodulatory cytokine synthesis, and affect the expression of cutaneous proteins (Baroni et al., 2001). A study done by same authors added to the evidence of its role in the hyperproliferation seen in psoriasis. Using western blot analysis they found that *Malassezia* can induce the overproduction of molecules involved in cell migration and hyperproliferation, thereby favoring the exacerbation of psoriasis. (Baroni et al., 2004).

Malassezia species differ in their ability to induce cytokine production by human keratinocytes, which is reflected in the different inflammatory responses in *Malassezia*-associated dermatoses, resulting in varied clinical and pathological manifestations.

A study examining the chemotaxis of neutrophils from psoriatic patients and controls demonstrated the presence of *Malassezia*-derived soluble components with chemo-attractant properties for polymorphonuclear leukocytes of psoriatic patients (Bunse & Mahrle, 1996).

Psoriatic lesions often develop at sites of trauma (the Koebner phenomenon) (Mohla & Brodell, 1999), and the increased chemotactic response of neutrophils to *Malassezia* was suggested to play a role in this event.

Kesavan et al. have shown that *Malassezia* yeasts significantly reduce the production of pro-inflammatory cytokines what is related to the presence of lipid-rich microfibrilar layer surrounding yeast cells (Kesavan et al., 1998) High quantity of lipid may prevent the yeast cell from inducing inflammation what is in consistent with their commensal status. Further study by the same group demonstrated that extraction of cell wall lipids reversed their capacity to reduce the level of pro-inflammatory cytokines (Kesavan et al., 2000). In psoriasis, however, these yeasts fail to posses lipid layer due to abnormalities in enzymes involved in lipid formation in stratum corneum of patients with psoriasis.

5. Conclusion

The role that *Malassezia* plays in psoriasis is, as yet, undetermined. Although it may contribute to the inflammation associated with the disease, via complement activation and neutrophil recruitment, convincing evidence that it is of prime importance in the pathogenesis of the disease is still lacking.

6. References

Alford RH., Vire CG, Cartwright BB, King LE. Ketoconazole's inhibition of fungal antigen-induced thymidine uptake by lymphocytes from patients with psoriasis. Am J Med Sci 1986;291:75-80.

Amaya M, T ajima M, Okubo Y, et al. Molecular analysis of *Malassezia* microflora in the lesional skin of psoriasis patients. J ournal of Dermatology 2007;34:619-24.

Ashbee HR. Recent developments in the immunology and biology of Malassezia species. FEMS Immunol Med Microbiol. 2006 Jun;47(1):14-23.

Ashbee HR. Update on the genus Malassezia. Med Mycol 2007; 45: 287-303.

Baker BS, Bokth S, Powles A, Garioch JJ, Lewis H, A, Valdimarsson H, *et al.* Group A streptococcal antigen-specific T lymphocytes in guttate psoriasis lesions. Br J Dermatol 1993;128:493-9.

Baker BS, Powles A, Garioch JJ, Hardman C, Fry L. Differential T-cell reactivity to the round and oval forms of Pityrosporum in the skin of patients with psoriasis. Br J Dermatol 1997;136:319-25.

Baroni A, Perfetto B, Paoletti I, Ruocco E, Canozo N, Orlando M, Buommino E. Malassezia furfur invasiveness in a keratinocyte cell line (HaCat): effects on cytoskeleton and on adhesion molecule and cytokine expression. Arch Dermatol Res. 2001 Aug;293(8):414-9.

Baroni A, Paoletti I, Ruocco E, Agozzino M, Tufano MA, Donnarumma G. Possible role of Malassezia furfur in psoriasis: modulation of TGF-beta1, integrin, and HSP70 expression in human keratinocytes and in the skin of psoriasis-affected patients. J Cutan Pathol. 2004 Jan;31(1):35-42.

Baroni A, Orlando M, Donnarumma G, Farro P, Iovene MR, Tufano MA, Buommino E. Toll-like receptor 2 (TLR2) mediates intracellular signalling in human keratinocytes in response to Malassezia furfur. Arch Dermatol Res. 2006 Jan;297(7):280-8.

Batra R, Boekhout T, Guého E, Cabañes FJ, Dawson TL Jr, Gupta AK. *Malassezia* Baillon, emerging clinical yeasts. FEMS Yeast Res. 2005 Dec;5(12):1101-13.

Blanco JL, Garcia ME. Immune response to fungal infections. Vet Immunol Immunopathol 2008; 125(1-2): 47-70.

Boekhout T, Gueho E. Basidiomycetous yeast. In: Pathogenic Fungi in Humans and Animals (Howard, DH,., ED.), 2nd edn, pp 537-542, Marcel Dekker, Inc., New York, USA.

Bunse T, Mahrle G. Soluble Pityrosporum-derived chemoattractant for polymorphonuclear leukocytes of psoriatic patients. Acta Derm Venereol. 1996 Jan;76(1):10-2.

Cabañes FJ, Theelen B, Castellá G, Boekhout T. Two new lipid-dependent *Malassezia* species from domestic animals. FEMS Yeast Res 2007; 7: 1064-1076.

Cabañes FJ, Vega S, Castellá G. *Malassezia* cuniculi sp. nov., a novel yeast species isolated from rabbit skin. Med Mycol. 2011 Jan;49(1):40-8.

Cafarchia C, Gasser RB, Figueredo LA, Latrofa MS, Otranto D. Advances in the identification of *Malassezia*. Mol Cell Probes. 2011 Feb;25(1):1-7.

Cannon PF. International Commission on the Taxonomy of Fungi (ICTF): name changes in fungi of microbiological, industrial and medical importance. Part 1. Microbiol Sci. 1986 Jun;3(6):168-71.

Crespo Erchiga V, Ojeda Martos A, Vera Casano A, Crespo Erchiga A, Sanches Fajardo F, Gueho E. Mycology of pityriasis versicolor. J Mycol Med 1999; 9: 143-8.

Elewski B. Does *Pityrosporum ovale* have a role in psoriasis? Arch Dermatol 1990;126:1111-2.

Flytström I, Bergbrant IM, Bråred J, Brandberg LL. Microorganisms in intertriginous psoriasis: no evidence of Candida. Acta Derm Venereol. 2003;83(2):121-3.

Fry L, Baker BS. Triggering psoriasis: the role of infections and medications. Clin Dermatol. 2007 Nov-Dec;25(6):606-15.

Gudjonsson JE, Thorarinsson AM, Sigurgeirsson B, Kristinsson KG, Valdimarsson H. Streptococcal throat infections and exacerbation of chronic plaque psoriasis: a prospective study. Br J Dermatol. 2003;149:530–4.

Gudmundsdottir AS, Sigmundsdottir H, Sigurgeirsson B, Good MF, Valdimarsson H, Jonsdottir I. Is an epitope on keratin 17 a major target for autoreactive T lymphocytes in psoriasis? Clin Exp Immunol. 1999 Sep;117(3):580-6.

Gueho E. Midgley G. Guillot J. The Genus *Malassezia* with description of four new species. Antonie van Leeuwenhoek 1996;69:337-55.

Guillot J, Bond R. *Malassezia pachydermatis*: a review. Med Mycol 1999; 37:295-306.

Guillot J, Gueho E, Lesourd M, Midgley G, Chevrier G, Dupont B. Identification of *Malassezia* species. A practical approach. J Mycol Med 1996;6:103-10.

Gupta AK, Kohli Y, Li A, Faergemann J, Summerbell RC. In vitro susceptibility of the seven *Malassezia* species to ketoconazole, voriconazole, itraconazole and terbinafine. Br J Dermatol 2000;142:758-65.

Gupta AK, Kohli Y, Faergemann J, Summerbell RC. Epidemiology of *Malassezia* yeasts associated with pityriasis versicolor in Ontario, Canada. Med Mycol 2001; 39: 199-206.

Gupta AK, Batra R, Bluhm R, Boekhout T, Dawson TL. Skin diseases associated with *Malassezia* species. J Am Acad Dermatol 2004; 51: 789-98.

Hernandez Hernandez F, Mendez T ovar Lj, Bazan Mora E , et al. Species of *Malassezia* associated with various dermatose and healthy skin in the Mexican population. Rev I beroam Micol 2003;20:141-4.

Hirai A, Kano R, Makimura K, *et al. Malassezia nana* sp. nov., a novel lipid-dependent yeast species isolated from animals. Int J Syst Evol Microbiol 2004; 54: 623-627.

Juntachai W, Oura T, Murayama SY, Kajiwara S. The lipolytic enzymes activities of *Malassezia* species. Med Mycol. 2009;47(5):477-84.

Jones DA, Yawalkar N, Suh KY, Sadat S, Rich B, Kupper TS. Identification of autoantigens in psoriatic plaques using expression cloning. J Invest Dermatol. 2004 Jul;123(1):93-100.

Kallioinen M, Koivukangas V, Järvinen M, Oikarinen A. Expression of cytokeratins in regenerating human epidermis. Br J Dermatol. 1995 Dec;133(6):830-5.

Kanda N, Tani K, Enomoto U, Nakai K, Watanabe S. The skin fungus-induced Th1- and Th2-related cytokine, chemokine and prostaglandin E2 production in peripheral blood mononuclear cells from patients with atopic dermatitis and psoriasis vulgaris. Clin Exp Allergy. 2002 Aug;32(8):1243-50.

Kesavan S, Walters CE, Holland KT, Ingham E. The effects of Malassezia on pro-inflammatory cytokine production by human peripheral blood mononuclear cells in vitro. Med Mycol. 1998 Apr;36(2):97-106.

Kesavan S, Holland KT, Ingham E. The effects of lipid extraction on the immunomodulatory activity of Malassezia species in vitro. Med Mycol. 2000 Jun;38(3):239-47.

Lee MR. Cooper AJ. Immunopathogenesis of psoriasis. Australas J Dermatol, 2006;47:151-9.

Leibovici V, Alkalay R, Hershko K, Ingber A, Westerman M, Leviatan-Strauss N, Hochberg M. Prevalence of Candida on the tongue and intertriginous areas of psoriatic and atopic dermatitis patients. Mycoses. 2008 Jan;51(1):63-6.

Liang YS, Wen HQ, Xiao R. Serum levels of antibodies for IgG, IgA, and IgM against the fungi antigen in psoriasis vulgaris. Hunan Yi Ke Da Xue Xue Bao. 2003 Dec;28(6):638-40.

Lintu P, S avolainen J , K alimo K. I gE antibodies to protein and mannan antigens of Pityrosporum ovale in atopic dermatitis. Clin Exp Allergy 1997;27:87-95.

Lober CW, Belew PW, Rosenberg EW, Bale G. Patch test with killed sonicated microflora in patients with psoriasis. Arch Dermatol 1982;118:322-5.

Macias ES, Pereira FA, Rietkerk W, Safai B. Superantigens in dermatology. J Am Acad Dermatol. 2011 Mar;64(3):455-72;

Mathov I , Plotkin L, Abatangelo C, Galimberti R , S quiquera L. Antibodies from patients with psoriasis recognize N -acetylglucosamine terminals in glycoproteins from *Pityrosporum ovale*. Clin Exp I mmunol 1996;105:79-83.

McFadden JP, Baker BS, Powles AV, & Fry L. 2009. Psoriasis and streptococci: the natural selection of psoriasis revisited. Br J Dermatol. 2009 May 160(5):929-37.

Midgley G. The lipophilic yeasts: state of the art and prospects. Med Mycol. 2000;38 Suppl 1:9-16.

Mohla G, Brodell RT . K oebner phenomenon in psoriasis. A common response to skin trauma. Postgrad Med 1999;106:39-40.

Nazzaro Porro M, Passi S, Picardo M, Mercantini R, Breathnach AS. Lipoxygenase activity of *Pityrosporum* in vitro and in vivo. J Invest Dermatol 1986; 87: 108-112.

Nissen D, Pedersen LJ, Skov PS, Vejlsgaard GL, Poulsen LK, Jarløv JO, Karlsmark T, Nolte H. IgE-binding components of staphylococcal enterotoxins in patients with atopic dermatitis. Ann Allergy Asthma Immunol. 1997 Nov;79(5):403-8.

Prohic A. I dentification of Malassezia species isolated from scalp skin of patients with psoriasis and healthy subjects. Acta Dermatovenereol Croat 2003;11:11-8.

Prohic A, Ozegovic L. Malassezia species isolated from lesional and non-lesional skin in patients with pityriasis versicolor. Mycoses. 2007 Jan;50(1):58-63.

Rebora A. Candida and psoriasis. Acta Derm Venereol. 2004;84(2):175.

Rivolta S. Parasiti vegetali. In: Di Giulio Speirani F, editor. 1st ed . Torino: 1873. p. 469-71.

Rosenberg EW, Belew PW, Bale G. Effect of topical applications of heavy suspensions of killed *Malassezia* ovalis on rabbit skin. Mycopathologia 1980;72:147-54.

Rosenberg EW, Belew PW. Improvement of psoriasis of the scalp with ketoconazole. Arch Dermatol 1982;118:370-1.

Saadatzadeh MR., Ashbee HR, Holland KT, Ingham E. Production of the mycelial phase of Malassezia in vitro. Med Mycol 2001; 38; 487-493.

Sandström Falk MH, T engvall Linder M, J ohansson C, *et al.* The prevalence of *Malassezia* yeasts in patients with atopic dermatitis, seborrhoeic dermatitis and healthy controls. Acta Derm Venereol 2005;85:17-23.

Simmons RB, Gueho E. A new species of *Malassezia.* Mycol Res. 1990; 94: 1146-1149.

Squiquera L, Galimberti R, Morelli L, Plotkin L, Milicich R, Kowalckzuk A, Leoni J. Antibodies to proteins from *Pityrosporum ovale* in the sera from patients with psoriasis. Clin Exp Dermatol. 1994 Jul;19(4):289-93.

Sugita T, Takashima M, Shinoda T, *et al.* New yeast species, *Malassezia dermatis,* isolated from a patient with atopic dermatitis. J Clin Microbiol 2002; 40: 1363-1367.

Sugita T, Takashima M, Kodama M, Ryoji T, Nishikawa A. Description of a new species *Malassezia japonica* and its detection in patients with atopic dermatitis and healthy subjects. J Clin Microbiol 2003; 41: 4695-4699.

Sugita T, Tajima M, Takashima M, *et al.* A new yeast, *Malassezia yamatoensis,* isolated from a patient with seborrheic dermatitis, and its distribution in patients and healthy subjects. Microbiol Imunol 2004; 48: 579-483.

Tokura Y, Mori T, Hino R. Psoriasis and other Th17-mediated skin diseases. J UOEH. 2010 Dec 1;32(4):317-28.

Trabelsi S, Oueslati J, Fekih N, Kammoun MR, Khaled S. Identification of *Malassezia* species from Tunisian patients with pityriasis versicolor. Tunis Med. 2010 Feb;88(2):85-7.

Tragiannidis A, Bisping G, Koehler G, Groll AH. Minireview: *Malassezia* infections in immunocompromised patients. Mycoses 2010; 53(3): 187-195.

Valdimarsson H, Baker BS, Jonsdottir I, Powlws A, Fry L. Psoriasis: a T-cell mediated autoimmune disease produced by streptococcal superantigens? Immunol Today 1995;16:145-9.

Waldman A, Gilhar A, Duek L, Berdicevsky I. Incidence of *Candida in psoriasis*-a study on the fungal flora of psoriatic patients. Mycoses. 2001 May;44(3-4):77-81.

Van Muijen GN, Warnaar SO, Ponec M. Differentiation-related changes of cytokeratin expression in cultured keratinocytes and in fetal, newborn, and adult epidermis. Exp Cell Res. 1987 Aug;171(2):331-45.

Zomorodian K , Mirhendi H, Tarazooie B, *et al.* Distribution of *Malassezia* species in patients with psoriasis and healthy individuals in I ran. J Cutan Pathol 2008;35:1027-31.

5

SAPHO Syndrome

Gunter Assmann
University Medical School of Saarland
Germany

1. Introduction

In 1987, Chamot et al attempted to unify the various descriptions of osteoarticular disease associated with skin manifestations into a syndrome with the acronym SAPHO: synovitis, acne, pustulosis, hyperostosis, and osteitis (Chamot et al., 1987). Furthermore, the clinical feature of aseptic chronic recurrent multiple osteomyelitis (CRMO) accompanied by pustulosis with its typical presentation in the pediatric population justifies the inclusion of CRMO into the same nosologic group as the SAPHO syndrome according to several authors (Juri et al., 1988, Kahn et al., 1994). The differentiating clinical features of pediatric CRMO and adult hyperostosis with osteitis in patients with SAPHO syndrome seem to be mainly in localization of inflammation: in pediatric CRMO more often the extremities, in adults the axial skeleton preferentially with costosternoclavicular region (Rohekar et al., 2006). The wide spectrum of SAPHO syndrome describes overlapping clinical radiologic and pathologic characteristics that SAPHO shares with well-defined rheumatologic and dermatologic disorders, such as psoriatic arthritis (PsA) and ankylosing spondylitis (AS). Against this background the SAPHO syndrome has been often controversially discussed and more than 50 competing terms have been proposed for these or for very similiar entities, among others pustulotic arthro-osteitis and acquired hyperostosis syndrome (AHS) (Kirchhoff et al., 2003). With the increase in reports dealing with growing numbers of patients with SAPHO syndrome, this disease entity should be suspected in patients who fulfil one of the following diagnostic criteria (Assmann et al., 2011): (1) Osteoarticular manifestations with dermatosis like acne conglobata, acne fulminans, or palmoplantar pustulosis (PPP); (2) axial or appendicular osteitis and hyperostosis with or without dermatosis; (3) CRMO involving the axial or appendicular skeleton with or without dermatosis. However, in this broad spectrum of osteoarticular and chronic dermatological manifestations, osteitis seems to be the leading characteristic finding to determine the entity of SAPHO syndrome.

2. Epidemiologic data

The question of the frequency of the SAPHO syndrome is first of all an issue of history: In the 1960s, there were several reports of patients with musculoskeletal disorders and associated dermatologic lesions that were related to neutrophilic dermatitis (acne, PPP, pyoderma gangrenosum) (Windom et al., 1961). In 1972, a very rare pathological entity of unknown aetiology, CRMO, was first described – with or without PPP (Giedion et al., 1972; Bjorksten et al., 1978). Subsequently, several similar cases of pustulotic arthro-osteitis have been reported and have been called by a variety of different terms such as Koehler`s disease, pyogenic sterile arthritis, or PAPA syndrome. However, only with the introduction of the acronym SAPHO as a unifying concept adequate data about the prevalence of this syndrome have been available: in the beginning of 1990, only 225 cases of SAPHO were described in Germany, Austria and Switzerland, and about 400 cases in France. Astonishingly enough, in 2009 there were estimates that the prevalence of SAPHO syndrome was probably no greater then 1 in 10,000 based on several reports about the disease from Japan and north-western Europe (Kahn et al., 1994a, 2009b). SAPHO can occur at any age, but demographic data show that it is a disease of children, young adults or middle-aged individuals, with a female predilection (Mueller-Richter et al., 2009). The disease has been reported mainly from Japan and Northern Europe, rarely from Anglo-Saxon countries. It rarely occurs beyond the sixth decade of life (Van Doornum et al., 2000). However, it is difficult to determine whether this observation of geographic characteristics is related to immunogenic or ethnic differences or just to the failure to clinically recognize this syndrome in other areas than Japan or Europe.

3. Etiology

The aetiology of SAPHO syndrome is still not known but various theories have been postulated including genetic considerations, a possible link with an infectious agent and/or immune dysfunction.

3.1 Genetics

Several genetic abnormalities have been identified in patients with SAPHO syndrome. The association with the positivity for HLA B27 is only evident in cases with SAPHO syndrome and AS for the overall observation any association is not firmly established (Colina et al., 2009; Earwaker et al., 2003, Kahn et al., 1994). A murine model developed for displaying the characteristic chronic multifocal aseptic osteomyelitis seen in SAPHO syndrome showed a mutation mapped to chromosome 18 affecting the proline-serine-threonine phosphatase interacting protein 2 (PSTPIP2). These results were confirmed by the localisation of the susceptibility gene from CRMO patients to chromosome 18q21.3-18q22 (Ferguson et al., 2006; Golla et al., 2002). Similarly, pyogenic sterile arthritis, pyoderma gangrenosum, and acne syndrome (PAPA syndrome) has characteristics that may lend insight to the pathogenesis of SAPHO syndrome. PAPA has been found to be transmitted in an autosomal dominant fashion, and the predisposing genetic variation is located on chromosome 15 affecting CD2-binding protein/PSTPIP1 (Yeon et al., 2000; Wise et al., 2002). The Majeed syndrome, an inherited disease first described in 1989, is characterized by neutrophilic dermatosis, multiple osteitic lesions, and abnormalities of erythropoesis (Majeed et al., 1989). It is caused by a mutation on gene LPIN2, which encodes lipin 2. Lipin 2 may be involved in the apoptosis of polymorphonuclear neutrophiles (PMN) (Ferguson et al., 2005). Another pathway of putative importance is the NOD2/CARD15 system leading to an exaggerated response to intestinal bacteria through an up-regulation of the pro-inflammatory transcription factor NFκB (Hayem et al., 2007). Recent studies have shown that p53 as an important negative regulator of NFκB can in turn be blocked by its own negative regulator, the E3 ubiquitin ligase human murine double minute Mdm2 (Gudkov et al., 2007). In this context, one of these studies reported susceptibility for SAPHO syndrome due to the Mdm2 SNP T309G allele causing higher Mdm2 levels and thus a less efficient p53 response with possibly higher NFκB activity (Assmann et al., 2010).

3.2 Infectious agent

Numerous investigations have brought forth the theory that osteitis and its dermatologic manifestations in patients with SAPHO syndrome are results of persisting pathogen of low virulence, or that the syndrome is triggered by a pathogen and sustained by an autoimmune response subsequent to that infectious challenge (Rohekar et al., 2006; Kahn et al., 1995). The infectious theory has long been proposed with conflicting reports, most of them implicating *Propionibacterium acnes (P acnes),* a slowly growing anaerobic microorganism usually found in acne lesions and considered to be a normal inhabitant of the skin (Kotilainen eta al., 1996). Furthermore, a part of coagulase negative *staphylococcus aureus, haemophilus parainfluenzae,* and *actinomyces* were reported to be associated with SAPHO syndrome (Rozin et al., 2007; Eyrich et al., 2000). However, positive cultures could not be found in all procedures of bone biopsy specimen. A possible explanation might be the ability of *P. acnes* to persist in bone lesions in a form that does not permit culturing. Although the bone lesions are often sterile, several recent studies have reported an association between SAPHO and *P. acnes* in 42% of the cases in total (Assmann et al., 2011). In particular, a recent study by Assmann et al. (2009) showed positive microbiological cultures for *P. acnes* in 67% of the bone biopsies. However, the mechanism that potentially leads to osteitis or arthritis by microbes is still unknown. The *ex vivo* effect of *P. acnes* on blood PMN isolated from patients with SAPHO syndrome was found to be dose dependant but impaired compared with rheumatoid arthritis (RA) or PsA patients. Interestingly, the PMN capacity for interleukin (IL-8) and tumor necrosis factor α (TNFα) production upon *P. acnes* stimulation was drastically lower in SAPHO patients, suggesting hyporeactivity to *P. acnes,* probably related to chronic exposure to this semi-pathogenic bacterium. In which way this potential desensitization to bacterial challenge plays a pathological role in the etiology of osteitis and/or dermatitis (acne, PPP) remains to be proved (Amital et al., 2008; Hurtado-Nedelec et al., 2008).

3.3 Immune dysfunction

According to this observation the SAPHO syndrome seems to be associated with inflammatory cytokine release and global neutrophil activation. In comparison with other rheumatologic disorders the SAPHO syndrome suggests a comparable hyperstimulation of innate immune response, as reflected by increased levels of IL-8 and TNFα by neutrophils in response to *ex vivo* stimulation (Magrey et al., 2009; Hurtado-Nedelec et al., 2008). Furthermore, elevated plasma levels of IL-8 and IL-18, but not IL-10 could be observed.

Together with the above outlined hyporeactivity to *P. acnes* the scenario indicates an altered immune mechanism in patients with SAPHO syndrome. With regard to the characteristic lesion of the SAPHO syndrome, osteitis with hyperostosis and/or CRMO, respectively, bone biopsy showed hypercellular bone marrow with large numbers of plasma cells and neutrophile polymorphs in different samples (Gikas et al., 2009). However, a paucity of inflammation with predominant sclerosis and fibrosis frequently occurs in the chronic phase. Wagner et al. (2002) demonstrate an elevated level of TNFα expression in bone biopsy specimens. Generally, the bone lesions in SAPHO syndrome have to be described as a histologically nonspecific inflammation. Accordingly, osteitic lesions may preferentially occur due to auto-amplified reaction to a low-virulence infection (Edlund et al., 1988). In this context, a comparison of T-cell stimulatory activity in skin lesions showed that *P. acnes* may trigger the non-specific activation of cell-mediated immunity, an immunological response that may be an attempt to eliminate the germ perpetuating the inflammation (Jappe et al., 2004); a comparable investigation with bone specimens has not been conducted so far. In conclusion, the autoimmune inflammatory situation especially the one concerning the bone, bone marrow, and the skin cannot be classified into a predominately B-cell, plasma cell or T-cell mediated disease.

4. Clinical features

The clinical features of SAPHO can approximately be summarized by its descriptive acronym: synovitis, acne, pustulosis, hyperostosis, and osteitis.

4.1 Skin manifestations

The tyical skin lesions seen in patients with SAPHO syndrome include PPP and acne (Kahn et al., 1994). Acne often manifests itself in its severe form with acne conglobata, acne fulminans or hidradenitis suppuratica. In addition, pyoderma gangrenosum, particularly in patients with concomitant Crohn`s disease, Sweet syndrome and other neutrophilic disorders are observed (Yamasaki et al., 2003). The association of SAPHO syndrome with different manifestations of psoriasis is typical, predominately the pustular psoriasis that shows the same histological pattern as the PPP (Hayem et al., 1999). Approximately two-thirds of the patients with osteoarthritic lesions developed skin manifestions which could be defined as SAPHO syndrome. However, in some cases, the osteoarticular manifestations precede the skin features by years, making the clinical picture more suggestive of different rheumatologic disorders than of the SAPHO syndrome. In most cases, the time interval between the onset of skin and osteoarticular manifestations is less than two years, however, intervals of more than 20 years have been recorded as well (Sugimoto et al., 1998; Davies et al., 1999).

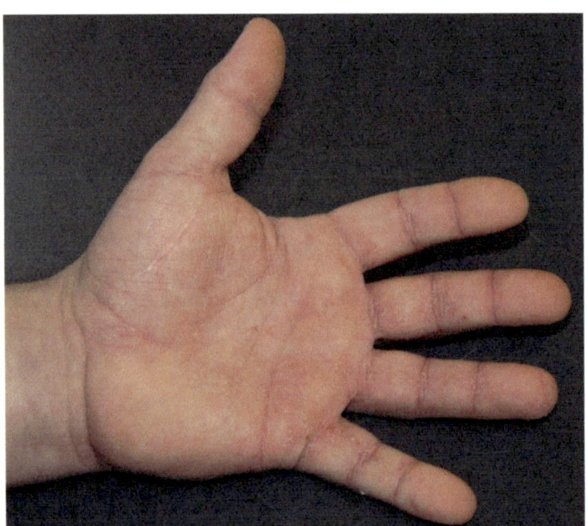

Fig. 1. 53 year old female SAPHO patient: hand with pustulosis palmoplantaris

4.2 Osteoarticular manifestations

The osteoarticular manifestations in patients with SAPHO syndrome implicate synovitis, hyperostosis and osteitis. Synovitis manifests in oligo- or polyarthritis; a monarthritis seems to be a rare clinical rheumatologic symptom. In terms of peripheral arthritis concerning the knees, hips and ankles synovitis is a frequent manifestation. Moreover, the axial arthritis is more common, reported in up to 91% of cases. In the same patients the clinically appearing arthritis of the mandibular joint is seen as well as a unilateral sacroileitis (Earwaker et al., 2003). Colina et al. (2009) presented data of peripheral arthritis in patients preferentially younger than 25 years.

However, the characteristic features of SAPHO syndrome are the aseptic osteitis and hyperostosis. The proof of the *P. acnes* in bone biopsies did not change the character of an inflammation missing typically histological signs of the bacterial septic osteomyelitis. Osteitis refers to inflammation of bone, which may involve the cortex and the medullary cavity. Clinically, the patient complains bone pain and tenderness. The anterior chest wall is a classic location of involvement in adult patients, in particular, the clavicles, sternum, and sterno-costo-clavicular (SCC) joints. The pattern of osteoarticular involvement seems to be age dependent and more frequently occurring in young and middle-aged adults (Hayem et al., 1999). The hyperostosis and osteitis often cause a tumor with hyperthermia of the skin in this region (Kahn et al., 1991). Although the SCC manifestation is typical, it is not exclusive

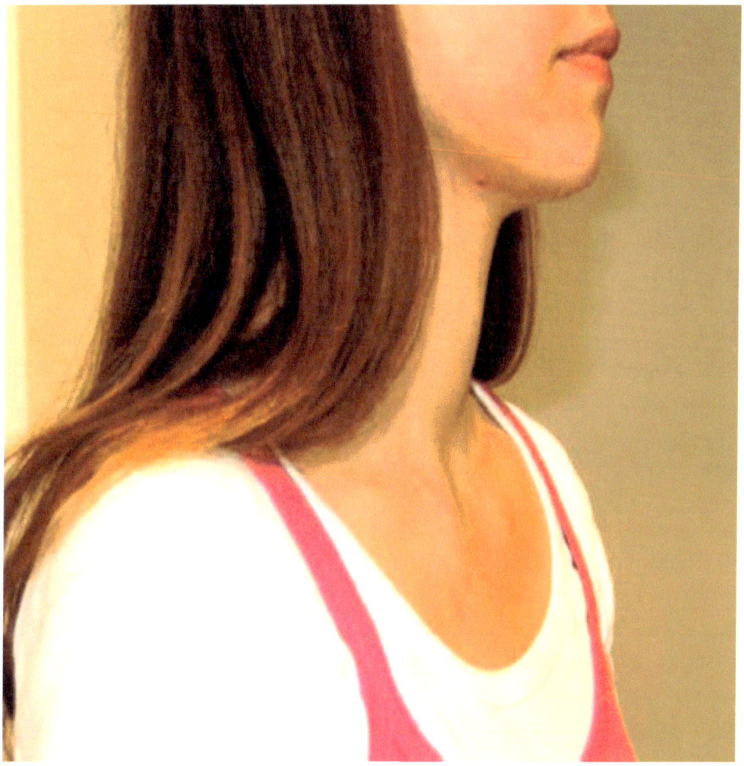

Fig. 2. 23 year old female SAPHO patient: bilateral sternocostoclavicular osteitis and hyperostosis

nor pathognomonic (Kahn, 2002). The singular or multiple involvement of the spine, pelvic girdle, sacroiliac joint, peripheral joint, long bones, and the mandibles is frequent, but not common (Mueller-Richter et al, 2009; Gikas et al., 2009). The clinical presentation of synovitis and osteitis in axial manifestation can not clearly distinguish between the two different entities. The CRMO, as manifestation of the SAPHO syndrome more common in children, appears often in the long bones, followed by clavicle and the spine. In those cases, the patients usually show localized swelling and pain accompanied by commonly generalized inflammation signs like fever and grippal symptoms.

5. Radiological findings

The predominant radiologic features of SAPHO syndrome include osteitis and hyperostosis with cortical thickening, periostitis, and cortical erosions in the concerned area. A variety of imaging tests are basically available for diagnosis and follow up SAPHO patients.

Plain radiographs reveal nonspecific features suggestive of osteomyelitis in the regions of osteitis and hyperostosis. Imaging of osteitis and hyperostosis - typically located in the clavicle bone - reveals a characteristic poorly defined, moth-eaten, destructive lesion typically involving the medial and middle third of the bone, with expansion, sclerosis, and a solid or multi-laminated periosteal reaction. Flat bones, such as the ileum and mandible, also can be involved, displaying predominantly diffuse sclerosis. Peripheral arthritis is seen, but radiographic joint destruction as it occurs in RA is rare. However, early radiographic changes including juxtaarticular osteoporosis may be seen; as well as later changes such as joint space narrowing (Rohekar et al., 2006; Earwaker et al., 2003). With regard to osteitis and hyperostosis, the manifestation in the typical region of the SCC joint is commonly not clearly detectable by conventional radiographic imaging.

Bone scintigraphy by technetium-99m phosphate is highly sensitive to detect the anterior chest wall lesions, and the characteristic "bull`s head" pattern of increased inflammatory activity. Furthermore, this tool of imaging is also suitable to detect occult and asymptomatic osteitis lesions in the skeletal system; the procedure is basically recommended to exclude multiple appearances of osteitis manifestations in the bones. Performing this investigation a highly detectable activity is commonly seen in the early phase of application of the technetium-99 isotope. However, the scintigraphy can not achieve a reliable differentiation between bacterial ostemyleitis, malignat tumor or osteitis/CRMO.

X-ray computed tomography (CT) nicely demonstrates the osteoarticular lesions. The value of CT is that it demonstrates the location of the lesion and pattern of destruction in an area that may be poorly demonstrated radiographically as well as the nature of the periosteal response (Gikas et al., 2009). On CT, the mentioned pathological changes in osteitis lesions and hyperostosis appear as sharply defined hyperdense osteosclerosis of the periarticular bone, in some cases with lytic areas. CT can be clearly recommended as the primary diagnostic tool in cases of complications caused by osteitis and hyperostosis in the anterior chest wall, such as compression of the large vessels in the thoracic aperture; furthermore, the CT is basically employed for the imaging-guided bone biopsy of osteitis lesions if required.

The magnetic resonance imaging (MRI) is in wide use to identify the osteitis in its exact enlargement and inflammatory activity. MRI using fat-suppressed, T2-weighted, or short-t inversion recovery sequences reveals bone marrow edema as well as arthritis changes, and helps differentiate active from chronic less active lesions. MRI demonstrates bone expansion, marrow heterogeneity with bone, and adjacent soft tissue edema resulting in reduced T1-weighted signal intensity and increased T2-weighted modus. Furthermore, the MRI can be employed to identify the bone regions with the most pronounced inflammatory changes in order to carry out further diagnostic such as CT-guided bone biopsy (Kirchhoff et al., 2003). In addition, the MRI is supposed to be the most reliable diagnostic tool in the follow-up of osteitis activity under anti-inflammatory treatment.

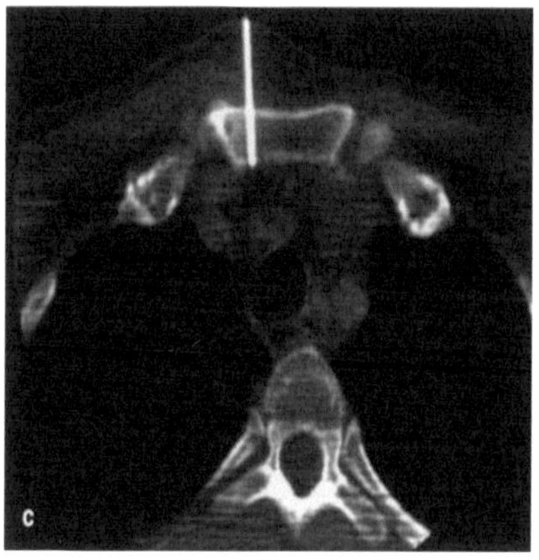

Fig. 3. 58 year old male SAPHO patient with osteitis of the right sterno-clavicular region and CT-guided biopsy of the sclerotic region (Kirchhoff et al, 2003)

6. Laboratory diagnostic

Patients with SAPHO syndrome often show symptoms of humoral inflammatory activity. C reactive protein (CRP) and erythrocyte sedimentation rate (ESR) are usually normal or slightly elevated during exacerbations. Abnormal levels are observed in only one third of the cases (Colina et al., 2009). Apart from reports of positive anti nuclear antibody (ANA) in 30% of patients with CRMO (Janson et al., 2007) and anti-thyroid antibodies in 28% of patients with SAPHO, the data on autoimmunity in SAPHO is rather scant. A recent study investigated the prevalence of the autoantibody patterns classically associated with RA and PsA. Though their prevalence was increased compared to the general population, a specific antibody-profile could not be found (Grosjean et al., 2010). Extended investigations of numerous antibodies found that RA markers (rheumatoid factor (RF) and anti-cyclic citrulline peptides antibodies (anti-CCP2) were absent in SAPHO (Hurtado-Nedelec et al., 2008). A pathway that might play a role in the bone damage observed in SAPHO syndrome is TNFα and RANKL-mediated osteoclast differentiation (Ritchlin et al., 2003). Jansson et al. recently reported elevated TNFα levels in two thirds of patients with CRMO. Furthermore, a different pattern of immunoglobulins with significantly higher levels of immunoglobulin A was observed compared to healthy controls. In conclusion the observed laboratory findings are somewhat contradictory. Nevertheless the co-occurrence of other immune-mediated conditions like psoriasis vulgaris, inflammatory bowel disease (IBD) and pyoderma gangrenosum suggest a self-amplifying inflammatory response, possibly involving autoimmune mechanisms (Assmann et al., 2011). The possible role of infectious agents in SAPHO was already considered in the 1980's when pathogens were isolated from different sites, namely anterior chest wall, spine, synovial fluid, bone tissue and skin pustules. A range of bacteria have been identified, including *Staphylococcus aureus, Haemophilus parainfluenzae, Actinomyces,* and even *Treponema pallidum.* However, it may be supposed that *P. acnes* play the major role, because they have been found more often than other microorganisms (Assmann et al., 2009). However, an extensive bacterial diagnostic procedure for detecting microbes like the *P. acnes* out of blood specimen, skin lesions, or bone-biopsy could not be recommended so far.

7. SAPHO syndrome and psoriasis

Regarding the definition of SAPHO syndrome as an arthro-osteo-cutaneus disease it is clear that SAPHO is an entity that fits into a variety of already established disease categories. There are aspects of SAPHO that are common in AS, in particular, the most frequently involvement of the axial skeleton. Furthermore, the radiologic findings often show sacroileitis which cannot be distinguished from typical AS in 13-52% cases (Earwaker eta al., 2003). In addition, the skin osteoarticular manifestations could often lead to the diagnosis of PsA with axial skeleton manifestation and pustular psoriasis, a special subgroup of psoriatic disease. Furthermore, the PPP is histologically identical to that of the pustular psoriasis. However, the radiographic signs of osteitis with hyperostosis are not often seen in PsA (Rohekar et al., 2006). On the other hand, Kahn et al. (1994) have already demonstrated in a

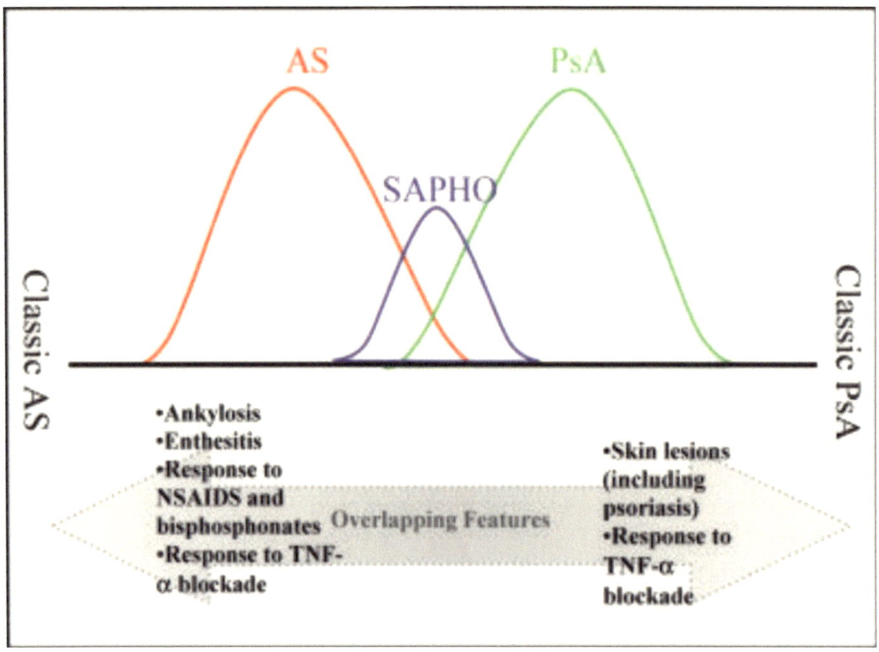

Fig. 4. Model of overlapping features in a spectrum of disease. (AS: ankylosing spondylitis; PsA: psoriatic arthritis; NSAIDs: nonsteroidal anti-inflammatory drugs; TNFα: tumor necrosis factor α) (Rohekar et al., 2006)

multicenter study that the amount of psoriasis among the SAPHO patients is three times as much, compared with the general population. In some cases, psoriasis vulgaris has developed months or years after initial skin lesions with PPP together with osteoarthritic manifestations. With regard to clinical presentations of SAPHO patients figure four demonstrates a model for overlapping features in a spectrum of disease between AS and PsA.

8. Strategy for management

The knowledge of the clinical and the radiographic characteristics of SAPHO syndrome allows a relatively prompt and correct diagnosis; however, the observation of the long-term follow-up of SAPHO patients demonstrates that patients have often been diagnosed first for other rheumatologic disorders such as RA, PsA, or AS - commonly with the additional remark "seronegative" and/or "atypical". The key to a correct diagnosis of SAPHO is the diagnosis of osteitis and, in addition, in most of the cases, the observation of an interrelation or connection with cutaneous and osteoarticular manifestations. The diagnosis can be particularly difficult in patients with an isolated symptomatic bone lesion, when multiple differential diagnoses such as bacterial osteomyelitis, Langerhans cell histiocytosis, benign or malignant bone tumors (e.g. Ewing's sarcoma), Paget's disease, infectious arthritis or AS have to be taken into consideration. Further diagnostic problems may arise due to other incomplete manifestations of SAPHO. In addition to a careful physical examination, a total body skeleton scintigraphy is therefore strongly advised in patients with pain in the anterior chest wall and suspicion of SAPHO. Completing the reasonable diagnostic procedure includes laboratory tests with ESR and CRP, RA markers (rheumatoid factor (RF) and anti-CCP2 antibodies); with regard to diagnostic imaging X-radiograph of the bone region concerned (clavicle, vertebral column, iliosacral joints, skeleton regions with peripheral arthritis) should be performed. In case of osteitis suspicious lesions further imaging with MRI in specific technical setting modalities is recommended. (see above).

9. Treatment options

Although the classification of SAPHO syndrome exists as a distinct disease entity, the overlap and similarities with other rheumatic diseases form the basis for trials investigating anti-rheumatic drugs that are the accepted standard for the treatment of PsA and other spondyloarthritides. Studies have been published with small numbers of patients treated with NSAIDs (Girschick et al., 1998), steroids (Benhamou et al., 1988; Schultz et al., 1999), and immunosuppressive agents that showed only partial efficacy. In detail, the SAPHO specific lesions like osteitis and/or CRMO often show therapeutic resistance against the established anti-rheumatic drugs including the disease modifying anti rheumatic drugs (DMARDs), whereas an accompanying arthritis and/or spondylarthritis seems to respond positively to the therapy. Investigations of methotrexate and azathioprine yielded no convincing results (Handrik et al., 1998; Kalke et al., 2001). However, several reports presenting promising results, obtained with bisphosphonates (Marshall et al., 2002; Kopterides et al., 2004; Just et al., 2008) or biologicals like TNFα-blockers (Olivieri et al., 2002; Wagner et al., 2002 , Magrey 2009), have recently been published. In this context, it has been found that infliximab could show good therapeutic efficacy. Some cases, however, were reported with an amelioration of skin manifestations together with improvement of osteoarticular symptoms. With regard to a possible link to an infectious etiology of SAPHO syndrome, several studies with small numbers of patients treated with antibiotics reported contradictory results (Schilling et al., 2000; Wagner et al., 1997). However, recently published data based on a prospective interventional study in 27 SAPHO patients show an effect of a four-month treatment with the antibiotic azithromycin (also with doxycycline and clindamycin in one patient each) with respect to MRI findings and to the activity of skin disease and osteitis (Figure 5). Three months after the end of antibiotic treatment, however, these effects had disappeared (Assmann et al., 2009). In rare cases SAPHO syndrome develops serious complications mostly based on vascular compression followed by blood stasis and venous thrombosis. In these cases a surgical intervention is often required. There are no data for the efficacy of radiation therapy available.

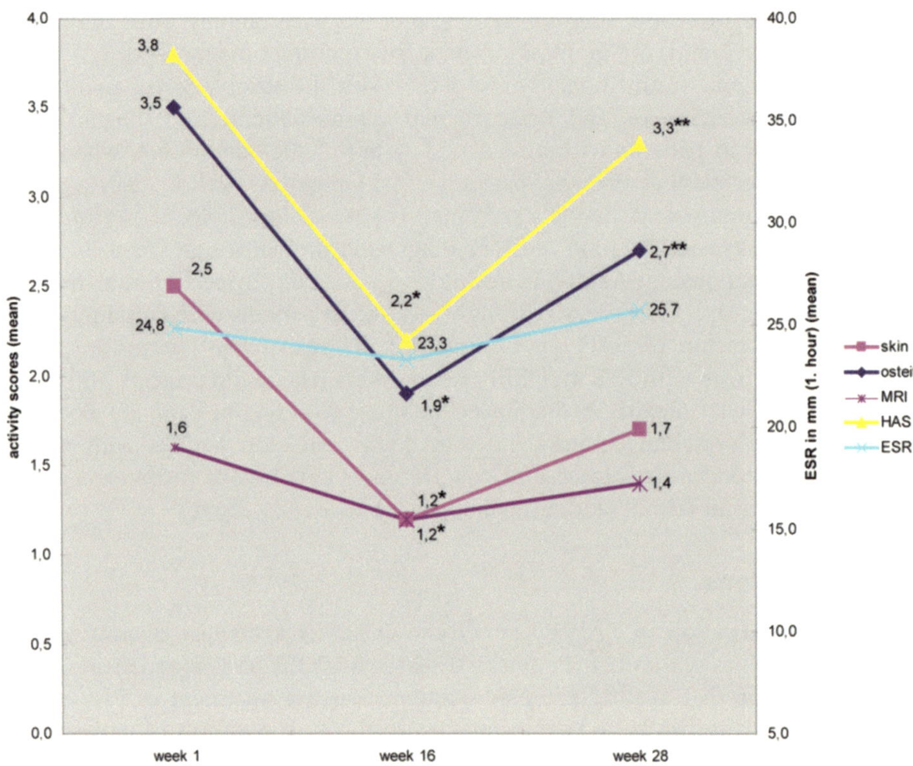

Fig. 5. Activity scores and erythrocyte sedimentation rate (ESR) values (mean) of SAPHO patients treated with antibiotics. * differences of values between week 1 and week 16: $p<0.05$; ** differences of values between week 16 and week 28: $p<0.05$; HAS=health assessment score; MRI=magnet resonance imaging) (Assmann at al, 2009)

10. Conclusions

The SAPHO syndrome represents a constellation of overlapping osteoarticular and cutaneous manifestations. Its clinical presentation is heterogeneous and often incomplete, resulting in diagnostic difficulties. Although controversy still exists regarding its relation to the spondylarthropathies, SAPHO is now recognized as a distinct clinical entity. However, SAPHO continues to represent a nosologic enigma. Further examinations and a better understanding of the underlying pathogenetic mechanisms are essential for the development of appropriate therapies. Especially with regard to osteitis as the characteristic manifestation of the SAPHO syndrome, data concerning the existing treatment options are conflicting. The use of antibiotics has shown contradictory results in several reports although some patients are obviously responsive to this therapy.

11. References

Amital H, Govoni M, Maya R, Meroni PL, Ori B, Shoenfeld Y, Tincani A, Trotta F, Sarzi-Puttini P, Atzeni F. Role of infectious agents in systemic rheumatic diseases. Clin Exp Rheumatol. 2008 Jan-Feb;26(1 Suppl 48):S27-32.

Assmann G, Wagner AD, Monika M et al. Single-nucleotide polymorphisms p53 G72C and Mdm2 T309G in patients with psoriasis, psoriatic arthritis and SAPHO syndrome. Rheumatol Int 2010 Aug;30(10):1273-6

Assmann G, Kueck O, Kirchhoff T et al. Efficacy of antibiotic therapy for SAPHO syndrome is lost after its discontinuation: Interventional study. Arthritis Res Ther. 2009;11:R140

Assmann G, Simon P. The SAPHO syndrome - Are microbes involved. Best Practice and Research Clinical Rheumatology 2011, doi:10.1016/j.berh.2011.01.0017

Benhamou CL, Chamot AM, Kahn MF: Synovitis - acne - pustulosis hyperostosis - osteomyelitis syndrome (SAPHO). A new syndrome among the spondyloarthropathies? Clin Exp Rheumatol 1988, 6:109-112.

Björkstén B, Gustavson KH, Eriksson B, Lindholm A, Nordström S. Chronic recurrent multifocal osteomyelitis and pustulosis palmoplantaris. J Pediatr. 1978 Aug;93(2):227-31.

Chamot AM, Benhamou CL, Kahn MF, Beraneck L, Kaplan G, Prost A. Acne-pustulosis-hyperostosis-osteitis

Colina M, Govoni M, Orzincolo C, Trotta F. Clinical and radiologic evolution of synovitis, acne, pustulosis, hyperostosis, and osteitis syndrome: a single center study of a cohort of 71 subjects. Arthritis Rheum. 2009 Jun 15;61(6):813-21.

Davies AM, Marins AJ, Evans N et al. SAPHO syndrome: 20 year follow up. Skeletal Radiol 1999;28:159–162

Earwaker JW, Cotten A. SAPHO: syndrome or concept? Imaging findings Skeletal Radiol. 2003 Jun;32(6):311-27. Epub 2003 Apr 29

Edlund E, Johnsson U, Lidgren L, Pettersson H, Sturfelt G, Svensson B, Theander J, Willén H. Palmoplantar pustulosis and sternocostoclavicular arthro-osteitis. Ann Rheum Dis. 1988 Oct;47(10):809-15

Eyrich GK, Langenegger T, Bruder E, Sailer HF, Michel BA: Diffuse chronic sclerosing osteomyelitis and the synovitis, acne, pustolosis, hyperostosis, osteitis (SAPHO) syndrome in two sisters. Int J Oral Maxillofac Surg. 2000, 29:49-53.

Ferguson PJ, Bing X, Vasef MA, Ochoa LA, Mahgoub A, Waldschmidt TJ, Tygrett LT, Schlueter AJ, El-Shanti H. A missense mutation in pstpip2 is associated with the murine autoinflammatory disorder chronic multifocal osteomyelitis. Bone. 2006 Jan;38(1):41-7. Epub 2005 Aug 24.

Ferguson PJ, Chen S, Tayeh MK et al. Homozygous mutations in LPIN2 are responsible for the syndrome of CRMO and congenital dyserythropoietic anaemia (Majeed Syndrome). J Med Genet 2005;42:551-7

Giedion A, Holthusen W, Masel LF, Vischer D.Subacute and chronic "symmetrical" osteomyelitisAnn Radiol (Paris). 1972 Mar-Apr;15(3):329-42

Gikas PD, Islam L, Aston W, Tirabosco R, Saifuddin A, Briggs TW, Cannon SR, O'Donnell P, Jacobs B, Flanagan AM. Nonbacterial osteitis: a clinical, histopathological, and imaging study with a proposal for protocol-based management of patients with this diagnosis. J Orthop Sci. 2009 Sep;14(5):505-16. Epub 2009 Oct 3.

Girschick HJ, Krauspe R, Tschammler A, Huppertz HI: Chronic recurrent osteomyelitis with clavicular involvement in children: diagnostic value of different imaging techniques and therapy with non-steroidal anti-inflammatory drugs. Eur J Pediatr 1998, 157:28-33.

Golla A, Jansson A, Ramser J, Hellebrand H, Zahn R, Meitinger T, Belohradsky BH, Meindl A. Chronic recurrent multifocal osteomyelitis (CRMO): evidence for a susceptibility gene located on chromosome 18q21.3-18q22 Eur J Hum Genet. 2002 Mar;10(3):217-21

Grosjean C, Hurtado-Nedelec M, Nicaise-Roland P et al. Prevalence of autoantibodies in SAPHO syndrome: a single-center study of 90 patients. J Rheumatol March 2010;37:639-643

Gudkov AV, Komarova EA. Dangerous habits of a security guard: the two faces of p53 as a drug target. Hum Mol Genet 2007;16:67-72

Handrick W, Hörmann D, Voppmann A, Schille R, Reichardt P, Tröbs RB, Möritz RP, Borte M: Chronic recurrent multifocal osteomyelitis - report of eight patients. Pediatr Surg Int 1998, 14:195-198.

Hayem G. Valuabale lesson from SAPHO syndrome. Joint Bone Spine 2007;74:123-6

Hayem G, Bouchaud-Chabot A, Benali K, Roux S, Palazzo E, Silbermann-Hoffman O, Kahn MF, Meyer O. SAPHO syndrome: a long-term follow-up study of 120 cases. Semin Arthritis Rheum. 1999 Dec;29(3):159-71

Hurtado-Nedelec M, Chollet-Martin S, Nicaise-Roland P, Grootenboer-Mignot S, Ruimy R, Meyer O, Hayem G. Characterization of the immune response in the synovitis, acne, pustulosis, hyperostosis, osteitis (SAPHO) syndrome. Rheumatology (Oxford). 2008 Aug;47(8):1160-7. Epub 2008 Jun 17.

Jansson A, Renner ED, Ramser J et al. Classification of nonbacterial osteitis: retrospective study of clinical, immunological and genetic aspects in 89 patients. Rheumatology (Oxford) 2007;46:154-60

Jappe U, Boit R, Farrar MD, Ingham E, Sandoe J, Holland KT. Evidence for diversity within Propionibacterium acnes: a comparison of the T-cell stimulatory activity of isolates from inflammatory acne, endocarditis and the laboratory.J Eur Acad Dermatol Venereol. 2004 Jul;18(4):450-4.

Jurik AG, Helmig O, Ternowitz T, Møller BN. Chronic recurrent multifocal osteomyelitis: a follow-up study. J Pediatr Orthop. 1988 Jan-Feb;8(1):49-58.

Just A, Adams S, Brinkmeier T, Barsegian V, Lorenzen J, Schilling F, Frosch P: Successful treatment of primary chronic osteomyelitis in SAPHO syndrome with bisphosphonates. J Dtsch Dermatol Ges 2008, 6:657-660.

Kahn MF. Why the "SAPHO" syndrome? J Rheumatol. 1995 Nov;22(11):2017-9.

Kahn MF, Hayem F, Hayem G, Grossin M. Is diffuse sclerosing osteomyelitis of the mandible part of the synovitis, acne, pustulosis, hyperostosis, osteitis (SAPHO) syndrome? Analysis of seven cases. Oral Surg Oral Med Oral Pathol. 1994 Nov;78(5):594-8.

Kahn MF, Bouvier M, Palazzo E, Tebib JG, Colson F. Sternoclavicular pustulotic osteitis (SAPHO). 20-year interval between skin and bone lesions. J Rheumatol. 1991 Jul;18(7):1104-8.

Kahn MF, Khan MA. The SAPHO syndrome. Baillieres Clin Rheumatol. 1994 May;8(2):333-62.

Kalke S, Perera SD, Patel ND, Gordon TE, Dasgupta B: The sternoclavicular syndrome: experience from a district general hospital and results of a national postal survey. Rheumatology (Oxford) 2001, 40:170-177.

Khan MA. Udate on spondylarthropathies. Ann Int Med 2002;135:896-907

Kirchhoff T, Merkesdal S, Rosenthal H, Prokop M, Chavan A, Wagner A, Mai U, Hammer M, Zeidler H, Galanski M. Diagnostic management of patients with SAPHO syndrome: use of MR imaging to guide bone biopsy at CT for microbiological and histological work-up. Eur Radiol. 2003 Oct;13(10):2304-8. Epub 2003 Mar 13.

Kopterides P, Pikazis D, Koufos C: Successful treatment of SAPHO syndrome with zoledronic acid. Arthritis Rheum 2004, 50:2970-2973.

Kotilainen P, Merilahti-Palo R, Lehtonen OP, Manner I, Helander I, Möttönen T, Rintala E. Propionibacterium acnes isolated from sternal osteitis in a patient with SAPHO syndrome. J Rheumatol. 1996 Jul;23(7):1302-4.

Majeed HA, Kalaawi M, Mohanty D et al. Congenital dyserytrhopoietic anemia and chronic recurrent multifocal osteomyelitis in three related children and the association with Sweet syndrome in two siblings. J Pediatr 1989;115:730-4

Magrey M, Khan MA. New insights into synovitis, acne, pustulosis, hyperostosis, and osteitis (SAPHO) syndrome. Curr Rheumatol Rep. 2009 Oct;11(5):329-33

Marshall H, Bromilow J, Thomas AL, Arden NK: Pamidronate: a novel treatment for the SAPHO syndrome? Rheumatology (Oxford) 2002, 41:231-233.

Muller-Richter UDA, Roldan JC, Mortl M et al. SAPHO syndrome with ankylosis of the temporomandibular joint. Int J Oral Maxill of Surg 2009:38:1335–1341

Olivieri I, Padula A, Ciancio G, Salvarani C, Niccoli L, Cantini F: Successful treatment of SAPHO syndrome with infliximab: report of two cases. Ann Rheum Dis 2002, 61:375-376.

Ritchlin CT, Haas-Smith SA, Li P et al. Mechanisms of TNF-alpha and RANKL mediated osteoclastogenesis and bone resorption in psoriatic arthritis. J Clin Invest 2003;111:821-31

Rohekar G, Inman RD. Conundrums in nosology: synovitis, acne, pustulosis, hyperostosis, and osteitis syndrome and spondylarthritis. Arthritis Rheum. 2006 Aug 15;55(4):665-9.

Rozin AP, Nahir AM: Is SAPHO syndrome a target for antibiotic therapy? Clin Rheumatol. 2007, 26: 817-820.

Schilling F, Wagner AD: Azithromycin: an anti-inflammatory effect in chronic recurrent multifocal osteomyelitis? A preliminary report. Z Rheumatol 2000, 59:352-353.

Schultz C, Holterhus PM, Seidel A, Jonas S, Barthel M, Kruse K, Bucsky P: Chronic recurrent multifocal osteomyelitis in children. Pediatr Infect Dis J 1999, 18:1008-1013.

Sugimoto H, Tamura K, Fujii T. The SAPHO syndrome: defining the radiological spectrum of disease comprising the syndrome. Eur Radiol 1998;8:800–806

Van Doornum S, Barraclough D, McColl G, Wicks I. SAPHO: rare or just not recognized? Semin Arthritis Rheum 2000;30:70-7

Wagner AD, Andresen J, Huelsemann J, Zeidler H: Long-term antibiotic therapy successful in patients with SAPHO-syndrome [abstract]. Arthritis Rheum 1997, 40:S62.

Wagner AD, Andresen J, Jendro MC, Hülsemann JL, Zeidler H. Sustained response to tumor necrosis factor alpha-blocking agents in two patients with SAPHO syndrome. Arthritis Rheum. 2002 Jul;46(7):1965-8. No abstract available.

Windom RE, Sanford JP, Ziff M. Acne conglobata and arthritis. Arthritis Rheum. 1961 Dec;4:632-5. Results of a national survey. 85 cases. Rev Rhum Mal Osteoartic. 1987 Mar;54(3):187-96.

Wise CA, Gillum JD, Seidman CE, Lindor NM, Veile R, Bashiardes S, Lovett M. Mutations in CD2BP1 disrupt binding to PTP PEST and are responsible for PAPA syndrome, an autoinflammatory disorder. Hum Mol Genet. 2002 Apr 15;11(8):961-9.

Yamasaki O, Iwatsuki K, Kaneko F. A case of SAPHO syndrome with pyoderma gangrenosum and inflammatory bowel disease masquerading as Behçet's disease.Adv Exp Med Biol. 2003;528:339-41

Yeon HB, Lindor NM, Seidman JG, Seidman CE Pyogenic arthritis, pyoderma gangrenosum, and acne syndrome maps to chromosome 15q Am J Hum Genet. 2000 Apr;66(4):1443-8. Epub 2000 Mar 21.

6

Peptidylarginine Deiminases and Protein Deimination in Skin Physiopathology

Shibo Ying[1], Michel Simon[2], Guy Serre[2] and Hidenari Takahara[1]
[1]*Ibaraki University*
[2]*CNRS-University of Toulouse III*
[1]*Japan*
[2]*France*

1. Introduction

Post-translational modifications of proteins are crucial because they may alter the physical and chemical properties, folding, distribution, stability, activity, and consequently the functions of the targets, some of which being involved into diseases. Recently, one of these post-translational modifications, deimination (also called citrullination), became of an increasing concern. It corresponds to the conversion of protein-bound arginine residues to citrulline residues in the presence of calcium ions (Figure 1). This modification dramatically alters the charge of residues from positive to neutral, probably resulting for the targets in loss of conformation, in aggregation ability, or in depolymerization tendency. Peptidylarginine deiminases (PADs, EC 3.5.3.15) have been found as the enzymes that catalyze deimination (Rogers and Taylor, 1977; Sugawara et al., 1982; Takahara et al., 1983). These enzymes belong to the family of hydrolases, those acting on carbon-nitrogen bonds other than peptide bonds, specifically in linear amidines.

Protein deimination has been demonstrated to be implicated in several skin physiological and pathological processes in human. PADs have long been suspected to be responsible for protein citrullination in the epidermis, as well as in some skin appendages, and their biological roles to be important. Thereby, there is an increasing interest about PAD research in dermatology and biomedicine. However, the molecular mechanisms controlling their expression and activity in human skin are still not fully understood.

In this chapter, we review PAD gene family, the regulation of their expression in keratinocytes, their known skin substrates, their physiological roles in the epidermis and skin appendages, and their associations with skin diseases. It is anticipated that these investigations will provide novel therapeutic and prophylactic targets for future approaches to the treatment or prevention of severe psoriasis and other skin diseases.

Peptidylarginine deiminases (PAD) hydrolyze arginine residues within proteins to create the non-native amino acid citrulline (see Figure 1, next page). Calcium ion is essential for the enzyme activation. Enzymatic deimination abolishes positive charges of native protein molecules, inevitably causing significant alterations in their structures and functions.

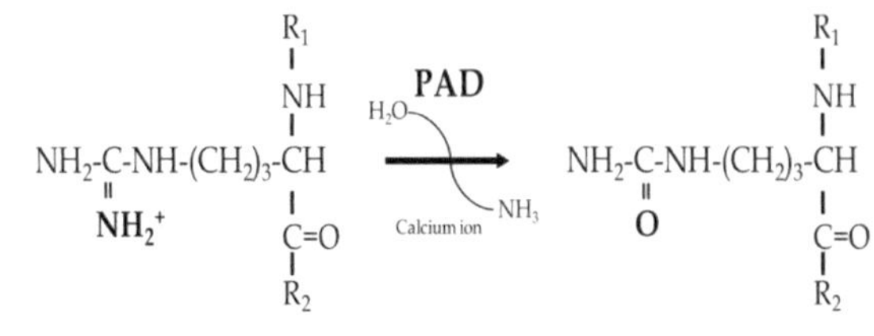

Fig. 1. Schematic representation of the deimination reaction catalyzed by a peptidylarginine deiminase.

2. Peptidylarginine deiminase family

Recently, vertebrate PADs were categorized into five isotypes, named PAD type I (PAD1), type II (PAD2), type III (PAD3), type IV (PAD4), and type VI (PAD6), based on their amino acid sequences, substrate specificities and tissue location (Chavanas et al., 2004; Méchin et al., 2005; Nachat et al., 2005a, 2005b). PAD4 has been previously designated as PAD5 (Vossenaar et al., 2003). Three isotypes are known in birds (*Gallus gallus*), whereas only one seems to exist in amphibians (*Xenopus laevis*) and fish (*Danio rerio, Takifugu rubripes, Tetraodon nigroviris,* and *Oncorhynchus mykiss*) (Vossenaar et al., 2003; Ying et al., 2009; Rebl et al., 2010). In mammals, all five isotypes of PADs have definitely been found in mouse (*Mus musculus*), rat (*Rattus norvegicus*) and human (*Homo sapiens*) (Terakawa, et al., 1991; Vossenaar et al., 2003). The five mammalian PADs are highly conserved at the amino acid sequence level with 59-71% of homology between human paralogs (45-55% identity). In addition, the genes (named *PADI*) encoding each mammalian PAD type are clustered on single chromosomal locus, and they display the same exon/intron structure and a high nucleotide sequence homology in exons.

In human, all *PADI* genes are located at a single cluster which spans an about 334.7 kb region on the short arm of Chromosome 1 near the telomere (1p36.1). Conservation has been demonstrated at the levels of nucleotide sequences and organization of the human and murine *PADI* gene loci (Chavanas et al., 2004; Balandraud et al. 2005). Human PADs are proteins of 74.1-77.7 kDa predicted molecular mass (663-694 amino acids) with a rather acidic pI (4.97-6.15). Human PAD1 is mainly found in the epidermis and hair follicles. This isotype is involved in the late stages of epidermal differentiation. In corneocytes, it deiminates filaggrin and keratin K1, which maintains hydration of the stratum corneum, and hence the epidermal barrier function. This enzyme may also play a role in hair follicle formation (Chavanas et al., 2006). Human PAD2 enzyme is the most widely expressed family member (Ishigami et al., 2002, 2005). In particular, PAD2 is the only one among PAD isotypes to be expressed at a high level in central nervous system. Myelin basic protein, glial fibrillary acidic protein and vimentin are its known substrates. PAD2 is thought to play a role in the onset and progression of neurodegenerative human disorders, including Alzheimer disease and multiple sclerosis, and it has also been implicated in glaucoma pathogenesis (Bhattacharya et al., 2006; Moscarello et al., 2007; Cafaro et al., 2010). Human PAD3 modulates hair follicle structural proteins, such as trichohyalin and S100A3 in the inner root sheath (Rogers et al., 1997; Kanno et al., 2000; Kizawa et al., 2008). Together with the PAD1 enzyme, PAD3 may also play a role in terminal differentiation of the epidermis (Senshu et al., 1996; Méchin et al., 2007). Human PAD4 was first identified from the myeloid leukaemia cell line, HL-60 (Nakashima et al., 1999). It is normally found in the nucleus and in cytoplasmic granules of eosinophils and neutrophils. It has been reported to be involved in granulocyte and macrophage development leading to inflammation and the immune response (Wang et al., 2004). PAD4 is also expressed in rheumatoid arthritis synovial tissues (Vossenaar et al., 2003; Foulquier et al., 2007). Moreover, PAD4 is important for epigenetics, since the deimination of arginines and/or monomethylated arginines on histones 3 and 4 can act to antagonise arginine methylation (Kouzarides, 2007). Human PAD6, also known as ePad in mouse, was first identified in the year of 2004 (Chavanas et al., 2004). PAD6 mRNAs have been detected in ovary, testis, peripheral blood leucocytes, oocytes and early cleavage stage embryos (Chavanas et al., 2004; Esposito, et al., 2007; Yurttas, et al., 2008). However, the detail functions of PAD6/ePad are not well-known yet, even if it is essential for mouse fertility. Indeed, its absence induces an early zygote/embryo developmental defect (Esposito et al., 2007).

3. Expression of peptidylarginine deiminases in human skin

Although all *PADI* genes share significant identities at the level of their coding nucleotide sequences, the mechanisms responsible for their patterns of expression have been suspected to diverge. As described in section 2, each *PADI* gene has its own specific pattern of expression depending on the considered tissue, cell type or differentiation stage of the cells. Among the human PADs, only PAD1, PAD2 and PAD3 are expressed in the skin (Kanno et al., 2000; Ishigami et al., 2002; Guerrin et al., 2003). Here, we will sum up the actual findings on PAD expression in the human epidermis and skin appendages.

3.1 Peptidylarginine deiminases in the epidermis

Using RT-PCR experiments we have shown that only three PAD genes are expressed in human skin and epidermis at the mRNA level, namely the *PADI*1, 2 and 3 genes (Kanno et al., 2000; Ishigami et al., 2002; Guerrin et al., 2003). Messenger RNAs encoding PAD 4 and 6 are not detected in the normal tissue. Using anti-peptide antibodies specific for each isoform, we have confirmed this result at the protein level (Nachat et al., 2005a; Chavanas et al., 2006). Moreover, PAD1 is localized in the cytoplasm of keratinocytes throughout the whole human epidermis, with a higher expression in the granular layer, and in the corneocytes. PAD2 has been detected in the cytoplasm of the spinous keratinocytes and at the periphery of the granular ones, with a more intense staining of the latter. Anti-PAD3 antibodies have produced a punctate staining in the cytosol of the granular keratinocytes. PAD3 has also been observed in the matrix of the lower corneocytes, colocated with filaggrin, but could not be detected beyond the third or fourth corneocyte layer. Immunoelectron microscopy analyses have been used to specify the location at the ultrastructural level: PAD1 and PAD3 are located in the keratohyalin granules, together with profilaggrin, and in the fibrous matrix of the corneocytes together with filaggrin. PAD1 is also associated with the keratin intermediate filaments in the granular cells. Immunoblottings carried out on samples obtained from the superficial horny layer using adhesive tape stripping, confirmed that only PAD1 persists in the upper corneocytes, where keratins K1 and K10 are deiminated. Based on their biochemical properties and location within the fibrous matrix of the lower corneocytes, we have proposed PAD1 and PAD3 as the isoforms responsible for the deimination of filaggrin (Méchin et al., 2005; Nachat et al., 2005a; Chavanas et al., 2006). Therefore, PAD1 and 3 may participate in, and possibly control, the production of the amino acid components of the Natural Moisturizing Factor (NMF). In the upper cornified layer, the NH_2- and COOH-termini of keratins K1 and K10 are deiminated by PAD1 since it is the only PAD isoform detected there. In agreement, PAD1 is less sensitive than the other isoforms to a pH of 5.2, closed to the acidic pH of the upper stratum corneum (Méchin et al., 2007). The effect of keratin deimination is not really known, but it is concomitant with and therefore could be involved in the modifications of the intracorneocyte fibrous matrix observed at the ultrastructural level. In addition, PAD1 and/or PAD3 could be involved in the deimination of filaggrin-2, a recently described protein of the S100-fused type protein family that may participate in the formation of the NMF (Hsu et al, 2011). The epidermal targets and the function of PAD2 in the epidermis have not been identified so far.

3.2 Peptidylarginine deiminases in skin appendages

We have also been able to localize PADs in human skin appendages using the same specific antibodies (Nachat et al., 2005b). PAD1 has been observed, together with PAD2, in the secretory and myoepithelial cells of the sweat glands, and in the arrector pili muscles (Nachat et al., 2005b; Urano, et al.; 1990). However, no deiminated proteins have been detected in these appendages. For the moment, the role of PADs in cells of sweat glands and arrector muscles is completely unknown. So far, no PADs have been detected in human sebaceous glands.

PADs have also been detected in hair follicles in the anagen stage. PAD1 is expressed in the cytoplasm of keratinocytes in the concentric epithelial sheaths forming the hair follicles: first (starting from the hair bulb) the cuticle of the inner root sheath, then the Huxley's layer of the inner root sheath and finally the companion layer between the inner and the outer root sheaths. PAD3 is present within the inner root sheath and the medulla of the hair follicles. PAD3 has been shown to be perfectly colocalized with trichohyalin, which is the first protein shown to be deiminated. Trichohyalin is a major structural protein of cells in the inner root sheath and in the medulla of the hair shaft. Moreover, *in vitro* deimination by PAD3 of this alpha-helix-rich insoluble protein makes it more soluble and renders it available for efficient cross-linking by transglutaminase 3 (Tarca et al., 1997; Kanno et al., 2000). This strongly suggests that *in vivo* deimination by PAD3 allows trichohyalin to be solubilized from cytoplasmic granules where it is aggregated and then to be associated with hair keratins and other cornified cell components through covalent cross-links carried out by transglutaminases. Interestingly, some of these hair keratins, namely the inner root sheath-specific type-I keratin 27 and its mouse ortholog, are also deiminated before being cross-linked (Steinert et al., 2003). Therefore, PAD3 plays a major role in the establishment of the mechanical resistance of cells in the hair follicles and particularly in the hair shaft. PAD3 is also colocalized with S100A3, a calcium-binding protein of the S100 protein family supposed to be involved in hair cell differentiation. *In vitro* deimination by PAD3 of S100A3 at the Arg-51 promotes the assembly of a homotetramer, and increases its affinity for calcium ions (Kizawa et al., 2008).

4. Regulation of peptidylarginine deiminase expression in keratinocytes

As the specific expression and distribution of PADs in human epidermis and skin appendages became clear, it appeared another question "how is the PAD gene expression controlled?" In fact, the *PADI* gene locus represents an interesting model to study the mechanisms which direct the spatial and temporal expression of genes in the epidermis. Indeed *PADI* gene expression is accurately regulated during the keratinocyte differentiation steps. PAD1 is detected throughout the epidermis with an increased expression in differentiated cells, PAD2 in the suprabasal layers, and PAD3 only in the terminally differentiated keratinocytes. Therefore PAD expression clearly depends upon the keratinocyte differentiation state. Until 2010, several original papers, shown in Figure 2 for a chronologic study, were published by our groups on *PADI* gene regulations at the transcriptional level.

These publications support the hypothesis of multiple DNA/transcription factor chromatin modules regulating PAD expression in normal human epidermal keratinocytes (NHEK), at the transcriptional level through a complex and original mechanism. The following sections will review what is known about the transcriptional regulation of *PADI*1-3 expression, remark the multiple regulatory modules, and highlight their significant features.

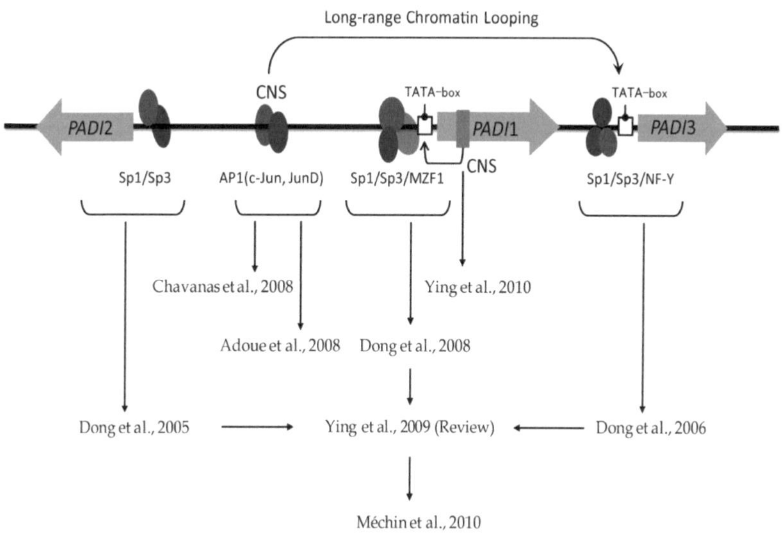

Fig. 2. History of transcriptional regulation of *PADI*1-3

Until 2010, the promoters of *PADI*1, 2 and 3, including the transcriptional factors and their binding sites, have been identified (Dong et al., 2005; Dong et al., 2006; Dong et al., 2008). Moreover, conserved non-coding sequences (CNSs) have been found in the *PADI* gene locus. They have been shown to contribute to long-distance transcriptional regulations of *PADI*1 and *PADI*3 promoters. One is an intronic enhancer located in the first intron of *PADI*1. Driven by NF-κB, it is able to enhance the *PADI*1 promoter activity (Ying et al., 2010). The other one located between *PADI*2 and *PADI*3 regulates *PADI*3 transcription by a long-range chromatin looping (86-kb) during keratinocyte differentiation (Chavanas et al., 2008; Adoue et al., 2008). See detail in the text. Note that the scale is not respected.

4.1 Basal regulation of proximal promoters

Proximal promoter elements are required for basal expression of all *PADI*1, 2 and 3 genes. The characterization of the *PADI*1-3 promoters has revealed several *cis*-elements for a number of distinct transcription factors. In the case of *PADI*1, chromatin immunoprecipitation (ChIP) assays have demonstrated that MZF1 and Sp1/Sp3 bind to its promoter region *in vivo*. Furthermore, either MZF1 or Sp1, but not Sp3, small interfering RNAs have effectively diminished the *PADI*1 expression in NHEK cultured in both low- and high-calcium containing medium (Dong et al., 2008). In addition, it also has been found that the expression of MZF1 and PAD1 increases synchronously during epidermal keratinocyte differentiation *in vivo*. Probably, MZF1 acts as an activator of the basic transcriptional activity, in response to the extracellular Ca^{2+} signaling cascades that lead to *PADI*1 expression during cell early differentiation (Dong et al., 2008). Although it lacks canonical TATA and CAAT boxes, the minimal promoter region of *PADI*2 contains some typical eukaryotic promoter elements, including four canonical GC boxes. Electrophoretic mobility-shift assays and super-shift analyses have demonstrated that both Sp1 and Sp3 actually bind to the GC boxes, and shown their marked involvement in the transcription regulation of *PADI*2. *PADI*3 proximal promoter has two CCAAT boxes, two GC boxes and a typical TATA box (Dong et al., 2005, 2006). Electrophoretic mobility-shift and ChIP assays have revealed that nuclear factor Y (NF-Y) present in keratinocyte nuclear extracts actually bind the two CCAAT boxes, while Sp1/Sp3 bind the two GC boxes both *in vitro* and *in vivo*. Either deletion or site-directed mutagenesis of one of the CCAAT or GC boxes dramatically decreases the promoter activity (Dong et al., 2006). Furthermore, Sp1 or NF-YA (one of the three subunits of NF-Y) small interfering RNAs effectively diminish *PADI*3 gene expression in NHEK cultured in both low- and high-calcium medium. Therefore, both Sp1 and NF-Y are necessary for the expression of *PADI*3.

In the transcriptional regulation of *PADI*1, 2 and 3 in NHEK, Sp1/Sp3 is a common basic transcriptional factor. Sp-family of ubiquitous transcription activators is known to regulate the constitutive expression of a considerable number of genes, and to take part in virtually all aspects of cellular functions, including proliferation, apoptosis and differentiation (Kaczynski et al., 2003). Our results suggest that the ratio of Sp1 and Sp3 factors bound to the promoter of *PADI* genes is responsible for the basal regulation of PAD1-3 in the upper keratinocyte layers of the epidermis (Ying et al., 2009).

4.2 Enhancer activity of conserved non-coding sequences

Eukaryotic gene transcription is controlled not only by promoters but also by intragenic *cis*-elements. More recently, a number of CNSs in vertebrate genomes have been shown to be transcriptional regulatory regions (Adams, 2005; Pennacchio, et al., 2006). Curiously, some highly conserved *cis*-regulatory regions are preferentially linked to developmental regulatory genes such as transcription factors and certain cell communication signals (Strähle & Rastegar, 2008). Regarding to *PADI* genes, nineteen CNSs are clustered in an 8-kb region between *PADI*1 and *PADI*2. Interestingly, this region shows remarkable sequence conservation between several species, further suggesting its functional relevance (Chavanas et al, 2004). Subsequently, this region has been shown to contain a calcium responsive enhancer called CNS2 or PIE (for PAD intergenic enhancer segment), which dramatically triggers the activity of the *PADI*3 gene promoter upon epidermal keratinocyte differentiation, and links *PADI3* expression to the AP-1 transcription factors c-Jun and JunD (Chavanas et al., 2008; Adoue et al., 2008). AP1 and Sp families have been suggested to play a central role in the regulation of epidermal gene expression during keratinocyte differentiation.

Moreover, except *PADI6* gene, each of the human *PADI* genes contains a long first intron (10-23 kb), suggesting the first introns of these *PADI* genes are conserved during the speciation. In past, it has generally been assumed that the introns correspond to junk DNA without any function. More recently, however, this was disputed: more and more evidences revealed that introns are involved in transcriptional regulation and other functions (Eckert and Welter, 1996; Eckert et al., 1997). In particular, *in silico* analysis identified a conserved putative enhancer region within the first intron of *PADI1*. This region contains several consensus binding motifs for transcription factors, such as NF-κB, ELK1 and CREL. Furthermore, ChIP results provided powerful evidence that both p50 and p65 NF-κB subunits directly bind to a *cis*-element (named CNSi) identified within the first intron of the *PADI1* gene, and are critical for the *in vivo* expression of this gene via transcriptional regulatory mechanisms (Ying et al., 2010).

4.3 Regulatory mechanism by an intra-chromatin loop

Of great interest, chromosome conformation capture (3C) technique recently testified that distant enhancers co-localize and thus that chromatin has necessary to form loops to put them in contact within the nucleus (Dekker et al., 2002, 2006). The 3C technique has confirmed that the enhancer CNS2 described above, is physically close to the *PADI3* gene promoter, thanks to a chromatin loop formation. Indeed, as shown in Figure 2, the enhancer is located 86 kb away from the *PADI3* promoter (Chavanas et al., 2008; Adoue et al., 2008). Afterwards, 3C has also provided conclusive evidence for a potential interaction between the intronic CNSi, including the NF-κB *cis*-element, and the *PADI1* gene promoter by way of chromatin looping (Ying et al., 2010). Long-range *cis*-elements are recently known as important regulators of gene transcription, particularly for paralogous genes clustered on a unique chromosomal region (for examples, see Ying et al., 2010). Such a contact between chromatin regions in calcium-stimulated keratinocytes suggests that intra-chromatin loopings govern the specific expression of *PADI1* and 3 genes in a dynamic and united mechanism. Since long-range enhancers have been identified in a variety of other chromosomal regions distant from their cognate promoters and shown to be functional in keratinocytes (Carter et al. 2002; Li et al., 2002; Fraser, 2006; Bartkuhn et al., 2008), such a gene regulation at a distance might be a key feature in keratinocytes. These intrachromosomal chromatin loops constitute an important element in the architecture of the nucleus and in the regulatory control of a number of genes.

4.4 Other modules

Calcium ion has long been suspected as a major regulator of *PADI* genes at the transcriptional level. Similarly to the increased detection of PAD1-3 in the epidermis in the course of differentiation (Ying et al., 2009), the expression of *PADI1*-3 mRNAs is enhanced about two fold in NHEK cultured in 1.2 mM calcium (differentiating conditions) as compared to 0.15 mM (proliferating conditions). Local calcium ion concentrations could also regulate the subcellular localization of PADs, and their activity (Ying et al., 2009). In addition, high NHEK density increases PAD1 (threefold) and 3 (fivefold), but not PAD2, at the mRNA and protein levels, and up-regulates protein deimination (Méchin et al., 2010). By contrast, vitamin D increases PAD1–3 mRNA amounts, with distinct kinetics, but neither the corresponding enzymes nor the deimination rate (Méchin et al., 2010).

5. Peptidylarginine deiminases in skin physiology and diseases

As well-known, the skin provides a mechanical protection and is an important barrier for preventing the invasion of pathogens, the unintentional entrance of exogenous substances, and the uncontrolled loss of water and solutes (Madison, 2003). More and more evidence indicate that protein deimination and PADs are involved in several epidermal physiological and pathological processes. Thus, the identification of the targets of PADs is considered critical for advancing research on skin physiology and diseases.

5.1 Deimination and peptidylarginine deiminases in skin physiology

In human skin, all known substrates of PADs are cytoskeletal and cytoskeleton-associated proteins, crucial components for human skin homeostasis involved in forming rigid structures and keeping moisturizing of the horny layer. It has been found that filaggrin, filaggrin-2, keratin 1 (K1) and keratin 10 (K10) in the epidermis (Senshu et al., 1996; Kamata et al., 2009; Hsu et al, 2011), as well as trichohyalin and S100A3 in the hair follicles are the major deiminated proteins (Rogers et al., 1997; Tarcsa et al., 1996, 1997). The presence of deiminated proteins mainly in the stratum corneum suggests a function for deimination during cornification, the last steps of terminal differentiation of keratinocytes.

Deimination of filaggrin is a critical step in the production of a pool of amino acids necessary for the epidermal barrier functions (Kamata et al., 2009). Filaggrin is one of structural basic proteins found in abundance in the epidermis, and produced by the keratinocytes for organizing the keratin matrix. Filaggrin is synthesized by keratinocytes of the granular layer as a large precursor (400 kDa in human) called profilaggrin, an essential component of type F keratohyalin granules. During the granular keratinocyte to corneocyte transition, profilaggrin is proteolysed into filaggrin units. These histidine- and arginine-rich units associate with the keratin intermediate filaments facilitating their aggregation and the resulting formation of the intracorneocyte fibrous matrix. After its deimination in the stratum corneum, each filaggrin unit is thought to dissociate from the matrix and to be fully proteolysed to generate free amino acids of the NMF, a complex mixture of osmotic agents essential to maintain 10–15% water in the stratum corneum (Rawlings & Matts, 2005; Méchin et al., 2007; Kamata et al., 2009). The NMF is composed of glycerol, urea, lactate, ions and free amino acids (52%), of which two derivatives have been characterized: pyrrolidone carboxylic acid and trans-urocanic acid. The amino acid content of NMF are nearly all produced from the degradation of filaggrin, their relative proportion being closely related to the filaggrin composition (Méchin et al., 2007; Simon et al., 2008; Kamata et al., 2009). However, filaggrin-2 degradation is strongly suspected to participate to the NMF formation (Hsu et al., 2011). Deimination of both filaggrin and filaggrin-2 increases the rate of their degradation by calpain 1 ad bleomycin hydrolases (Kamata et al., 20009; Hsu et al., 2011). Recently, non-sense mutations of the filaggrin gene have been defined as very strong pre-disposing factors for atopic dermatitis (OMIM 603165) and causative factors of ichtyosis vulgaris (OMIM 146700) (Irvine & McLean, 2006; Palmer et al., 2006; Smith et al., 2006; Nomura et al., 2007; Sandilands et al., 2007). We have demonstrated the capacity of purified recombinant PADs to deiminate human filaggrin *in vitro* with different calcium and pH sensitivities according to the isotype of the used enzymes. These differences could regulate filaggrin deimination *in vivo* as calcium- and pH-gradients are known to exist in the stratum corneum (Méchin et al., 2005, 2007). The exact role of keratin deimination is not well known. We can suspect an effect on the structure of the intracorneocyte filamentous matrix, or on their partial proteolysis in the upper part of the stratum corneum.

As mentioned in Section 3.2, trichohyalin is a structural protein of cells in the inner root sheath and in the medulla of the hair shaft. The deimination of trichohyalin catalyzed by PAD3 is crucial for the properties of trichohyalin, as well as for S100A3, another major protein of the hair follicles (Tarcsa et al., 1996, 1997; Steinert et al., 2003; Kizawa et al., 2008). Thereby, PAD3 is likely to play a major role in the establishment of the mechanical resistance of cells in the hair follicles and particularly in the hair shaft. However, the exact function of PAD1 and PAD2 in the hair follicles, including their targeted proteins, remains unknown.

5.2 Deimination and peptidylarginine deiminases in skin diseases

In recent years, more and more evidences suggested that the deimination and PADs are associated with skin diseases, especially with psoriasis. For example, decreased levels of keratin, in particular K1, deimination were observed in the epidermis of patients with bullous congenital ichthyosiform erythroderma (OMIM 113800) and psoriasis (OMIM 177900) (Ishida-Yamamoto, et al., 2000, 2002). Moreover, the PAD inhibitor paclitaxel, a well known molecule for cancer therapy, has been shown to improve severe psoriasis in a prospective phase II pilot study (Ehrlich et al., 2004). Furthermore, since vitamin D is beneficial in the treatment of psoriasis (Durakovic et al., 2004), it is tempting to speculate that the three PADs (PAD1, 2 and 3) expressed in the epidermis are possible therapeutic targets in the disease.

Interestingly, it is also thought that PADs might be involved in skin cancer. Indeed, PAD4 is abnormally expressed in some cutaneous cancers, as skin malignant melanoma (Chang et al., 2006, 2009). Especially, expression of PAD4 has been observed in some malignant tumors including skin carcinomas, with a concominant increased in deiminated keratins, and in extramammary Paget's disease (OMIM#167300) (Urano et al., 1990; Chang et al., 2006, 2009). PAD4 expression is not detected in the corresponding human normal tissues. In agreement with the hypothesis of a possible involvement of PADs in tumorigenesis, inhibition or depletion, in osteosarcoma U2OS cells, of PAD4, the isotype responsible for the deimination of histones and involved in gene-expression regulation, has recently been shown to result in cell cycle arrest and apoptosis (Li, et al., 2008). So, PAD4 is becoming a target for an epigenetic cancer therapy (Slack et al., 2011). As a new finding, differential expression of the *PADI*1 gene has been claimed as a hallmark of squamous cell carcinomas of the oral cavity and oropharynx (Chen et al., 2008).

6. Conclusion

Nowadays, PADs are more and more considered as important in cellular physiology and human diseases. Over-expression of PAD and accumulation of citrullinated proteins could have a negative role. As we know, citrulline produced by PADs is a "non-natural" amino acid. Thereby, citrulline may stimulate the immune system and induce immune responses. More and more reports claim that citrullinated autoantigens are the possible cause of several autoimmune inflammatory diseases, including neurodegenerative disorders (multiple sclerosis and Alzheimer disease) and rheumatoid arthritis. Indeed, the current knowledge attests that multiple sclerosis is strongly linked to overcitrullination of the myelin basic protein (reviewed in Méchin et al., 2007). As another similar example, the patients with Alzheimer's disease have significantly elevated rate of citrullination (vimentin and glial fibrillary acidic protein) in their central nervous system, mainly in the hippocampus, which is the region of the brain mostly affected by the disease (Ishigami et al., 2005). Therefore PADs are now taken as potential drug targets.

Because of the description of their involvement in the late steps of keratinocyte terminal differentiation and the stratum corneum barrier functions, dermatologists are expected to take a great interest in these enzymes. In future, some approaches should provide new insight into *PADI* gene regulatory networks and discover the elaborate mechanisms of their signalling pathways upon cell dynamic state. More work is of great significance to definitively conclude on their contribution to skin diseases, especially in psoriasis and other inflammatory disorders.

7. Acknowledgment

The authors would like to thank all members of the Laboratory of Biochemistry and Molecular Biology of Ibaraki University (especially Prof. Toshio Kojima and Dr. Sijun Dong); and of the UMR5165 of the CNRS and Toulouse University (especially Dr. Marie-Claire Méchin, Rachida Nachat, Stéphane Chavanas, Fanny Coudane and Véronique Adoue) for their contributions to the research discussed in this review. The authors' laboratories were supported in part by the Ministry of Education, Culture, Sports, Science and Technology of Japan, the French Society for Dermatology (SFD) and by Pierre Fabre Dermo-Cosmétique (Toulouse, France).

8. References

Adams, M.D. (2005) Conserved sequences and the evolution of gene regulatory signals. *Current Opinion in Genetics & Development*, Vol.15, No.6 (December 2005), pp.628-633, ISSN 0959-437X

Adoue, V.; Chavanas, S.; Coudane, F.; Méchin, M.; Caubet, C.; Ying, S.; Dong, S; Duplan, H.; Charveron, M.; Takahara, H.; Serre, G.; & Simon, M. (2008). Long-range enhancer differentially regulated by c-Jun and JunD controls peptidylarginine deiminase-3 gene in keratinocytes. *Journal of Molecular Biology*, Vol.384, No.5, (December 2008), pp.1048-1057, ISSN 0022-2836

Balandraud, N.; Gouret, P.; Danchin, E.; Blanc, M.; Zinn, D. & Roudier, J. (2005). A rigorous method for multigenic families' functional annotation: the peptidyl arginine deiminase (PADs) proteins family example. *BMC Genomics*, Vol.4, No.6, (November 2005), pp. 153, ISSN 1471-2164

Bartkuhn, M. & Renkawitz, R. (2008). Long range chromatin interactions involved in gene regulation. *Biochimica et Biophysica Acta - Molecular Cell Research*, Vol.1783, No. 11, (November 2008), pp. 2161-2166, ISSN 0167-4889

Bhattacharya, S.; Crabb, J.; Bonilha, V.; Gu, X.; Takahara, H. & Crabb, J. (2006). Proteomics implicates peptidyl arginine deiminase 2 and optic nerve citrullination in glaucoma pathogenesis. *Investigative Ophthalomolgy and Visual Sciences*, Vol.47, No. 6 (June 2006), pp. 2508-2514, ISSN 0146-0404

Cafaro, T.; Santo, S.; Robles, L.; Crim, N.; Urrets-Zavalia, J. & Serra, H. (2010) Peptidylarginine deiminase type 2 is over expressed in the glaucomatous optic nerve. *Molecular Vision*, Vol.16 (August 2010), pp. 1654-1658, ISSN 1090-0535

Carter, D.; Chakalova, L.; Osborne, C.; Dai, Y. & Fraser, P. (2002). Long-range chromatin regulatory interactions *in vivo*. *Nature Genetics*, Vol.32, No. 6 (December 2002), pp. 623-626, ISSN 1061-4036

Chang, X. & Han, J. (2006) Expression of peptidylarginine deiminase type 4 (PAD4) in various tumors. *Molecular Carcinogenesis*, Vol.45, No.3 (March 2006), pp. 183-196, ISSN 0899-1987

Chang, X.; Han, J.; Pang, L.; Zhao, Y.; Yang, Y. & Shen, Z. (2009) Increased *PADI4* expression in blood and tissues of patients with malignant tumors. *BMC Cancer*, Vol.9 (January 2009), pp. 40-51, ISSN 1471-2407

Chavanas, S.; Adoue, V.; Méchin, M.; Ying, S.; Dong, S.; Duplan, H.; Charveron, M.; Takahara, H.; Serre, G. & Simon, M. (2008). Long-range enhancer associated with chromatin looping allows AP-1 regulation of the peptidylarginine deiminase 3 gene in differentiated keratinocyte. *PLoS One*, Vol.3, No. 10 (October 2008), e3408, ISSN 1932-6203

Chavanas, S.; Méchin, M.; Nachat, R.; Adoue, V.; Coudane, F.; Serre, G. & Simon, M. (2006). Peptidylarginine deiminases and deimination in biology and pathology: Relevance to skin homeostasis. *Journal of Dermatological Science*, Vol.44, No.2, (November 2006), pp. 63-72, ISSN 0923-1811

Chavanas, S.; Méchin, M.; Takahara, H.; Kawada, A.; Nachat, R.; Serre, G. & Simon, M. (2004). Comparative analysis of the mouse and human peptidylarginine deiminase gene clusters reveals highly conserved non-coding segments and a new gene, *PADI6*. *Gene*, Vol.330, No.1 (April 2004), pp. 19-27, ISSN 0378-1119

Chen, C.; Méndez, E.; Houck, J.; Fan, W.; Lohavanichbutr, P.; Doody, D.; Yueh, B.; Futran, N.D.; Upton, M.; Farwell, D.G.; Schwartz, S.M. & Zhao, L.P. (2008) Gene expression profiling identifies genes predictive of oral squamous cell carcinoma. *Cancer Epidemiology Biomarkers & Prevention*, Vol.17, No.8 (August 2008), pp. 2152-2162, ISSN 1055-9965

Dekker, J., Rippe, K., Dekker, M. & Kleckner N (2002) Capturing chromosome conformation. *Science*. Vol.295, No.5558 (Febuary 2002), pp. 1306-1311, ISSN 0036-8075

Dekker, J. (2006), The three 'C' s of chromosome conformation capture: controls, controls, controls. *Nature Methods*, Vol.3, No.1, (January 2006), pp. 17-21, ISSN 1548-7091

Dong, S.; Kanno, T.; Yamaki, A.; Kojima, T.; Shiraiwa, M.; Kawada, A.; Méchin, M.; Chavanas, S.; Serre, G.; Simon, M. & Takahara, H. (2006). NF-Y and Sp1/Sp3 are involved in the transcriptional regulation of the peptidylarginine deiminase type III gene (*PADI3*) in human keratinocytes. *Biochemical Journal*, Vol.397, No.3 (August 2006), pp. 449-459, ISSN 0264-6021

Dong, S.; Kojima, T.; Shiraiwa, M.; Méchin, M.; Chavanas, S.; Serre, G.; Simon, M.; Kawada, A. & Takahara, H. (2005). Regulation of the expression of peptidylarginine deiminase type II gene (*PADI2*) in human keratinocytes involves Sp1 and Sp3 transcription factors. *Journal of Investigative Dermatology*, Vol.124, No.5 (May 2005), pp. 1026-1033, ISSN 0022-202X

Dong, S.; Ying, S.; Kojima, T.; Shiraiwa, M.; Kawada, A.; Méchin, M.; Adoue, V.; Chavanas, S.; Serre, G.; Simon, M. & Takahara, H. (2008) Crucial roles of MZF1 and Sp1 in the transcriptional regulation of the peptidylarginine deiminase type I gene (*PADI1*) in Human Keratinocytes. *Journal of Investigative Dermatology*, Vol.128, No.3 (March 2008), pp. 549-557, ISSN 0022-202X

Durakovic, C.; Ray, S. & Holick, M.F. (2004) Topical paricalcitol (19-nor-1 alpha,25-dihydroxyvitamin D2) is a novel, safe and effective treatment for plaque psoriasis: a pilot study. *British Journal of Dermatology*, Vol.151, No.1 (July 2004), pp. 190-195, ISSN 0007-0963

Eckert, R.L. & Welter, J.F. (1996) Transcription factor regulation of epidermal keratinocyte gene expression. *Molecular Biology Reports*, Vol. 23, No.1 (January 1996), pp. 59-70, ISSN 0301-4851

Eckert, R.L.; Crish, J.F.; Banks, E.B. & Welter, J.F. (1997) The epidermis: genes on - genes off. *Journal of Investigative Dermatology*, Vol.109, No.4 (October 1997), pp. 501-509, ISSN 0022-202X

Ehrlich, A.; Booher, S.; Becerra, Y.; Borris, D.L.; Figg, W.D.; Turner, M.L. & Blauvelt, A.(2004) Micellar paclitaxel improves severe psoriasis in a prospective phase II pilot study. *Journal of the American Academy of Dermatology*, Vol.50, No.4 (April 2004), pp. 533-540, ISSN 0190-9622

Esposito, G.; Vitale, A.M.; Leijten, F.P.; Strik, A.M.; Koonen-Reemst, A.M.; Yurttas, P.; Robben, T.J.; Coonrod, S. & Gossen J.A. (2007) Peptidylarginine deiminase (PAD) 6 is essential for oocyte cytoskeletal sheet formation and female fertility. *Molecular and Cellular Endocrinology*, Vol. 273, No. 1, pp. 25-31, ISSN 0303-7207

Fraser, P. (2006) Transcriptional control thrown for a loop. *Current Opinion in Genetics & Development*, Vol. 16, No. 5 (October 2006), pp. 490-495, ISSN 0959-437X

Foulquier, C.; Sebbag, M.; Clavel, C.; Chapuy-Regaud, S.; Al Badine, R.; Méchin, M.-C.; Vincent, C.; Nachat, R.; Yamada, M.; Takahara, H.; Simon, M.; Guerrin, M. & Serre, G. (2007) Peptidyl arginine deiminase type 2 (PAD-2) and PAD-4 but not PAD-1, PAD-3, and PAD-6 are expressed in rheumatoid arthritis synovium in close association with tissue inflammation. *Arthritis and Rheumatism*, Vol. 56, No.11 (November 2007), pp. 3541-53, ISSN 1529-0131

Guerrin, M.; Ishigami, A.; Méchin, M.; Nachat, R.; Valmary, S.; Sebbag, M.; Simon, M.; Senshu, T. & Serre, G. (2003) cDNA cloning, gene organization and expression analysis of human peptidylarginine deiminase type I. *Biochemical Journal*, Vol.15, No.1 (February 2003), pp. 167-174, ISSN 0264-6021

Hsu, C.Y.; Henry, J.; Raymond, A.A.; Méchin, M.C.; Pendaries, V.; Nassar, D.; Hansmann, B.; Balica, S.; Burlet-Schiltz, O.; Schmitt, A.M.; Takahara, H.; Paul, C.; Serre, G. & Simon, M. (2011) Deimination of human filaggrin-2 promotes its proteolysis by calpain 1. *Journal of Biological Chemistry*, Vol. 286, No.26 (July 2011), pp. 23222-23233, ISSN 0021-9258

Irvine, A.D. & McLean, W.H. (2006) Breaking the (un)sound barrier: filaggrin is a major gene for atopic dermatitis. *Journal of Investigative Dermatology*, Vol.126, No.6 (June 2006), pp.1200-1202, ISSN 0022-202X

Ishigami, A.; Ohsawa, T.; Asaga, H.; Akiyama, K.; Kuramoto, M. & Maruyama, N. (2002) Human peptidylarginine deiminase type II: molecular cloning, gene organization, and expression in human skin. *Archives of Biochemistry and Biophysics*, Vol.407, No.1 (November 2002), pp. 167-174, ISSN 0003-9861

Ishigami, A.; Ohsawa, T.; Hiratsuka, M.; Taguchi, H.; Kobayashi, S.; Saito, Y.; Murayama, S.; Asaga. H.; Toda, T.; Kimura, N. & Maruyama N. (2005) Abnormal accumulation of citrullinated proteins catalyzed by peptidylarginine deiminase in hippocampal extracts from patients with Alzheimer's disease. *Journal of Neuroscience Research*, Vol. 80, No.1 (April 2005), pp.120-128, ISSN 0360-4012

Ishida-Yamamoto, A.; Eady, R.A.; Takahashi, H.; Shimizu, H.; Akiyama, M. & Iizuka, H. (2002) Sequential reorganization of cornified cell keratin filaments involving filaggrin-mediated compaction and keratin 1 deimination. *Journal of Investigative Dermatology*, Vol.118, No.2 (February 2002), pp. 282-287, ISSN 0022-202X

Ishida-Yamamoto, A.; Senshu, T.; Takahashi, H.; Akiyama, K.; Nomura, K. & Iizuka, H. (2000) Decreased deiminated keratin K1 in psoriatic hyperproliferative epidermis. *Journal of Investigative Dermatology*, Vol.114, No.4 (April 2000), pp. 701-705, ISSN 0022-202X

Kaczynski, J.; Cook, T. & Urrutia, R. (2003) Sp1- and Krüppel-like transcription factors. *Genome Biology*, Vol.4, No.2 (November 2003), pp.206, ISSN 1474-760X

Kamata, Y.; Taniguchi, A.; Yamamoto, M.; Nomura, J.; Ishihara, K.; Takahara, H.; Hibino, T. & Takeda, A. (2009) Neutral cysteine protease bleomycin hydrolase is essential for the breakdown of deiminated filaggrin into amino acids. *Journal of Biological Chemistry*, Vol.284, No.19 (May 2009), pp. 12829-12836, ISSN 0021-9258

Kanno, T.; Kawada, A.; Yamanouchi, J.; Yosida-Noro, C.; Yoshiki, A.; Shiraiwa, M.; Kusakabe, M.; Manabe, M.; Tezuka, T.; & Takahara, H. (2000) Human peptidylarginine deiminase type III: molecular cloning and nucleotide sequence of the cDNA, properties of the recombinant enzyme, and immunohistochemical localization in human skin. *Journal of Investigative Dermatology*, Vol.115, No.5 (November 2000), pp. 813-823, ISSN 0022-202X

Kouzarides, T. (2007) Chromatin modifications and their function. *Cell*, Vol.128, No.4 (February 2007), pp. 693-705, ISSN 0092-8674

Kizawa, K.; Takahara, H.; Troxler, H.; Kleinert, P.; Mochida, U. & Heizmann, C. (2008) Specific citrullination causes assembly of a globular S100A3 homotetramer: a putative Ca^{2+} modulator matures human hair cuticle. *Journal of Biological Chemistry*, Vol.283, No.8 (February, 2008), pp. 5004-5013, ISSN 0021-9258

Li, P.; Yao, H.; Zhang, Z.; Li, M.; Luo, Y.; Thompson, P.R.; Gilmour, D.S. & Wang, Y.(2008) Regulation of p53 target gene expression by peptidylarginine deiminase 4. *Molecular and Cellular Biology*, Vol.28, No.15 (August 2008), pp. 4745-4758, ISSN 0270-7306

Li, Q.; Peterson, K.R.; Fang, X. & Stamatoyannopoulos, G. (2002) Locus control regions. *Blood*, Vol.100, No.9 (November 2002), pp. 3077-3086, ISSN 0006-4971

Madison, K.C. (2003) Barrier function of the skin: "la raison d'être" of the epidermis. *Journal of Investigative Dermatology*, Vol.121, No.2 (Augest 2003), pp.231-241, ISSN 0022-202X

Méchin, M.; Coudane, F.; Adoue, V.; Arnaud, J.; Duplan, H.; Charveron, M.; Schmitt, AM.; Takahara, H.; Serre, G. & Simon, M. (2010) Deimination is regulated at multiple levels including auto-deimination of peptidylarginine deiminases. *Cellular and Molecular Life Sciences*, Vol.67, No.9 (May 2010), pp.1491-1503, ISSN 1420-682X

Méchin, M.; Enji, M.; Nachat, R.; Chavanas, S.; Charveron, M.; Ishida-Yamamoto, A.; Serre, G.; Takahara, H. & Simon M. (2005) The peptidylarginine deiminases expressed in human epidermis differ by their substrate specificities and subcellular locations. *Cellular and Molecular Life Sciences*, Vol.62, No.17 (September 2005), pp.1984-1995, ISSN 1420-682X

Méchin, M.; Sebbag, M.; Arnaud, J.; Nachat, R.; Foulquier, C.; Adoue, V.; Coudane, F.; Duplan, H.; Schmitt, A.; Chavanas, S.; Guerrin, M.; Serre, G. & Simon, M. (2007) Update on peptidylarginine deiminases and deimination in skin physiology and severe human diseases. *International Journal of Cosmetic Science*, Vol.29, No.3 (June 2007), pp.147-168, ISSN 0142-5463

Moscarello, M.; Mastronardi, F. & Wood, D. (2007) The role of citrullinated proteins suggests a novel mechanism in the pathogenesis of multiple sclerosis. *Neurochemical Research*, Vol.32, No.2, pp.251-256, ISSN 0364-3190

Nachat, R.; Méchin, M.; Takahara, H.; Chavanas, S.; Charveron, M.; Serre, G. & Simon, M. (2005a) Peptidylarginine deiminase isoforms 1-3 are expressed in the epidermis and involved in the deimination of K1 and filaggrin. *Journal of Investigative Dermatology*, Vol.124, No.2 (February, 2005), pp.384-393, ISSN 0022-202X

Nachat, R.; Méchin, M.; Charveron, M.; Serre, G.; Constans, J. & Simon, M. (2005b) Peptidylarginine deiminase isoforms are differentially expressed in the anagen hair follicles and other human skin appendages. *Journal of Investigative Dermatology*, Vol.125, No.1 (July, 2005), pp.34-41, ISSN 0022-202X

Nakashima, K.; Hagiwara, T.; Ishigami, A.; Nagata, S.; Asaga, H.; Kuramoto, M.; Senshu, T. & Yamada, M. (1999) Molecular characterization of peptidylarginine deiminase in HL-60 cells induced by retinoic acid and 1α, 25-dihydroxyvitamin D(3). *Journal of Biological Chemistry*, Vol.274, No.39 (September 1999), pp.27786-27792, ISSN 0021-9258

Nomura, T.; Sandilands, A.; Akiyama, M.; Liao, H.; Evans, A.T.; Sakai, K.; Ota, M.; Sugiura, H.; Yamamoto, K.; Sato, H.; Palmer, C.N.; Smith, F.J.; McLean, W.H. & Shimizu, H. (2007) Unique mutations in the filaggrin gene in Japanese patients with ichthyosis vulgaris and atopic dermatitis. *Journal of Allergy and Clinical Immunology*, Vol.119, No.2 (February 2007), pp.434-440, ISSN 0091-6749

Palmer, C.N.; Irvine, A.D.; Terron-Kwiatkowski. A.; Zhao, Y.; Liao, H.; Lee, S.P.; Goudie, D.R.; Sandilands, A.; Campbell, L.E.; Smith, F.J.; O'Regan, G,M.; Watson, R.M.; Cecil, J.E.; Bale, S.J.; Compton, J.G.; DiGiovanna, J.J.; Fleckman, P.; Lewis-Jones, S.; Arseculeratne, G.; Sergeant, A.; Munro, C.S.; El Houate, B.; McElreavey, K.; Halkjaer, L.B.; Bisgaard, H.; Mukhopadhyay, S. &McLean, W.H. (2006) Common loss-of-function variants of the epidermal barrier protein filaggrin are a major predisposing factor for atopic dermatitis. *Nature Genetics*, Vol.38, No.4 (April, 2006), pp.441-446, ISSN 1061-4036

Pennacchio, L.A.; Ahituv, N.; Moses, A.M.; Prabhakar, S.; Nobrega, M.A.; Shoukry, M.; Minovitsky, S.; Dubchak, I.; Holt, A.; Lewis, K.D.; Plajzer-Frick, I.; Akiyama, J.; De Val, S.; Afzal, V.; Black, B.L.; Couronne, O.; Eisen, M.B.; Visel, A. & Rubin

E.M.(2006) . In vivo enhancer analysis of human conserved non-coding sequences. *Nature*, Vol.444, No.7118 (November 2006), pp.499-502, ISSN 0028-0836

Rawlings, A.V. & Matts, P.J. (2005) Stratum corneum moisturization at the molecular level: an update in relation to the dry skin cycle. *Journal of Investigative Dermatology*, Vol.124, No.6 (June 2005), pp. 1099-1110, ISSN 0022-202X

Rebl, A.; Köllner, B.; Anders, E.; Wimmers, K. & Goldammer, T. (2010) Peptidylarginine deiminase gene is differentially expressed in freshwater and brackish water rainbow trout. *Molecular Biology Reports*, Vol.37, No.5 (June 2010), pp.2333-2339, ISSN 0301-4851

Rogers, G.; Winter, B.; McLaughlan, C.; Powell, B. & Nesci, T. (1997) Peptidylarginine deiminase of the hair follicle: characterization, localization, and function in keratinizing tissues. *Journal of Investigative Dermatology*, Vol.108, No.5 (May 1997), pp.700–707, ISSN 0022-202X

Rogers, G. & Taylor, L. (1977) The enzymic derivation of citrulline residues from arginine residues in situ during the biosynthesis of hair proteins that are cross-linked by isopeptide bonds. *Advances in Experimental Medicine and Biology*, Vol.86A, (January 1977), pp.283-294, ISSN 0065-2598

Sandilands, A.; Terron-Kwiatkowski, A.; Hull, PR.; O'Regan, G.M.; Clayton, T.H.; Watson, R.M.; Carrick, T.; Evans, A.T.; Liao, H.; Zhao, Y.; Campbell, L.E.; Schmuth, M.; Gruber, R.; Janecke, A.R.; Elias, P.M.; van Steensel M.A.; Nagtzaam, I.; van Geel, M.; Steijlen, P.M.; Munro, C.S.; Bradley, D.G.; Palmer, C.N.; Smith, F.J.; McLean, W.H. & Irvine, A.D. (2007) Comprehensive analysis of the gene encoding filaggrin uncovers prevalent and rare mutations in ichthyosis vulgaris and atopic eczema. *Nature Genetics*, Vol.39, No.5 (May, 2007), pp.650-654, ISSN 1061-4036

Senshu, T.; Kan, S.; Ogawa, H.; Manabe, M. & Asaga, H. (1996) Preferential deimination of keratin K1 and filaggrin during the terminal differentiation of human epidermis. *Biochemical and Biophysical Research Communications*, Vol.225, No.3 (August 1996), pp.712-719, ISSN 0006-291X

Simon, M.; Takahara, H. & Serre, G. (2008). Peptidylarginine deiminases, In: *Skin Moisturization*, Rawlings, A. & Leyden, J. (Ed.), pp.69-82, Informa Healthcare, ISBN 142-007-0940, London, United Kingdom

Slack, J.L.; Causey, C.P. & Thompson, P.R. (2011) Protein arginine deiminase 4: a target for an epigenetic cancer therapy. *Cellular and Molecular Life Sciences*, Vol.68, No.4 (February 2011), pp.709-720, ISSN 1420-682X

Smith, F.J.; Irvine, A.D.; Terron-Kwiatkowski, A.; Sandilands, A.; Campbell, L.E.; Zhao, Y.; Liao, H.; Evans, A.T.; Goudie, D.R.; Lewis-Jones, S.; Arseculeratne, G.; Munro, C.S.; Sergeant, A.; O'Regan, G.; Bale, S.J.; Compton, J.G.; DiGiovanna, J.J.; Presland, R.B.; Fleckman, P. & McLean, W.H. (2006) Loss-of-function mutations in the gene encoding filaggrin cause ichthyosis vulgaris. *Nature Genetics*, Vol.38, No.3 (March, 2006), pp.337-342, ISSN 1061-4036

Steinert, P.M.; Parry, D.A. & Marekov, L.N. (2003) Trichohyalin mechanically strengthens the hair follicle: multiple cross-bridging roles in the inner root shealth. *Journal of Biological Chemistry*, Vol.278, No.42 (Octomber 2003), pp.41409-41419, ISSN 0021-9258

Strähle, U. & Rastegar, S. (2008) Conserved non-coding sequences and transcriptional regulation. *Brain Research Bulletin*, Vol.75, No.2 (March 2008), pp.225-230, ISSN 0361-9230

Sugawara, K., Oikawa, Y. & Ouchi, T. (1982) Identification and properties of peptidylarginine deiminase from rabbit skeletal muscle. *Journal of Biochemistry*, Vol. 91, No.3 (March 1982), pp.1065-1071, ISSN 0021-924X

Takahara, H., Oikawa, Y. & Sugawara, K. (1983) Purification and characterization of peptidylarginine deiminase from rabbit skeletal muscle. *Journal of biochemistry*,Vol. 94, No.6 (December 1983), pp.1945-1953, ISSN 0021-924X

Tarcsa, E.; Marekov, L.; Andreoli, J.; Idler, W.; Candi, E.; Chung, S. & Steinert, P. (1997) The fate of trichohyalin. Sequential post-translational modifications by peptidylarginine deiminase and transglutaminases. *Journal of Biological Chemistry*, Vol.272, No.44 (October 1997), pp. 27893-27901, ISSN 0021-9258

Tarcsa, E.; Marekov, L.; Mei, G.; Melino, G.; Lee, S.; & Steinert, P. (1996) Protein unfolding by peptidylarginine deiminase. Substrate specificity and structural relationships of the natural substrates trichohyalin and filaggrin. *Journal of Biological Chemistry*, Vol.271, No.48 (November 1996), pp.30709-30716, ISSN 0021-9258

Terakawa, H.; Takahara, H. & Sugawara, K. (1991) Three types of mouse peptidylarginine deiminase: characterization and tissue distribution. *Journal of Biochemistry*, Vol.110, No.4 (October 1991), pp. 661-666, ISSN 0021-924X

Urano, Y.; Watanabe, K.; Sakaki, A.; Arase, S.; Watanabe, Y.; Shigemi, F.; Takeda, K.; Akiyama, K. & Senshu, T. (1990). Immunohistochemical demonstration of peptidylarginine deiminase in human sweat glands. *American Journal of Dermatopathology*, Vol.12, No.3 (June 1990), pp. 249-55, ISSN 0193-1091

Vossenaar, E.; Zendman, A.; van Venrooij, W. & Pruijn, G. (2003) PAD, a growing family of citrullinating enzymes: genes, features and involvement in disease. *BioEssays*, Vol.25, No.11 (November, 2003), pp.1106-1118, ISSN 1521-1878

Wang, Y.; Wysocka. J.; Sayegh. J.; Lee, Y.H.; Perlin, J.R.; Leonelli, L.; Sonbuchner, L.S; McDonald, C.H.; Cook, R.G.; Dou, Y.; Roeder, R.G.; Clarke, S.; Stallcup, M.R.; Allis , C.D.; & Coonrod, S.A. (2004) Human PAD4 regulates histone arginine methylation levels via demethylimination. *Science*. Vol. 306, No. 5694 (October 2004), pp. 279-283, ISSN 0036-8075

Ying, S.; Dong, S.; Kawada, A.; Kojima, T.; Chavanas, S.; Méchin, M.; Adoue, V.; Serre, G.; Simon, M. & Takahara, H. (2009) Transcriptional regulation of peptidylarginine deiminase expression in human keratinocytes. *Journal of Dermatological Science*, Vol.53, No.1 (January 2009), pp. 2-9, ISSN 0923-1811

Ying, S.; Kojima, T.; Kawada, A.; Nachat, R.; Serre, G.; Simon, M. & Takahara, H. (2010) An intronic enhancer driven by NF-κB contributes to transcriptional regulation of peptidylarginine deiminase type I gene in human keratinocytes. *Journal of Investigative Dermatology*, Vol.130, No.11 (November 2010), pp.2543-2552, ISSN 0022-202X

Yurttas, P.; Vitale, A.M.; Fitzhenry, R.J.; Cohen-Gould L.; Wu, W.; Gossen, J.A. & Coonrod, S.A. (2008) Role for *PADI*6 and the cytoplasmic lattices in ribosomal storage in oocytes and translational control in the early mouse embryo. *Development*, Vol. 135, No.15 (August 2008), pp. 2627-2636, ISSN 0950-1991

7

Insights into the Pathogenesis and Treatment of Psoriasis

Robyn S. Fallen[1], Aupam Mitra[2] and Hermenio C. Lima[3]

[1]*Michael G. DeGroote School of Medicine - Waterloo Regional Campus - McMaster University*

[2]*UC Davis School of Medicine, Allergy and Clinical Immunology, Hospital Way, Mather, CA*

[3]*Department of Medicine - Division of Dermatology Michael G. DeGroote School of Medicine - McMaster University -*

[1,3]*Canada*

[2]*USA*

1. Introduction

By virtue of the dynamic nature of the scientific process, the description of the pathogenesis of a disease is always a work in progress. Each day new research shapes and refines our understanding of disease processes; an attempt to describe the current scientific understanding provides merely a snapshot of a body of knowledge that is constantly changing. However, characterizing a disease using homeostatic and physiological terms allows the creation of a framework to convey the most up-to-date theories while maintaining the potential for their evolution.

The complex nature of psoriasis can similarly be unveiled through understanding the historical context of our current understanding, examining prevailing hypotheses, and extrapolating horizons for new research. To develop a framework for understanding the pathogenesis of psoriasis and its evolution, the first perception to be changed is the prevalent view of the immune system. The general notion of the immune system as a defense arrangement that protects us against the microorganisms must be changed. This view results from a reduction of the process itself and, as mentioned by Dr. Nelson Vaz, are features derived from the birth of the immunology (Vaz et al., 2006). Immunology, as scientific field, is new in the history of medicine. Immunology developed in a century marked by the First and Second World War and Cold War tension. Hence, many models to exemplify the immunological concepts were simplified and described in relation to war affairs to facilitate the understanding of this science. In this model, if a microorganism attacks a human being, the individual advocates the use of the immune system to counteract. Another simple aspect is the teleology that prevails in the immune science. For example, the T lymphocyte exists to kill cells infected with intracellular parasites. This model full of logic and consequences does not apply in many other areas of medical and non-medical sciences. As such, it is necessary to move to a new approach to describing the relationship between the immune system and environment. In this new paradigm, the immune system does not react, but rather interacts with the environment, and this contact is made through the skin and mucous membranes. This interaction, causal or not, can have different results. In most cases, there is a balance, imperceptible to other sensory systems, which is characterized by the integrity of what we call health. Thus, homeostasis disorders or imbalances lead to disease. This seems obvious when written, but this search for stability has continuity for the duration of the life of a given organism. If we consider the immune system a sensorial system, it interacts with the modifications of the environment, detects this information of change, and responds with adjustments to maintain homeostasis. You might reduce this view by comparing it to an engine that runs under different types of fuel mixture. It detects the different fuel composition and changes the compression ratio of the cylinder for better efficiency to keep the car moving.

For better observation of this psoriasis pathogenesis, we will make a technical simulation of the immune system in a specific situation. This simulation will cover various aspects of immune response, spanning from the beginning of the inflammatory response, to specific immune response through the development of psoriasis. Here, under a historical perspective and comparing with a chess game, the main objective is to provide insights on the central role of some of these cytokines and immunological pathways in psoriasis pathophysiology. Through this, the aim is to explain some facts of modern immunodermatology that might be useful for clinicians to understand the basis of the immunology of psoriasis. Moreover, an important goal is to dispel some misinformation that might have a negative impact on the use of new immunomodulators and medications available for use by physicians. Treatment basis and therapeutic response experience strongly supports the use of immunomodulators as important modalities in the treatment of psoriatic arthritis and plaque psoriasis. Studies with these therapeutic agents, which act in different steps of the psoriatic inflammatory cascade, have also shown significant efficacy. (Scarpa et al., 2010).

Directly targeting this inflammatory cascade, blocking specific cytokines is a modern treatment option for psoriasis and other autoimmune diseases (Lima et al., 2009b). The rationale for this therapy arises from pathophysiology; in different autoimmune diseases there is an increase in production of proinflammatory cytokines by the immune system. Inflammatory cytokines, like many other cytokines, have an important role in both maintaining health and participating in disease manifestation (Feldmann et al., 1998). This chapter discusses the pivotal role of some of these cytokines in psoriasis pathophysiology, how our understanding of its mechanism evolved, and how blocking the effect of a specific cytokine might substantially improve the disease condition.

2. Pre-biologic immunological history of psoriasis

Psoriasis is a common skin disease with extra-cutaneous manifestations. It is characterized by chronic inflammation of the skin with changes in the maturation of keratinocytes, which is manifested by the hyperproliferation of the epidermis. Moreover, inflammatory reaction can be found in other systems of the same patient. However, this disease is mediated by T lymphocytes, orchestrated by orchestration multigenic and environmental factors. The altered immune system is essential for the inflammation present in both the skin and other organs. A concept of a multi-systemic disorder involving different organs of the patient is actual and reflects a better understanding of the complex pathophysiology of this disease (Scarpa et al., 2010).

The concept of biological therapy for psoriasis has been derived from its etiopathogenesis. As in a chess game, these new forms of treatment have evolved from an integration of the knowledge of interactions between the immune system cells (pieces) and its cytokines (movements) that initiates the pathologic processes and ultimately leads to the development of the clinical features of psoriasis.

In ancient records, the initial causes of psoriasis were attributed to multiple sources ranging from the divine power to racial associations (Squire, 1873). An unknown infectious organism was indicated as a source of psoriasis in 1927 (Heaney, 1927). Later, its etiology was described as primarily and essentially an epidermal problem, independent of immunologic phenomena (Ingram, 1953). The main objective of cytotoxic drugs developed in the 20th century, such as methotrexate, was to reduce keratinocyte proliferation. Immunological studies on psoriatic patients identified changes in humoral immune reactions as part of the overall problem but not the cause (Aswaq et al., 1960; Harber et al., 1962). Efficacy of the cytotoxic drugs in the late 1960s paved the road for ideas about the role of the immune system in psoriasis (Harris, 1971; Landau et al., 1965). Further investigations in the 1970s revealed the role of immunologic factors in psoriasis. However, the dominant thought was that psoriasis was a disease of faulty epidermopoiesis due to impaired autocontrol mechanisms (Shuster, 1971). Hunter *et al.* wrote "More work on cell turnover and its regulation will give the clue to psoriasis" (Hunter et al., 1974).

Other studies in the 1970s revealed the role of immunologic factors in psoriasis. Histopathologic examination of psoriatic lesions showed a striking resemblance to cellular inflammatory reactions observed in allergic contact dermatitis (Braun-Falco & Christophers, 1974). A selective immunosuppressant effect was the initial hypothesis used to describe the pathological cellular immune response (Krueger et al., 1978). Soon thereafter, the discovery of a soluble factor that played an important role in keratinocyte proliferation helped to form the cytokine-based theory for the induction/maintenance of the inflammatory and proliferative cascades of psoriatic lesions (Krueger & Jederberg, 1980). Subsequently, an integrated theory explaining the etiopathogenesis of psoriasis came into play: in a genetically susceptible patient, immunological factors trigger rapid turnover in the epidermis resulting in development of psoriasis (Champion, 1981).

The fundamental confirmation that any defect of the skin is not sufficient by itself to maintain a psoriatic lesion occurred in the subsequent decade. Some studies confirmed that T cells and soluble factors could stimulate keratinocyte proliferation. Immunophenotyping of psoriatic lesions showed mixed T lymphocyte (TL) cell populations (CD4 and CD8) and Langerhans cells (LCs) distinct from normal skin (Bos et al., 1983). This cellular infiltrate changed with topical or systemic treatment (Baker et al., 1985; Bos & Krieg, 1985). In another study, failure of plasma exchange and leukapheresis ruled out the major participation of humoral immune system in the pathogenesis of psoriasis (Lieden & Skogh, 1986). Thus, the cellular arm of the immune system was implicated in psoriasis for the first time during the 1980s (Valdimarsson et al., 1986).

During the 1990s, research on immunopathogenesis of psoriasis thus focused on the cellular and the cytokine components of the immune system. Researchers observed that an influx of activated T lymphocytes, mainly CD4+, HLA-DR+, Interleukin (IL)-2 receptor - CD25+ T cells, was one of the earliest events of psoriasis (Schlaak et al., 1994). Based on Mosmman and Coffman's publication (Mosmann et al., 1986), these T lymphocytes were classified as T helper (Th) type 1 cytokine producers (Th1) (Austin et al., 1999). They produce Interferon (IFN)-γ, IL-2, and Tumor Necrosis Factor (TNF)-α cytokines and implied that a cellular type 1 reaction was responsible for psoriasis (Figure 1). The observation of the historical evolution of the extra-cutaneous manifestations of psoriasis and their pathogenesis confirms the idea of a multi-organ disease with complex immunological pathways (Scarpa et al., 2010).

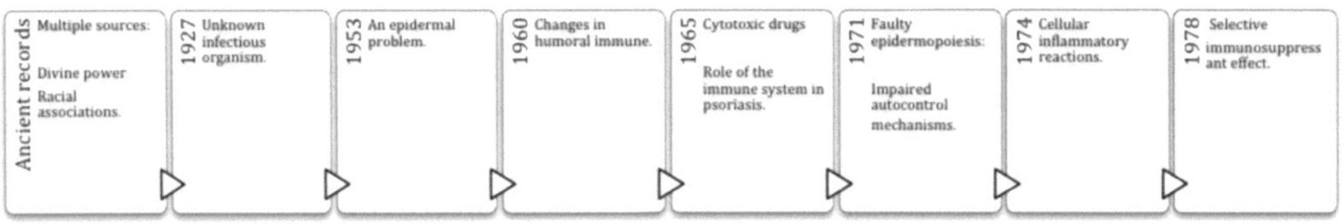

Fig. 1. Time line of development of psoriasis pathophysiology: From unknown by epidermal problem until Immunological disease.

3. Psoriasis: Many pieces and movements on a complex chessboard

Psoriasis plaque is induced and maintained by multiple interactions between cells of the skin and immune system. It seems that the pathogenesis of psoriasis could involve a stage of cellular infiltration resulting in epidermal (keratinocyte) proliferation. Each inflammatory pathway (IL-12/Th1, IL-23/Th17, and IL-22/Th22) has its impact on psoriasis development (Kagami et al., 2010). The different pathways are based on the fact that T helper cells can be skewed towards mutually exclusive subtypes on the basis of the cytokine environment (Abdi, 2002; Vanaudenaerde et al., 2010). The process of T lymphocyte reactivation results from interaction of T cells with the resident antigen presenting cells (APCs) found in plaque psoriasis, which in turn determines the cytokine environment and Th1/Th17/Th22 pathway.

The primary etiopathogenesis of an autoimmune disease, or the activation of Th1/Th17/Th22 pathways, is the dysregulation of immune system activation since the development of autoreactive lymphocytes occurs in the same basic manner as lymphocyte activation. The understanding of this process or processes is very important to maintain the balance of the normal performance of the immune system. Briefly, it is comparable to the process to find the moment where one player lost the chess game based on the retroactive analysis of his moves. Cytokines are the possible moves of different pieces of the game. Many pieces can produce the same movement but with different results. The moves are the key players in generating/establishment of a specific immune system reaction. Therefore, blocking cytokines that maintain autoimmune activity has become one the most successful strategies for autoimmunity therapy. A new balance can be established with the removal of a key piece or blocking of a lethal move so that the critical players are removed from the chessboard of an autoimmune response.

As with any other disease involving the immune system, psoriatic manifestation begins with Antigen-Presenting Cells (APC) activation by an unknown trigger. Different factors including infections, trauma, medications, and emotional stress can initiate the initial phase of the disease. Such factors can activate keratinocytes to release cytokines such as IL-1 and TNF-α, initiating the effector phase of psoriasis by activating resident skin macrophages and Dendritic Cells (DCs). DCs migrate to the regional lymph node, which initiates T lymphocyte activation in response to the stimuli. This is part of the working model of the immune synapse of T cells in psoriasis, integrating T cell signaling pathways in autoimmunity (Nickoloff & Nestle, 2004). This association leads to the production of IL-12/Th1/IFN-γ pathway. Many molecules in the plasma membrane of both cells, other than the Major Histocompatibility Complex (MHC) and T Cell Receptor (TCR), are involved in this phase and can be used as a target molecule for the treatment of psoriasis. The most important molecules are ICAM-1, LFA-3, and CD80/CD86 in the DC and LFA-1, CD2, and CD28 in the T cell, respectively. Alefacept, a fusion protein used for psoriasis treatment, blocks T cells activation by interfering with CD2 on the T cell membrane, thereby blocking the costimulatory molecule LFA-3/CD2 interaction (Kraan et al., 2002). Furthermore, it has recently been discovered that IL-27 suppressed macrophage responses to TNF-α and IL-1β, thus identifying an anti-inflammatory function of IL-27 (Kalliolias et al., 2010).

Continuing the evolving complex immunological chess game, the activated T lymphocyte Th1 cytokine producers leave the lymph node and migrate to the skin where cytokines like TNF-α, produced by keratinocytes and activated DCs, facilitate T lymphocyte diapedesis into the dermis and epidermis (Philipp et al., 2006). The TNF-α induces the skin immune cell infiltration by inducing chemokines and upregulating adhesion molecules on the endothelial cells of dermal vessels. Adhesion molecules such as CLA and LFA-1 on the T lymphocyte membrane and E-selectin and ICAM-1 on the endothelial cell membrane are involved in this process. Efalizumab, a Humanized Anti-CD11a, Anti-LFA-1 molecule has been used in psoriasis treatment by blocking the TL migration to the skin (Sobell et al., 2009). In summary, dendritic cells and effector T-cells are important in the development of the psoriastic lesion, and cytokines produced by these cells stimulate keratinocytes to proliferate and increase the migration of inflammatory cells into the skin, promoting epidermal hyperplasia and inflammation (Monteleone, G. et al., 2011).

3.1 The chessboard: The skin influence on psoriasis development

The primary cause of psoriasis was not found. Factors such as genetics and environmental exposure are now recognized to play a role in psoriasis development. Certainly, autoimmunity does not appear the only and necessary component to the development of psoriasis. However, psoriasis is a manifestation of skin immune reactions. Inflammation is a key feature of pathogenesis, with all inflammatory cell types implicated in psoriasis pathology by multiple interactions between cells of the skin or from other organs and immune system. Nonetheless, the etiology of psoriasis as an epidermal problem or a disease of faulty epidermopoiesis due to impaired autocontrol mechanisms is not completely wrong. Keratinocyte-derived inflammatory molecules amplificate skin immune responses associated with psoriasis, and contribute to the disease process and clinical phenotype (Albanesi & Pastore, 2010). Psoriatic keratinocytes respond aberrantly to cytokines and show altered intracellular signaling pathways (Endo et al., 2006).

Heterogeneous functions of other skin resident cells, such as fibroblasts and endothelial cells, may also contribute to the pathogenesis of psoriasis (Albanesi et al., 2007).

Furthermore, leukocytes that infiltrate skin lesions have been shown to be involved in the pathogenesis of this disease (Chen et al., 2010). Despite parallels to the chicken and egg causality dilemma, all of these accounts for what later clinicians observe in patients suffering from psoriasis.

4. The initial biologic treatments for psoriasis and implications on the understanding of immunological mechanism of psoriasis

Psoriasis was defined as Th1 type of disease based on the early understanding of the T helper subsets. The initial belief was that infiltrating T cell subpopulations derived from the draining lymph node regulated the development of the inflammatory responses in the skin by producing IFN-γ and TNF-α (Albanesi et al., 2005). The Th1-derived cytokines produced by these infiltrating Th1 favors further Th1 cell access, upregulates keratinocyte chemokine production, and supports dermal DC myeloid type (DC11c+) activation. In response to this cytokine activation, keratinocytes and other cells produce a plethora of immune mediators, which induce and amplify inflammatory responses in the skin (Lowes et al., 2007).

As a result, two logical biologic therapeutic approaches were tested: one was the administration of counter regulatory type 2 cytokines and the second was the blocking of type 1 cytokines. The use of monoclonal antibodies or fusion proteins to neutralize cytokines started to be used on a large scale because of their efficacy and practicality.

These studies have proved to be a useful biological model and test ground for evaluation of the skin immune system and psoriasis. Although these drugs were not initially developed in the treatment of psoriasis, but rather in rheumatoid arthritis and Crohn's disease, the observation that Crohn's disease patients with psoriasis were improving while on anti-TNF therapy profoundly influenced the studies that were to come (Schon & Boehncke, 2005).

Although clinical response to anti-TNF suggested a role for Th1 cells in psoriasis, evidence coming from other studies demonstrated that Th1/Th2 paradigm and key role of TNF were not sufficient to explain the full pathogenesis of psoriasis. At this point some academic resistance to an immunological pathogenesis for psoriasis was raised (Nickoloff et al., 2000). However, the main interpretation was that an important piece of the immunological cytokine puzzle was missing. Many other pieces would be involved in such a complex game.

5. The IL-12/23 and its role in the immunopathogenesis psoriasis

The initial quest for the missing cytokines was the search for pathway inducers. Researchers first noted that IL-12 is crucial for Th1-cell differentiation (Okamura et al., 1995). IL-12 signaling via its receptor activates Stat4 (signal transducer and activator of transcription 4), which upregulates IFN-γ. IFN-γ activates Stat1, which enhance T-bet (T-box expressed in T cells), the leading TH1 transcription factor, further enhancing IFN- γ production and downregulating IL-4 and IL-5 expression (Biedermann et al., 2004). IFN-γ mediates many of the pro-inflammatory activities of IL-12. Phagocytes and Dendritic Cells (DCs) are the main producers of IL-12 in response to microbial stimulation (Macatonia et al., 1995), and this relationship links innate resistance and adaptive immunity. The main function of IL-12 is resistance to infections with bacteria and intracellular parasites. However, it plays an important role in the Th1 response that sustains organ-specific autoimmunity (Trinchieri, 1998). The use of anti-IL-12 mAb (monoclonal antibody) in an experimental model of psoriasis also suggested the therapeutic value of blocking IL-12 in humans (Hong et al., 2001), although side effects of the drug limited further development in this area.

For many years, the IL-12-dependent Th1 cells were thought to be essential for the induction of autoimmunity. However, during the Th1/Th2 paradigm studies, an IFN-γ-independent mechanism responsible for the pathogenesis of many inflammatory diseases and psoriasis was found (Hong et al., 1999). IL-12 and IL-23, as discovered previously from human DNA sequence information, share the subunit p40 (Monteleone, I. et al., 2009). The use of anti-IL-12/23p40 and anti-IFN mAb ultimately established at least part of the solution to the riddle. Only neutralization of p40, but not of IFN-γ, ameliorated chronic inflammatory reactions. This finding suggested that the latter cytokine, IL-23, accounted for the IFN-γ-independent mechanism of inflammation.

Identified from human DNA sequence information, IL-23, like IL-12, is also a heterodimeric cytokine composed of the same subunit p40 paired with the unique p19 (Oppmann et al., 2000). It has been reported that IL-12 and IL-23 are up-regulated in psoriatic skin (Lee et al., 2004). Human studies with anti-IL-12p40 have shown that this treatment not only ameliorates psoriasis, but also down-regulates type 1 cytokines and IL-12/IL-23 in lesional skin (Toichi et al., 2006). Besides sharing the subunit p40 and signaling through similar receptors, IL-23 and IL-12 are responsible for driving different T-cell subsets. Moreover, presence of abundant $IL\text{-}23^{+}$ dendritic cells as well as elevated mRNA expression for both subunits of IL-23 (IL-23p19 and IL-23p40) in psoriatic lesions supports the role of IL-23 in the pathogenesis of psoriasis (Lee et al., 2004; Lillis et al., 2010; Piskin et al., 2006; Wilson et al., 2007). Genetic studies have revealed that polymorphisms in IL-23p19, IL-12/23p40, and IL-23R are associated with increased risk of psoriasis (Capon et al., 2007; Cargill et al., 2007; Nair et al., 2009). Furthermore, in an animal xenograft model of psoriasis, Tonel G *et al* showed that treatment with anti human IL-23 mAb causes statistically significant reduction of acanthosis and papillomatosis index in grafts of mice in comparison to isotype controlled mice. Moreover, they found comparable efficacy of anti human IL-23 mAb with anti TNF-α (infliximab) in blocking the development of psoriasis. They also showed a significant decrease in CD3+ T cells mainly in the epidermis of mice treated with anti human IL-23 mAb in comparison to control mice (Tonel et al., 2010).

IL-23 could also mediate and sustain late-stage chronic inflammation by the production of IL-17 by Th17 (Aggarwal et al., 2003). IL-23 plays an important role as a central growth factor (Korn et al., 2009; Miossec et al., 2009; Romagnani et al., 2009). In presence of TGF-β and IL-6, IL-23 helps in development of Th17 cells whereas TGF-β is inhibitory to production of IL-22 (Ghoreschi et al., 2010; Volpe et al., 2008; Zheng et al., 2007) (Figure 2).

The IL-23/Th17/IL-17 immune axis was initially elucidated when IL-17 gene expression was induced by *B. burgdorferi* independent of IL-12 (Infante-Duarte et al., 2000). The IL-17–producing CD4+ T cells distinct from those producing either IL-4 or IFN-γ were called Th17 (Harrington et al., 2005). Patients with psoriasis have increased Th17 cells as well as increased expression of mRNA for Th17 cytokines (IL-17A; IL-17F; TNF-α; IL-21 and IL-22) and chemokines (CCL20) (Boniface et al., 2007; Harper et al., 2009; Johansen et al., 2009; Lowes et al., 2008; Zaba et al., 2007). In psoriasis, Th17 cytokine IL-17A mainly induces cytokine and chemokine production by keratinocytes (Albanesi et al., 2000; Harper et al.,

2009; Nograles et al., 2008), whereas IL-22 induces proliferation of keratinocytes and production of antimicrobial peptides by keratinocytes (Liang et al., 2006; Sa et al., 2007; Wolk et al., 2006; Zheng et al., 2007). The role of IL-23 and IL-17 in psoriasis was further substantiated in some animal studies with recombinant IL-23 and anti IL-17A. In wild type (WT) mice, injection of recombinant murine (rm) IL-23 induces epidermal hyperplasia (Chan et al., 2006; Kopp et al., 2003), whereas, in IL-17 -/- mice showed less epidermal hyperplasia after repeated injection of rmIL-23. A recent publication by Rizzo et al showed that WT mice do not show epidermal hyperplasia to injection of rmIL-23 if they were treated with anti IL-17A antibodies (Rizzo et al., 2011). A redundant cytokine model has emerged as the evolving explanation for psoriasis pathogenesis. It is based on the IL-12/Th1/ IFN-γ - TNF-α and the IL-23/Th17/IL-17 immune pathways (Figure 3). The effectiveness of the anti-TNF treatment of psoriasis validated the first axis. The efficacy of anti-p40 (anti-IL12/23) treatment confirms the other (Nestle et al., 2009).

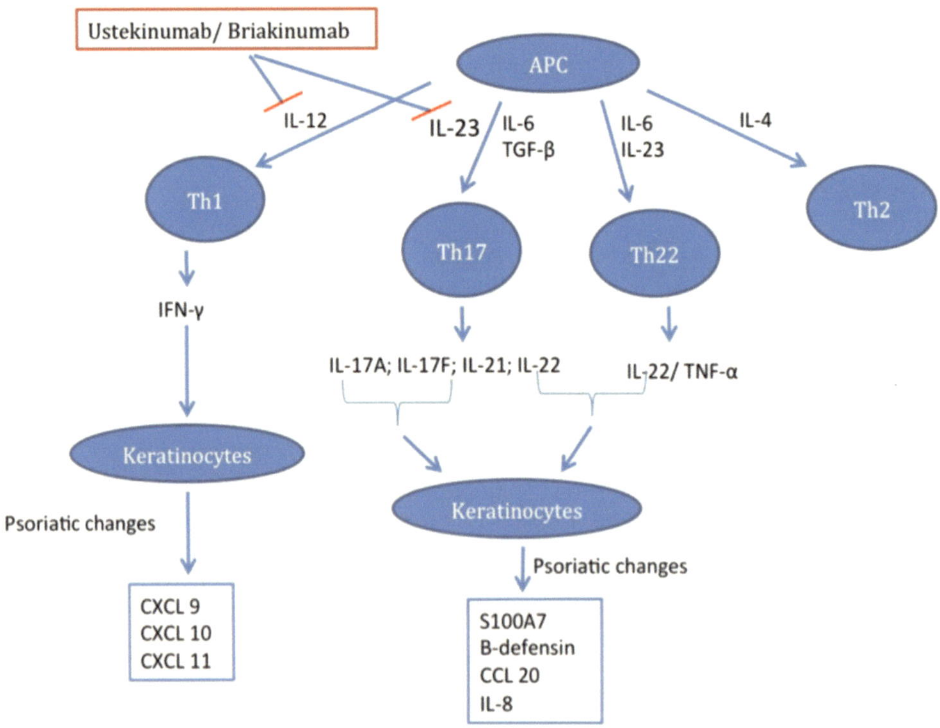

Fig. 2. The pivotal role of some of IL-12 and IL-23 in psoriasis etiopathogenesis: How blocking the effects of these cytokines substantially improve the disease condition.

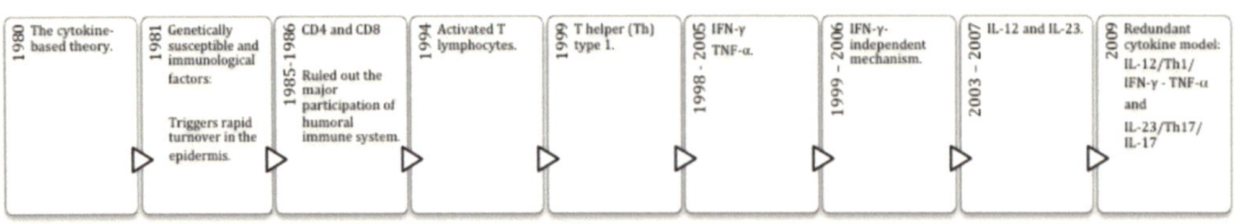

Fig. 3. Time line of development of psoriasis pathophysiology: From complex Immunological disease by genetic participation until recent advances.

6. Selective IL-23/Th17/IL-17 immune axis inhibition

IL-23 favors the proliferation of the Th17 subtype and consequent production of IL-22 and IL-6 that stimulates the proliferation of keratinocytes. IL-17 favors infiltration of neutrophils into the skin forming the typical Munro's micro-abscesses with some participation of IL-22 (Watanabe et al., 2009).

Studies have demonstrated that anti-p40 (anti-IL-12/23) treatment is highly efficacious for psoriasis. Ustekinumab anti IL-12/23 antibody showed its efficacy and safety in three phase III trials recruiting 2899 patients. From two placebo controlled trials, PHOENIX 1 and PHOENIX 2, ustekinumab showed its efficacy in ameliorating psoriatic plaques, pruritus, and nail psoriasis (Yeilding et al., 2011). (Table 1).

PASI scores	Placebo [n = 410]	Ustekinumab (45 mg) [n = 409]	Ustekinumab (90 mg) [n = 411]
PASI 50	41 (10%)	342 (83.6%)*	367 (89.3%)*
PASI 75	15 (3.7%)	273 (66.7%)*	311 (75.7%)*
PASI 90	3 (0.7%)	173 (42.3%)*	209 (50.9%)*
Physician's global assessment (Cleared)	0 (0.0%)	93 (22.7%)*	115 (28.0%)*
Physician's global assessment (Cleared or minimal)	20 (4.9%)	278 (68%)*	302 (73.5%)*
Physician's global assessment (marked or severe)	148 (36.1%)	15 (3.7%)*	10 (2.4%)*

* P <0.001 Adapted from: Papp KA, Langley RG, Lebwohl M, et al. Efficacy and safety of ustekinumab, a human interleukin-12/23 monoclonal antibody, in patients with psoriasis: 52-week results from a randomized, double-blind, placebo-controlled trial (PHOENIX 2). *Lancet.* 2008; 371(9625):1675-1684.

Table 1. Clinical improvement at week 12 (PHOENIX II)

Remarkably, in a phase II multicenter, randomized, double-blind, placebo-controlled trial briakinumab, another human monoclonal anti-IL-12/23 antibody, 90-93% of subjects in 4 dosing groups were able to achieve a PASI 75 (Lima et al., 2009a). This finding alone confirms the centrality of this pathway because these levels of efficacy have not been previously seen in studies with other agents (Leonardi et al., 2008). Safety data for both agents is limited, but to date has been favorable.

One issue with anti-p40 therapy is that it inhibits both the classical IL-12/Th1/IFN-γ and IL-23/Th17/IL-17 immune pathways. IL-12 and IL-23 are related cytokines with differences in their biological activities. After binding to their receptors, different intracellular transcription complexes are activated (Parham et al., 2002). IL-12 predominantly acts on naïve T cells and initiates the TH1 response. In contrast, IL-23 primarily affects memory T cells and expands the initiated Th1 inflammatory response by Th17 activity and maintains an adequate memory pool by compromising memory T cells (Oppmann et al., 2000; Parham et al., 2002; Trinchieri et al., 2003). Experimental studies suggest that IL-23/Th17/IL-17 immune axis blocking is sufficient to treat autoimmune inflammation (Monteleone, I. et al., 2009).

Another way to block both pathways is the immunoregulatory role of IFN-γ. It is well-known that the administration of anti-IFN-γ induces exacerbation of Experimental Autoimmune Encephalomyelitis (EAE) (Becher et al., 2002). One possible explanation is the inhibition of IL-12/Th1/IFN-γ axis may destroy the regulatory role of IFN-γ during chronic inflammation. TNF-α, like INF-γ, has a regulatory role in the immune system (Liu et al., 1998). This might explain the observation that anti-TNF therapies can induce psoriasis and other autoimmune diseases in some patients (Ramos-Casals et al., 2008).

An increase in efficacy and reduction of adverse events are the main drivers for new therapies. Infections, one type of adverse event, usually increase in patients receiving anti-cytokine therapy (Dinarello, 2003). Studies with anti-IL-23 therapy will require surveillance for the development of opportunistic infections. Reports from patients with IL-12 and/or IL-23 cytokine deficiency syndromes alert to these potential infections in individuals under anti-IL-23 therapy. Invasive salmonellosis and mycobacterial diseases were present more often in patients with IL-12/IL-23 deficiency indicating that immunity against these microorganisms appears to be dependent of IL-12 and/or IL-23 (MacLennan et al., 2004). However, antibodies against IL-12 and IL-23 may not cause a complete inactivity of these cytokines in a clinical scenario. For example, an experimental study showed that IL-23 plays a role in host defense against *P. carinii*, but it is not an essential one (Rudner et al., 2007). Clinical studies with anti-IL-12/23 treatment thus far have not increased the risk of non opportunistic or opportunistic infections (Shear et al., 2008). A recent study showed that blocking IL-23 with monoclonal antibodies during BCG infection does not appear to affect the bacterial burden in immunocompetent mice. In contrast, blocking TNF-α or both IL-23 and IL-12 with anti-p40 dramatically enhances mycobacterial growth. From this study, antibody blockade of IL-23 alone rather than IL-12 might be preferable in patients who have been, or may be, exposed to mycobacterial infection (Chackerian et al., 2006).

7. A new piece and a new move

As previously mentioned, the IL-23 favors the proliferation of the Th17 and consequent production of IL-22. IL-22 mRNA presence was initially described in IL-9 stimulated T-cell lines and in concanavalin A (Con-A)-activated murine spleen cells (Dumoutier et al., 2000). Further studies demonstrated that IL-22 expression can only be observed in activated immunological cells (Wolk et al., 2002). However, other reports have revealed that some T cells express IL-22 independently of IL-17 (Nograles et al., 2009). Finally, a new distinct human memory CD4+ T cell subset with skin-homing properties was identified and denominated Th22 (Duhen et al., 2009).

A preferential production of IL-22 cytokine by T cells (Th22, Th17, and Th1) is present in psoriasis lesions (Lowes et al., 2008). Many animal models indicate the role of IL-22 in psoriasis. IL-22 over-expressed transgenic mice developed psoriasis-like skin lesions (Wolk et al., 2009a). In IL-22 -/- mice, injection of IL-23 fails to induce epidermal hyperplasia indicating the role of IL-22 as a downstream mediator of tissue effects caused by IL-23 (Zheng et al., 2007). In a recent publication, Rizzo HL et al showed that to have IL-23 mediated epidermal hyperplasia, both IL-17 and IL-22 is required; any one of these is not sufficient to execute the effect of IL-23. They also showed that pre-treatment with anti IL-22 or anti IL-17A Abs block the rmIL-23 mediated epidermal hyperplasia in wild type mice (Rizzo et al., 2011). In reconstituted epidermis model, IL-22 produces acanthosis dose dependently, which resembles psoriasis and either one of these alone is not sufficient to execute the effect of IL-23. The effects of IL-20 subfamily cytokines on reconstituted human epidermis suggest potential roles in cutaneous innate defense and pathogenic adaptive immunity in psoriasis (Sa et al., 2007). In a study by Wolk K et al, a correlation was demonstrated between the plasma IL-22 levels and the severity of the disease (Wolk et al., 2006). IL-22 regulates the expression of genes responsible for antimicrobial defense, cellular differentiation, and mobility in keratinocytes and may play a: a potential role in psoriasis (Wolk et al., 2006). Moreover, IL-22 levels correlated with IL-20 levels, which is in accordance with the IL-22-induced keratinocyte IL-20 production (Wolk et al., 2009b). This suggests that IL-22 and its downstream mediator IL-20 play an important role in the final steps of psoriasis pathogenesis. Sabat R and his group in their studies showed that IL-22 regulates keratinocyte function in several ways: a. IL-22 helps form a biological barrier of the skin by producing antimicrobial proteins (AMPs) like β-defensins, and S100 proteins. This may be one of the reasons that psoriatic patients have less skin infections. b. IL-22 interferes with physiological desquamation process of skin by inhibiting the terminal differentiation of keratinocytes. c. IL-22 plays a role in recruiting neutrophilic granulocytes in skin by inducing the production of chemokines;. d. IL-22 indirectly helps in extracellular tissue degradation by inducing production of matrix metalloproteinases 1 and 3. IL-22 induces the production of IL-20, another IL-10 family cytokine which has similar effects as IL-22, thus resulting in amplification of the effects of IL-22 (Sabat & Wolk, 2011). In a transgenic mouse model, it has been showed that IL-22 causes acanthosis, hyperkeratosis, and hypogranulosis, which are hallmarks of psoriasis. IL-22 acts through STAT-3 to impact the differentiation of keratinocytes (Wolk et al., 2009a). IL-22 induces pro-inflammatory chemokines and antimicrobial proteins (AMPs) β-defensins (BDs), and promotes epidermal acanthosis and parakeratosis of keratinocytes (Boniface et al., 2005; Wolk et al., 2004; Wolk et al., 2006). Some synergistic effect was noted with other pro-inflammatory cytokines like TNF-α; IFN-γ; and IL-17 (Sabat & Wolk, 2011). Alone, TNF- α does not have much effect on terminal differentiation of keratinocytes, but when keratinocytes were co-cultured with IL-22 and TNF- α, the effects of IL-22 were amplified. This kind of synergism was also seen with CXCL8 and IL-20 expression in keratinocytes co-stimulated with IL-22 & TNF-α. One possible explanation of this may be that TNF-α increases the expression of IL-22 receptor complex and also affects the IL-22 signaling pathway (Wolk et al., 2009a). Thus, IL-22 and IL-20, but not IFN-γ or IL-17, are the key mediators of resulting epidermal proliferation. IL-22 acts through heterodimeric receptor complex composed of IL-22R1 and IL-10R2 (Kotenko et al., 2001). IL-10R2 chain is ubiquitously expressed in all cells and is important component of receptor complexes required for IL-22, IL-10, IL-26 and IL-28 and IL-29, whereas the IL-22R1 chain is present in epithelial cells and hepatocytes (Savan et al., 2011). Between the two subunits, IL-22 binds first to IL-22R1, the high-affinity receptor, and then IL-10R2, a lower affinity receptor (Jones et al., 2008). To produce its effect, IL-22 acts through different signaling pathways, mainly signal transducer and activator of transcription 3 (STAT-3) and mitogen activated protein kinase (Lejeune et al., 2002).

This final move induces the vicious cycle of proliferation and inflammation of the skin characterized by the hyper-proliferative phenotype of keratinocytes in psoriasis. An anti-IL-22/ IL-20 approach would have a complementary role to the neutralization of p40. However, there has not yet been a human study to demonstrate such a role or anti-IL-22 therapy in the treatment of psoriasis.

8. The other side of the chessboard: The role of Treg

Today, reading a book or scientific article on immunopathogensis, one will observe that suppressor T cells, renamed regulatory T cells (Tregs), have become a central concept in immunological vocabulary (Horwitz et al., 2002). Hundreds of publications on Tregs have validated the existence of this single line of T cells. The CD4+CD25+highFoxp3+ Treg subpopulation is developed in the thymus and may be peripherally induced during the course of a normal immune response. The model in which Tregs directly or indirectly modify activation and differentiation of pathogenic T cells by means of an effect on antigen-presenting cells is supported by *in vivo* analyses (Korn et al., 2010).

8.1 Regulatory T cells: Development of an immunological concept

Biological systems are subject to complex regulatory controls and the immune system is no exception. It is known that the immune system has the potential to generate lymphocytes against auto-antigens. Experiments, however, suggest that individuals cannot easily be immunized against their own tissues. Therefore, a suppression mechanism is necessary to control potentially pathogenic immune cells. Owen suggested that this tolerance against one's own tissues is acquired during the development of the immune system, and Burnet proposed that the clonal selective destruction of lymphocytes for auto-antigens occurs primarily in the thymus.

The destruction of auto-reactive lymphocytes is the primary mechanism that leads to tolerance, but we know that this system is not perfect. Self-reactive B and T lymphocytes can be isolated from normal individuals (Ramsdell & Fowlkes, 1990). Nishizuka and Sakakura proposed another mechanism for controlling auto-reactive cells. They observed that mice thymectomized between the second and fourth days of life developed an organ-specific autoimmune disease. This target-organ destruction can be prevented by restoring T cells from genetically identical individuals. The generation of regulator T cells was proposed in order to explain this mechanism of auto-tolerance attributed to the thymus (Sakaguchi et al., 1996).

Other studies observed that the prevention of autoimmune diseases was diminished by the reduction of CD4+ T cells, but not of CD8+ T cells, indicating that regulatory cells belonged to the CD4+ T cell class of lymphocytes. Sakaguchi subsequently characterized these regulatory cells as natural CD4+CD25+ Tregs that express Foxp3 (Sakaguchi et al., 2001).

8.2 Suppressor T cells: Regulatory T cells are suppressor T cells

Another control point of the immune response is established when the normal immune response is initiated. A different mechanism must be set off in order to control the magnitude of the response and its subsequent termination. This regulation should contribute to limiting clonal expansion and effector cell activity. Soon after the discovery that T lymphocytes function as helper cells for B-lymphocytes, RK Gershon proposed that they could also act as cells capable of suppressing the immune response (Gershon & Kondo, 1971). This subpopulation of suppressor T cells was considered a controller of both auto-reactive and effector cells. A suppressor cell was functionally defined as a lymphocyte that inhibits the immune response by influencing the activity of another type of cell involved in a cascade of suppression factors, a network of anti-idiotypic T cells, and counter-suppressive cells (Dorf & Benacerraf, 1984).

Many of the experiments carried out contain data that support the existence of suppressor T cells. However, the mechanism responsible for these suppressive phenomena was never clearly characterized, and consequently interest in the field of suppressor T cells has gradually dwindled. The discovery of Th1/Th2 cells led researchers to abandon the concept of suppressor T cells. Suppression was instead attributed to counter-regulatory cytokines. As pointed out by Green and Webb, the letter "S" started to resemble a foul word in cellular immunology, and its use was considered synonymous of scarce data with excessive interpretation or a mystic phenomenon (Green & Webb, 1993).

Suppressor T cells reappeared as regulatory T cells (Tregs) in the late 1990s when several subpopulations of T cells were identified as having the capacity to inhibit the proliferation of other cells. Shevach et al. were the first to call attention to the fact that regulatory T cells and suppressor T cells are the same (Shevach et al., 1998). Therefore, the term 'regulatory' gradually replaced the term 'suppressor'. The main problem, however, is not that cells are termed regulatory, but that they are considered to be suppressors. It is more appropriate to consider regulatory T cells as immune response directors instead of its suppressors.

9. Regulatory T cells and psoriasis

The regulation mechanism of the immune system by CD25+high Tregs is not well understood. Studies have not yet arrived at a simple mode of action. Whatever the mechanism, the homeostatic balance of the immune system is obtained by healthy cellular and humoral responses. Some inflammatory agents, whether physical, chemical, or infectious, induce an intense immune response. This immune response against them frequently results in tissue damage that could be more intense if it were not for the interference of regulatory mechanisms (Belkaid et al., 2006). As has already been specified, Treg cells help limit the damage caused by a vigorous immune response. Natural Treg cells may respond to an ample variety of auto-antigens, although there is evidence that they may also respond to antigens expressed by microbes. Induced regulatory T cells, such as TR1 or Th3, may develop from CD4+ T cells when exposed to specific conditions (Weiner et al., 2011).

Similarly, excessive activity of Treg cells may limit the magnitude of the immune response, which may result in failure to control an infection. On the other hand, the absence of the T regulator may result in intense inflammation and autoimmune dermatitis. Tissue damage may also result from the development of effector cells against their own auto-antigens (Figure 4).

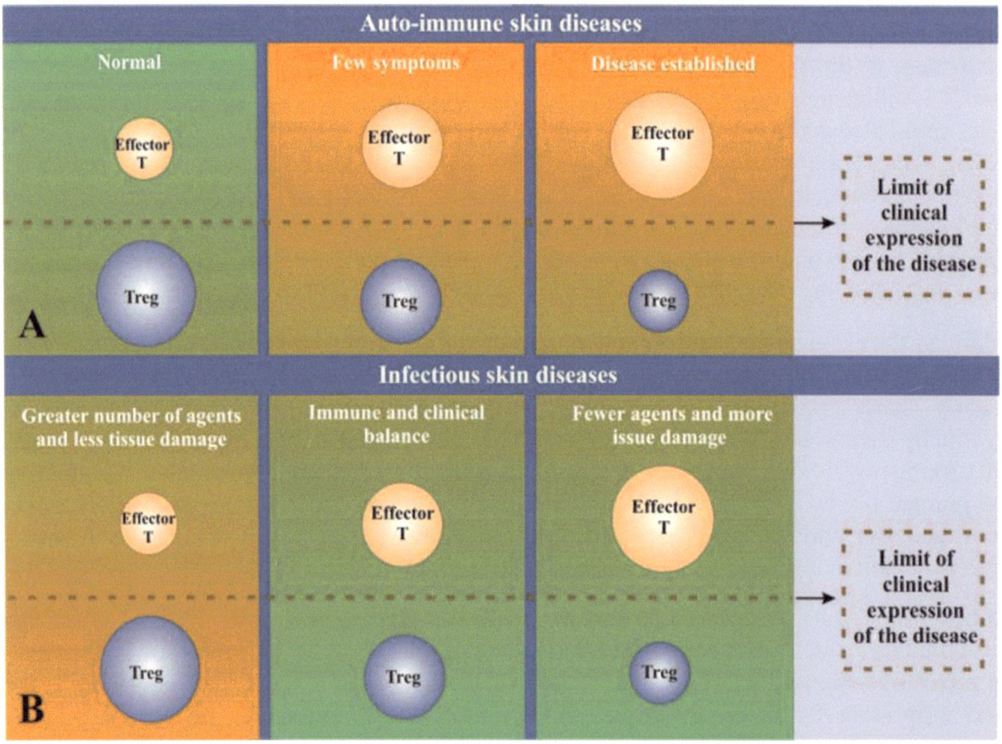

Fig. 4. Immune response regulation mechanisms. The force balance between Tregs and the effector T CD4+ cells may present in a different manner depending on being an autoantigen or a pathogen. In A portion, the clinical expression of autoimmune skin diseases is shown. In this case, there is clinical manifestation only when the number and function of Tregs are significantly reduced. B portion displays clinical manifestations that may occur in extreme cases. In case of excessive Treg function, the result shows reduction of effector lymphocytes against the pathogen, an increase in its number and less tissue damage. The contrary applies to effector cells against the pathogen that surpass the number and function of Treg. The ideal immune and clinical response occurs when there is a balance between functions

Psoriasis is sustained by the activation of pathogenic T cells. The regulatory expression of skin diseases discusses the action exerted by regulatory T cells, especially CD4+CD25+high Tregs on psoriasis. Various types of influence of these cells suggest that they may act by suppressing or augmenting immunity (Sabat et al., 2007; Shehata & Elghandour, 2007). The control of Treg cells may affect the results favorably or may be deleterious. There is no definitive view. In psoriasis, studies have shown that the subpopulation of CD4+ T lymphocytes in peripheral blood, phenotypically CD25+high, CTLA-4(+), Foxp3high, is deficient in its suppressor functions. This is associated with an accelerated proliferation of the CD4+ T cell response (Sugiyama et al., 2005). The presence of non-functional CD4+CD25+high Treg cells in peripheral blood and in tissues may lead to a reduced capacity to contain pathogenic T cells and to a hyperproliferation of the psoriatic plaque *in vivo*. These findings represent a critical component of this autoimmune disease and may have implications for potential therapy by manipulation of CD4+CD25+high Tregs *in vivo*. However, other factors, such as the immune status and genotype, and the presence of concomitant diseases or other infections may also have an influence. The manipulation of this balance can be explored therapeutically.

9.1 Clinical and therapeutic consequences of regulatory T cells

An improved understanding of the role of T regulators in psoriasis may lead to the identification of new targets for treatment. More specifically, the goal is to manipulate natural regulator cells or those induced by means of an increase or decrease of their function, depending on the circumstances.

Auto-injections of regulatory T cells are a promising approach to modulation of inflammation and autoimmune diseases (Wilhelm et al., 2010). Nevertheless, there is a significant decline in the function of natural CD4+CD25+high Treg cells of peripheral blood in patients with autoimmune diseases when compared to that of healthy individuals. In order to overcome this difficulty, cytokines were used to stimulate the growth of regulator T cells. IL-15 allows a significant *in vitro* expansion of regulator cells (Ortega et al., 2009). Natural CD4+CD25+high Treg cells obtained by *ex vivo* expansion through stimulation with allogeneic antigen-presenting cells and IL-2 were capable of modulating the graft-versus-host disease (GVHD). Induction of natural CD4+CD25+high Treg cells may facilitate the establishment and maintenance of immunological tolerance. Depletion of natural CD4+CD25+high Treg cells may be an effective way of reversing the tolerance induced by malignant tumors and increasing the activity of the immune system against cancer epitopes (Yu et al., 2005)

In the field of dermatology, the stimulation of Treg cells may be important in autoimmune diseases. For example, blockage of T lymphocyte stimulation, as in the use of the antibody associated with CTLA-4 (cytotoxic T lymphocyte-associated antigen 4-immunoglobulin, CTLA4Ig), reverts the development of psoriatic plaques (Abrams et al., 2000). In the clinical context, the effect of immunomodulator drugs on these cells warrants attention. For example, tacrolimus, an inhibitor of calcineurin, increases the inhibition of Treg cells in atopic dermatitis (Sewgobind et al., 2010; Vukmanovic-Stejic et al., 2005). Fludarabine reduces the frequency and suppressive function of natural CD4+CD25+high Treg cells (de Rezende et al., 2010). Low doses of cyclophosphamide induce the inhibition of natural CD4+CD25+high Treg cells and consequently increase the immune response in an apparently paradoxical effect (Lutsiak et al., 2005). Along the same line, cyclophosphamide decreases the function, proportion, and number of natural CD4+CD25+high Treg cells that suppress the induction of contact hypersensitivity (Cerullo et al., 2011; Ikezawa et al., 2005). Currently, topical corticosteroids constitute one of the most effective treatments for psoriasis and other inflammatory skin diseases. These drugs are effective in inhibiting the function of Th2 cells, eosinophils, and epithelial cells. However, treatment with these drugs during the presentation of the epitope may result in an increased tolerance by suppressing the development of dendrite cells that secrete IL-10, which are necessary for the induction of T regulators. Therefore, treatment with corticosteroids may increase the subsequent effect of the T response and aggravate, on the long run, the course of inflammatory diseases (Stock et al., 2005). This aspect may also be related to the rebound effect of inflammatory diseases once these drugs are removed.

10. Conclusion

In medicine, a gold standard is the intervention believed to be the best available option. Given the proven role of many cytokines in psoriasis, substantial interest exists in targeting them with neutralization immunotherapy. If Th1/Th17/Th22 pathways operate in different steps of psoriasis development, then targeted blockade place biologics as the standard-setting paradigm for therapy and understanding of the pathogenesis of psoriasis. However, large studies are needed to provide information on the therapeutic effects, adverse events of any anti-cytokine therapy, and their place in the treatment of psoriasis and other skin diseases. To complement this approach, a detailed comprehension of the associations among the various regulator cells may help in understanding the events leading to the genesis of skin diseases. Ultimately, an ability to manipulate the function of regulator T cells according to the desired therapeutic effect will be the goal. Together, an integrated immunologic approach to therapy holds great promise in reducing the burden of psoriatic disease.

11. References

Abdi, K. (2002). IL-12: the role of p40 versus p75. *Scand J Immunol* Vol. 56, No. 1, pp. 1-11, ISSN. 0300-9475

Abrams, J. R., Kelley, S. L., Hayes, E., Kikuchi, T., Brown, M. J., Kang, S., Lebwohl, M. G., Guzzo, C. A., Jegasothy, B. V., Linsley, P. S. & Krueger, J. G. (2000). Blockade of T lymphocyte costimulation with cytotoxic T lymphocyte-associated antigen 4-immunoglobulin (CTLA4Ig) reverses the cellular pathology of psoriatic plaques, including the activation of keratinocytes, dendritic cells, and endothelial cells. *J Exp Med* Vol. 192, No. 5, pp. 681-694, ISSN. 0022-1007

Aggarwal, S., Ghilardi, N., Xie, M. H., de Sauvage, F. J. & Gurney, A. L. (2003). Interleukin-23 promotes a distinct CD4 T cell activation state characterized by the production of interleukin-17. *J Biol Chem* Vol. 278, No. 3, pp. 1910-1914, ISSN. 0021-9258

Albanesi, C. & Pastore, S. (2010). Pathobiology of chronic inflammatory skin diseases: interplay between keratinocytes and immune cells as a target for anti-inflammatory drugs. *Curr Drug Metab* Vol. 11, No. 3, pp. 210-227, ISSN. 1875-5453

Albanesi, C., Scarponi, C., Cavani, A., Federici, M., Nasorri, F. & Girolomoni, G. (2000). Interleukin-17 is produced by both Th1 and Th2 lymphocytes, and modulates interferon-gamma- and interleukin-4-induced activation of human keratinocytes. *J Invest Dermatol* Vol. 115, No. 1, pp. 81-87, ISSN. 0022-202X

Albanesi, C., Scarponi, C., Giustizieri, M. L. & Girolomoni, G. (2005). Keratinocytes in inflammatory skin diseases. *Curr Drug Targets Inflamm Allergy* Vol. 4, No. 3, pp. 329-334, ISSN. 1568-010X

Aswaq, M., Farber, E. M., Moreci, A. P. & Raffel, S. (1960). Immunologic reactions in psoriasis. *Arch Dermatol* Vol. 82, No., pp. 663-666, ISSN. 0003-987X

Austin, L. M., Ozawa, M., Kikuchi, T., Walters, I. B. & Krueger, J. G. (1999). The majority of epidermal T cells in Psoriasis vulgaris lesions can produce type 1 cytokines, interferon-gamma, interleukin-2, and tumor necrosis factor-alpha, defining TC1 (cytotoxic T lymphocyte) and TH1 effector populations: a type 1 differentiation bias is also measured in circulating blood T cells in psoriatic patients. *J Invest Dermatol* Vol. 113, No. 5, pp. 752-759, ISSN. 0022-202X

Baker, B. S., Swain, A. F., Griffiths, C. E., Leonard, J. N., Fry, L. & Valdimarsson, H. (1985). The effects of topical treatment with steroids or dithranol on epidermal T lymphocytes and dendritic cells in psoriasis. *Scand J Immunol* Vol. 22, No. 5, pp. 471-477, ISSN. 0300-9475

Becher, B., Durell, B. G. & Noelle, R. J. (2002). Experimental autoimmune encephalitis and inflammation in the absence of interleukin-12. *J Clin Invest* Vol. 110, No. 4, pp. 493-497, ISSN. 0021-9738

Belkaid, Y., Blank, R. B. & Suffia, I. (2006). Natural regulatory T cells and parasites: a common quest for host homeostasis. *Immunol Rev* Vol. 212, No., pp. 287-300, ISSN. 0105-2896

Biedermann, T., Rocken, M. & Carballido, J. M. (2004). TH1 and TH2 lymphocyte development and regulation of TH cell-mediated immune responses of the skin. *J Investig Dermatol Symp Proc* Vol. 9, No. 1, pp. 5-14, ISSN. 1087-0024

Boniface, K., Bernard, F. X., Garcia, M., Gurney, A. L., Lecron, J. C. & Morel, F. (2005). IL-22 inhibits epidermal differentiation and induces proinflammatory gene expression and migration of human keratinocytes. *J Immunol* Vol. 174, No. 6, pp. 3695-3702, ISSN. 0022-1767

Boniface, K., Guignouard, E., Pedretti, N., Garcia, M., Delwail, A., Bernard, F. X., Nau, F., Guillet, G., Dagregorio, G., Yssel, H., Lecron, J. C. & Morel, F. (2007). A role for T cell-derived interleukin 22 in psoriatic skin inflammation. *Clin Exp Immunol* Vol. 150, No. 3, pp. 407-415, ISSN. 1365-2249

Bos, J. D., Hulsebosch, H. J., Krieg, S. R., Bakker, P. M. & Cormane, R. H. (1983). Immunocompetent cells in psoriasis. In situ immunophenotyping by monoclonal antibodies. *Arch Dermatol Res* Vol. 275, No. 3, pp. 181-189, ISSN. 0340-3696

Bos, J. D. & Krieg, S. R. (1985). Psoriasis infiltrating cell immunophenotype: changes induced by PUVA or corticosteroid treatment in T-cell subsets, Langerhans' cells and interdigitating cells. *Acta Derm Venereol* Vol. 65, No. 5, pp. 390-397, ISSN. 0001-5555

Braun-Falco, O. & Christophers, E. (1974). Structural aspects of initial psoriatic lesions. *Arch Dermatol Forsch* Vol. 251, No. 2, pp. 95-110, ISSN. 0003-9187

Capon, F., Di Meglio, P., Szaub, J., Prescott, N. J., Dunster, C., Baumber, L., Timms, K., Gutin, A., Abkevic, V., Burden, A. D., Lanchbury, J., Barker, J. N., Trembath, R. C. & Nestle, F. O. (2007). Sequence variants in the genes for the interleukin-23 receptor (IL23R) and its ligand (IL12B) confer protection against psoriasis. *Hum Genet* Vol. 122, No. 2, pp. 201-206, ISSN. 1432-1203

Cargill, M., Schrodi, S. J., Chang, M., Garcia, V. E., Brandon, R., Callis, K. P., Matsunami, N., Ardlie, K. G., Civello, D., Catanese, J. J., Leong, D. U., Panko, J. M., McAllister, L. B., Hansen, C. B., Papenfuss, J., Prescott, S. M., White, T. J., Leppert, M. F., Krueger, G. G. & Begovich, A. B. (2007). A large-scale genetic association study confirms IL12B and leads to the identification of IL23R as psoriasis-risk genes. *Am J Hum Genet* Vol. 80, No. 2, pp. 273-290, ISSN. 0002-9297

Cerullo, V., Diaconu, I., Kangasniemi, L., Rajecki, M., Escutenaire, S., Koski, A., Romano, V., Rouvinen, N., Tuuminen, T., Laasonen, L., Partanen, K., Kauppinen, S., Joensuu, T., Oksanen, M., Holm, S. L., Haavisto, E., Karioja-Kallio, A., Kanerva, A., Pesonen, S., Arstila, P. T. & Hemminki, A. (2011). Immunological Effects of Low-dose

Cyclophosphamide in Cancer Patients Treated With Oncolytic Adenovirus. *Mol Ther* Vol., No., pp., ISSN. 1525-0024

Chackerian, A. A., Chen, S. J., Brodie, S. J., Mattson, J. D., McClanahan, T. K., Kastelein, R. A. & Bowman, E. P. (2006). Neutralization or absence of the interleukin-23 pathway does not compromise immunity to mycobacterial infection. *Infect Immun* Vol. 74, No. 11, pp. 6092-6099, ISSN. 0019-9567

Champion, R. H. (1981). Psoriasis and its treatment. *Br Med J (Clin Res Ed)* Vol. 282, No. 6261, pp. 343-346, ISSN. 0267-0623

Chan, J. R., Blumenschein, W., Murphy, E., Diveu, C., Wiekowski, M., Abbondanzo, S., Lucian, L., Geissler, R., Brodie, S., Kimball, A. B., Gorman, D. M., Smith, K., de Waal Malefyt, R., Kastelein, R. A., McClanahan, T. K. & Bowman, E. P. (2006). IL-23 stimulates epidermal hyperplasia via TNF and IL-20R2-dependent mechanisms with implications for psoriasis pathogenesis. *J Exp Med* Vol. 203, No. 12, pp. 2577-2587, ISSN. 0022-1007

Chen, S. C., de Groot, M., Kinsley, D., Laverty, M., McClanahan, T., Arreaza, M., Gustafson, E. L., Teunissen, M. B., de Rie, M. A., Fine, J. S. & Kraan, M. (2010). Expression of chemokine receptor CXCR3 by lymphocytes and plasmacytoid dendritic cells in human psoriatic lesions. *Arch Dermatol Res* Vol. 302, No. 2, pp. 113-123, ISSN. 1432-069X

de Rezende, L. C., Silva, I. V., Rangel, L. B. & Guimaraes, M. C. (2010). Regulatory T cell as a target for cancer therapy. *Arch Immunol Ther Exp (Warsz)* Vol. 58, No. 3, pp. 179-190, ISSN. 1661-4917

Dinarello, C. A. (2003). Anti-cytokine therapeutics and infections. *Vaccine* Vol. 21 Suppl 2, No., pp. S24-34, ISSN. 0264-410X

Dorf, M. E. & Benacerraf, B. (1984). Suppressor cells and immunoregulation. *Annu Rev Immunol* Vol. 2, No., pp. 127-157, ISSN. 0732-0582

Duhen, T., Geiger, R., Jarrossay, D., Lanzavecchia, A. & Sallusto, F. (2009). Production of interleukin 22 but not interleukin 17 by a subset of human skin-homing memory T cells. *Nat Immunol* Vol. 10, No. 8, pp. 857-863, ISSN. 1529-2916

Dumoutier, L., Louahed, J. & Renauld, J. C. (2000). Cloning and characterization of IL-10-related T cell-derived inducible factor (IL-TIF), a novel cytokine structurally related to IL-10 and inducible by IL-9. *J Immunol* Vol. 164, No. 4, pp. 1814-1819, ISSN. 0022-1767

Feldmann, M., Brennan, F. M. & Maini, R. (1998). Cytokines in autoimmune disorders. *Int Rev Immunol* Vol. 17, No. 1-4, pp. 217-228, ISSN. 0883-0185

Gershon, R. K. & Kondo, K. (1971). Infectious immunological tolerance. *Immunology* Vol. 21, No. 6, pp. 903-914, ISSN. 0019-2805

Ghoreschi, K., Laurence, A., Yang, X. P., Tato, C. M., McGeachy, M. J., Konkel, J. E., Ramos, H. L., Wei, L., Davidson, T. S., Bouladoux, N., Grainger, J. R., Chen, Q., Kanno, Y., Watford, W. T., Sun, H. W., Eberl, G., Shevach, E. M., Belkaid, Y., Cua, D. J., Chen, W. & O'Shea, J. J. (2010). Generation of pathogenic T(H)17 cells in the absence of TGF-beta signalling. *Nature* Vol. 467, No. 7318, pp. 967-971, ISSN. 1476-4687

Green, D. R. & Webb, D. R. (1993). Saying the 'S' word in public. *Immunol Today* Vol. 14, No. 11, pp. 523-525, ISSN. 0167-5699

Harber, L. C., March, C. & Ovary, Z. (1962). Lack of passive cutaneous anaphylaxis in psoriasis. *Arch Dermatol* Vol. 85, No., pp. 716-719, ISSN. 0003-987X

Harper, E. G., Guo, C., Rizzo, H., Lillis, J. V., Kurtz, S. E., Skorcheva, I., Purdy, D., Fitch, E., Iordanov, M. & Blauvelt, A. (2009). Th17 cytokines stimulate CCL20 expression in keratinocytes in vitro and in vivo: implications for psoriasis pathogenesis. *J Invest Dermatol* Vol. 129, No. 9, pp. 2175-2183, ISSN. 1523-1747

Harrington, L. E., Hatton, R. D., Mangan, P. R., Turner, H., Murphy, T. L., Murphy, K. M. & Weaver, C. T. (2005). Interleukin 17-producing CD4+ effector T cells develop via a lineage distinct from the T helper type 1 and 2 lineages. *Nat Immunol* Vol. 6, No. 11, pp. 1123-1132, ISSN. 1529-2908

Harris, C. C. (1971). Malignancy during methotrexate and steroid therapy for psoriasis. *Arch Dermatol* Vol. 103, No. 5, pp. 501-504, ISSN. 0003-987X

Heaney, J. H. (1927). The Etiology and Treatment of Psoriasis. *Br Med J* Vol. 2
, No. Dec, pp. 1136-1137, ISSN.

Hong, K., Berg, E. L. & Ehrhardt, R. O. (2001). Persistence of pathogenic CD4+ Th1-like cells in vivo in the absence of IL-12 but in the presence of autoantigen. *J Immunol* Vol. 166, No. 7, pp. 4765-4772, ISSN. 0022-1767

Hong, K., Chu, A., Ludviksson, B. R., Berg, E. L. & Ehrhardt, R. O. (1999). IL-12, independently of IFN-gamma, plays a crucial role in the pathogenesis of a murine psoriasis-like skin disorder. *J Immunol* Vol. 162, No. 12, pp. 7480-7491, ISSN. 0022-1767

Horwitz, D. A., Gray, J. D. & Zheng, S. G. (2002). The potential of human regulatory T cells generated ex vivo as a treatment for lupus and other chronic inflammatory diseases. *Arthritis Res* Vol. 4, No. 4, pp. 241-246, ISSN. 1465-9905

Hunter, J. A., Ryan, T. J. & Savin, J. A. (1974). Diseases of the skin. Present and future trends in approaches to skin disease. *Br Med J* Vol. 1, No. 5902, pp. 283-284, ISSN. 0007-1447

Ikezawa, Y., Nakazawa, M., Tamura, C., Takahashi, K., Minami, M. & Ikezawa, Z. (2005). Cyclophosphamide decreases the number, percentage and the function of CD25+ CD4+ regulatory T cells, which suppress induction of contact hypersensitivity. *J Dermatol Sci* Vol. 39, No. 2, pp. 105-112, ISSN. 0923-1811

Infante-Duarte, C., Horton, H. F., Byrne, M. C. & Kamradt, T. (2000). Microbial lipopeptides induce the production of IL-17 in Th cells. *J Immunol* Vol. 165, No. 11, pp. 6107-6115, ISSN. 0022-1767

Ingram, J. T. (1953). The approach to psoriasis. *Br Med J* Vol. 2, No. 4836, pp. 591-594, ISSN. 0007-1447

Johansen, C., Usher, P. A., Kjellerup, R. B., Lundsgaard, D., Iversen, L. & Kragballe, K. (2009). Characterization of the interleukin-17 isoforms and receptors in lesional psoriatic skin. *Br J Dermatol* Vol. 160, No. 2, pp. 319-324, ISSN. 1365-2133

Jones, B. C., Logsdon, N. J. & Walter, M. R. (2008). Structure of IL-22 bound to its high-affinity IL-22R1 chain. *Structure* Vol. 16, No. 9, pp. 1333-1344, ISSN. 0969-2126

Kagami, S., Rizzo, H. L., Kurtz, S. E., Miller, L. S. & Blauvelt, A. (2010). IL-23 and IL-17A, but not IL-12 and IL-22, are required for optimal skin host defense against Candida albicans. *J Immunol* Vol. 185, No. 9, pp. 5453-5462, ISSN. 1550-6606

Kalliolias, G. D., Gordon, R. A. & Ivashkiv, L. B. (2010). Suppression of TNF-alpha and IL-1 signaling identifies a mechanism of homeostatic regulation of macrophages by IL-27. *J Immunol* Vol. 185, No. 11, pp. 7047-7056, ISSN. 1550-6606

Kopp, T., Lenz, P., Bello-Fernandez, C., Kastelein, R. A., Kupper, T. S. & Stingl, G. (2003). IL-23 production by cosecretion of endogenous p19 and transgenic p40 in keratin 14/p40 transgenic mice: evidence for enhanced cutaneous immunity. *J Immunol* Vol. 170, No. 11, pp. 5438-5444, ISSN. 0022-1767

Korn, T., Bettelli, E., Oukka, M. & Kuchroo, V. K. (2009). IL-17 and Th17 Cells. *Annu Rev Immunol* Vol. 27, No., pp. 485-517, ISSN. 0732-0582

Korn, T., Mitsdoerffer, M. & Kuchroo, V. K. (2010). Immunological basis for the development of tissue inflammation and organ-specific autoimmunity in animal models of multiple sclerosis. *Results Probl Cell Differ* Vol. 51, No., pp. 43-74, ISSN. 0080-1844

Kotenko, S. V., Izotova, L. S., Mirochnitchenko, O. V., Esterova, E., Dickensheets, H., Donnelly, R. P. & Pestka, S. (2001). Identification of the functional interleukin-22 (IL-22) receptor complex: the IL-10R2 chain (IL-10Rbeta) is a common chain of both the IL-10 and IL-22 (IL-10-related T cell-derived inducible factor, IL-TIF) receptor complexes. *J Biol Chem* Vol. 276, No. 4, pp. 2725-2732, ISSN. 0021-9258

Kraan, M. C., van Kuijk, A. W., Dinant, H. J., Goedkoop, A. Y., Smeets, T. J., de Rie, M. A., Dijkmans, B. A., Vaishnaw, A. K., Bos, J. D. & Tak, P. P. (2002). Alefacept treatment in psoriatic arthritis: reduction of the effector T cell population in peripheral blood and synovial tissue is associated with improvement of clinical signs of arthritis. *Arthritis Rheum* Vol. 46, No. 10, pp. 2776-2784, ISSN. 0004-3591

Krueger, G. G. & Jederberg, W. W. (1980). Alteration of HeLa cell growth equilibrium by supernatants of peripheral blood mononuclear cells from normal and psoriatic subjects. *J Invest Dermatol* Vol. 74, No. 3, pp. 148-153, ISSN. 0022-202X

Krueger, G. G., Jederberg, W. W., Ogden, B. E. & Reese, D. L. (1978). Inflammatory and immune cell function in psoriasis: II. Monocyte function, lymphokine production. *J Invest Dermatol* Vol. 71, No. 3, pp. 195-201, ISSN. 0022-202X

Landau, J., Gross, B. G., Newcomer, V. D. & Wright, E. T. (1965). Immunologic Response of Patients with Psoriasis. *Arch Dermatol* Vol. 91, No., pp. 607-610, ISSN. 0003-987X

Lee, E., Trepicchio, W. L., Oestreicher, J. L., Pittman, D., Wang, F., Chamian, F., Dhodapkar, M. & Krueger, J. G. (2004). Increased expression of interleukin 23 p19 and p40 in lesional skin of patients with psoriasis vulgaris. *J Exp Med* Vol. 199, No. 1, pp. 125-130, ISSN. 0022-1007

Lejeune, D., Dumoutier, L., Constantinescu, S., Kruijer, W., Schuringa, J. J. & Renauld, J. C. (2002). Interleukin-22 (IL-22) activates the JAK/STAT, ERK, JNK, and p38 MAP kinase pathways in a rat hepatoma cell line. Pathways that are shared with and distinct from IL-10. *J Biol Chem* Vol. 277, No. 37, pp. 33676-33682, ISSN. 0021-9258

Leonardi, C. L., Kimball, A. B., Papp, K. A., Yeilding, N., Guzzo, C., Wang, Y., Li, S., Dooley, L. T. & Gordon, K. B. (2008). Efficacy and safety of ustekinumab, a human interleukin-12/23 monoclonal antibody, in patients with psoriasis: 76-week results from a randomised, double-blind, placebo-controlled trial (PHOENIX 1). *Lancet* Vol. 371, No. 9625, pp. 1665-1674, ISSN. 1474-547X

Liang, S. C., Tan, X. Y., Luxenberg, D. P., Karim, R., Dunussi-Joannopoulos, K., Collins, M. & Fouser, L. A. (2006). Interleukin (IL)-22 and IL-17 are coexpressed by Th17 cells and cooperatively enhance expression of antimicrobial peptides. *J Exp Med* Vol. 203, No. 10, pp. 2271-2279, ISSN. 0022-1007

Lieden, G. & Skogh, M. (1986). Plasma exchange and leukapheresis in psoriasis--no effect? *Arch Dermatol Res* Vol. 278, No. 6, pp. 437-440, ISSN. 0340-3696

Lillis, J. V., Guo, C. S., Lee, J. J. & Blauvelt, A. (2010). Increased IL-23 expression in palmoplantar psoriasis and hyperkeratotic hand dermatitis. *Arch Dermatol* Vol. 146, No. 8, pp. 918-919, ISSN. 1538-3652

Lima, X. T., Abuabara, K., Kimball, A. B. & Lima, H. C. (2009a). Briakinumab. *Expert Opin Biol Ther* Vol. 9, No. 8, pp. 1107-1113, ISSN. 1744-7682

Lima, X. T., Seidler, E. M., Lima, H. C. & Kimball, A. B. (2009b). Long-term safety of biologics in dermatology. *Dermatol Ther* Vol. 22, No. 1, pp. 2-21, ISSN. 1529-8019

Liu, J., Marino, M. W., Wong, G., Grail, D., Dunn, A., Bettadapura, J., Slavin, A. J., Old, L. & Bernard, C. C. (1998). TNF is a potent anti-inflammatory cytokine in autoimmune-mediated demyelination. *Nat Med* Vol. 4, No. 1, pp. 78-83, ISSN. 1078-8956

Lowes, M. A., Bowcock, A. M. & Krueger, J. G. (2007). Pathogenesis and therapy of psoriasis. *Nature* Vol. 445, No. 7130, pp. 866-873, ISSN. 1476-4687

Lowes, M. A., Kikuchi, T., Fuentes-Duculan, J., Cardinale, I., Zaba, L. C., Haider, A. S., Bowman, E. P. & Krueger, J. G. (2008). Psoriasis vulgaris lesions contain discrete populations of Th1 and Th17 T cells. *J Invest Dermatol* Vol. 128, No. 5, pp. 1207-1211, ISSN. 1523-1747

Lutsiak, M. E., Semnani, R. T., De Pascalis, R., Kashmiri, S. V., Schlom, J. & Sabzevari, H. (2005). Inhibition of CD4(+)25+ T regulatory cell function implicated in enhanced immune response by low-dose cyclophosphamide. *Blood* Vol. 105, No. 7, pp. 2862-2868, ISSN. 0006-4971

Macatonia, S. E., Hosken, N. A., Litton, M., Vieira, P., Hsieh, C. S., Culpepper, J. A., Wysocka, M., Trinchieri, G., Murphy, K. M. & O'Garra, A. (1995). Dendritic cells produce IL-12 and direct the development of Th1 cells from naive CD4+ T cells. *J Immunol* Vol. 154, No. 10, pp. 5071-5079, ISSN. 0022-1767

MacLennan, C., Fieschi, C., Lammas, D. A., Picard, C., Dorman, S. E., Sanal, O., MacLennan, J. M., Holland, S. M., Ottenhoff, T. H., Casanova, J. L. & Kumararatne, D. S. (2004). Interleukin (IL)-12 and IL-23 are key cytokines for immunity against Salmonella in humans. *J Infect Dis* Vol. 190, No. 10, pp. 1755-1757, ISSN. 0022-1899

Miossec, P., Korn, T. & Kuchroo, V. K. (2009). Interleukin-17 and type 17 helper T cells. *N Engl J Med* Vol. 361, No. 9, pp. 888-898, ISSN. 1533-4406

Monteleone, G., Pallone, F., MacDonald, T. T., Chimenti, S. & Costanzo, A. (2011). Psoriasis: from pathogenesis to novel therapeutic approaches. *Clin Sci (Lond)* Vol. 120, No. 1, pp. 1-11, ISSN. 1470-8736

Monteleone, I., Pallone, F. & Monteleone, G. (2009). Interleukin-23 and Th17 cells in the control of gut inflammation. *Mediators Inflamm* Vol. 2009, No., pp. 297645, ISSN. 1466-1861

Mosmann, T. R., Cherwinski, H., Bond, M. W., Giedlin, M. A. & Coffman, R. L. (1986). Two types of murine helper T cell clone. I. Definition according to profiles of lymphokine activities and secreted proteins. *J Immunol* Vol. 136, No. 7, pp. 2348-2357, ISSN. 0022-1767

Nair, R. P., Ding, J., Duffin, K. C., Helms, C., Voorhees, J. J., Krueger, G. G., Bowcock, A. M., Abecasis, G. R. & Elder, J. T. (2009). Psoriasis bench to bedside: genetics meets immunology. *Arch Dermatol* Vol. 145, No. 4, pp. 462-464, ISSN. 1538-3652

Nestle, F. O., Kaplan, D. H. & Barker, J. (2009). Psoriasis. *N Engl J Med* Vol. 361, No. 5, pp. 496-509, ISSN. 1533-4406

Nickoloff, B. J. & Nestle, F. O. (2004). Recent insights into the immunopathogenesis of psoriasis provide new therapeutic opportunities. *J Clin Invest* Vol. 113, No. 12, pp. 1664-1675, ISSN. 0021-9738

Nickoloff, B. J., Schroder, J. M., von den Driesch, P., Raychaudhuri, S. P., Farber, E. M., Boehncke, W. H., Morhenn, V. B., Rosenberg, E. W., Schon, M. P. & Holick, M. F. (2000). Is psoriasis a T-cell disease? *Exp Dermatol* Vol. 9, No. 5, pp. 359-375, ISSN. 0906-6705

Nograles, K. E., Zaba, L. C., Guttman-Yassky, E., Fuentes-Duculan, J., Suarez-Farinas, M., Cardinale, I., Khatcherian, A., Gonzalez, J., Pierson, K. C., White, T. R., Pensabene, C., Coats, I., Novitskaya, I., Lowes, M. A. & Krueger, J. G. (2008). Th17 cytokines interleukin (IL)-17 and IL-22 modulate distinct inflammatory and keratinocyte-response pathways. *Br J Dermatol* Vol. 159, No. 5, pp. 1092-1102, ISSN. 1365-2133

Nograles, K. E., Zaba, L. C., Shemer, A., Fuentes-Duculan, J., Cardinale, I., Kikuchi, T., Ramon, M., Bergman, R., Krueger, J. G. & Guttman-Yassky, E. (2009). IL-22-producing "T22" T cells account for upregulated IL-22 in atopic dermatitis despite reduced IL-17-producing TH17 T cells. *J Allergy Clin Immunol* Vol. 123, No. 6, pp. 1244-1252 e1242, ISSN. 1097-6825

Okamura, H., Tsutsi, H., Komatsu, T., Yutsudo, M., Hakura, A., Tanimoto, T., Torigoe, K., Okura, T., Nukada, Y., Hattori, K. & et al. (1995). Cloning of a new cytokine that induces IFN-gamma production by T cells. *Nature* Vol. 378, No. 6552, pp. 88-91, ISSN. 0028-0836

Oppmann, B., Lesley, R., Blom, B., Timans, J. C., Xu, Y., Hunte, B., Vega, F., Yu, N., Wang, J., Singh, K., Zonin, F., Vaisberg, E., Churakova, T., Liu, M., Gorman, D., Wagner, J., Zurawski, S., Liu, Y., Abrams, J. S., Moore, K. W., Rennick, D., de Waal-Malefyt, R., Hannum, C., Bazan, J. F. & Kastelein, R. A. (2000). Novel p19 protein engages IL-12p40 to form a cytokine, IL-23, with biological activities similar as well as distinct from IL-12. *Immunity* Vol. 13, No. 5, pp. 715-725, ISSN. 1074-7613

Ortega, C., Fernandez, A. S., Carrillo, J. M., Romero, P., Molina, I. J., Moreno, J. C. & Santamaria, M. (2009). IL-17-producing CD8+ T lymphocytes from psoriasis skin plaques are cytotoxic effector cells that secrete Th17-related cytokines. *J Leukoc Biol* Vol. 86, No. 2, pp. 435-443, ISSN. 1938-3673

Parham, C., Chirica, M., Timans, J., Vaisberg, E., Travis, M., Cheung, J., Pflanz, S., Zhang, R., Singh, K. P., Vega, F., To, W., Wagner, J., O'Farrell, A. M., McClanahan, T., Zurawski, S., Hannum, C., Gorman, D., Rennick, D. M., Kastelein, R. A., de Waal Malefyt, R. & Moore, K. W. (2002). A receptor for the heterodimeric cytokine IL-23 is composed of IL-12Rbeta1 and a novel cytokine receptor subunit, IL-23R. *J Immunol* Vol. 168, No. 11, pp. 5699-5708, ISSN. 0022-1767

Philipp, S., Wolk, K., Kreutzer, S., Wallace, E., Ludwig, N., Roewert, J., Hoflich, C., Volk, H. D., Sterry, W. & Sabat, R. (2006). The evaluation of psoriasis therapy with biologics leads to a revision of the current view of the pathogenesis of this disorder. *Expert Opin Ther Targets* Vol. 10, No. 6, pp. 817-831, ISSN. 1744-7631

Piskin, G., Sylva-Steenland, R. M., Bos, J. D. & Teunissen, M. B. (2006). In vitro and in situ expression of IL-23 by keratinocytes in healthy skin and psoriasis lesions: enhanced expression in psoriatic skin. *J Immunol* Vol. 176, No. 3, pp. 1908-1915, ISSN. 0022-1767

Ramos-Casals, M., Brito-Zeron, P., Soto, M. J., Cuadrado, M. J. & Khamashta, M. A. (2008). Autoimmune diseases induced by TNF-targeted therapies. *Best Pract Res Clin Rheumatol* Vol. 22, No. 5, pp. 847-861, ISSN. 1532-1770

Ramsdell, F. & Fowlkes, B. J. (1990). Clonal deletion versus clonal anergy: the role of the thymus in inducing self tolerance. *Science* Vol. 248, No. 4961, pp. 1342-1348, ISSN. 0036-8075

Rizzo, H. L., Kagami, S., Phillips, K. G., Kurtz, S. E., Jacques, S. L. & Blauvelt, A. (2011). IL-23-mediated psoriasis-like epidermal hyperplasia is dependent on IL-17A. *J Immunol* Vol. 186, No. 3, pp. 1495-1502, ISSN. 1550-6606

Romagnani, S., Maggi, E., Liotta, F., Cosmi, L. & Annunziato, F. (2009). Properties and origin of human Th17 cells. *Mol Immunol* Vol. 47, No. 1, pp. 3-7, ISSN. 1872-9142

Rudner, X. L., Happel, K. I., Young, E. A. & Shellito, J. E. (2007). Interleukin-23 (IL-23)-IL-17 cytokine axis in murine Pneumocystis carinii infection. *Infect Immun* Vol. 75, No. 6, pp. 3055-3061, ISSN. 0019-9567

Sa, S. M., Valdez, P. A., Wu, J., Jung, K., Zhong, F., Hall, L., Kasman, I., Winer, J., Modrusan, Z., Danilenko, D. M. & Ouyang, W. (2007). The effects of IL-20 subfamily cytokines on reconstituted human epidermis suggest potential roles in cutaneous innate defense and pathogenic adaptive immunity in psoriasis. *J Immunol* Vol. 178, No. 4, pp. 2229-2240, ISSN. 0022-1767

Sabat, R., Philipp, S., Hoflich, C., Kreutzer, S., Wallace, E., Asadullah, K., Volk, H. D., Sterry, W. & Wolk, K. (2007). Immunopathogenesis of psoriasis. *Exp Dermatol* Vol. 16, No. 10, pp. 779-798, ISSN. 0906-6705

Sabat, R. & Wolk, K. (2011). Research in practice: IL-22 and IL-20: significance for epithelial homeostasis and psoriasis pathogenesis. *J Dtsch Dermatol Ges* Vol., No., pp., ISSN. 1610-0387

Sakaguchi, S., Sakaguchi, N., Shimizu, J., Yamazaki, S., Sakihama, T., Itoh, M., Kuniyasu, Y., Nomura, T., Toda, M. & Takahashi, T. (2001). Immunologic tolerance maintained by CD25+ CD4+ regulatory T cells: their common role in controlling autoimmunity, tumor immunity, and transplantation tolerance. *Immunol Rev* Vol. 182, No., pp. 18-32, ISSN. 0105-2896

Sakaguchi, S., Toda, M., Asano, M., Itoh, M., Morse, S. S. & Sakaguchi, N. (1996). T cell-mediated maintenance of natural self-tolerance: its breakdown as a possible cause of various autoimmune diseases. *J Autoimmun* Vol. 9, No. 2, pp. 211-220, ISSN. 0896-8411

Savan, R., McFarland, A. P., Reynolds, D. A., Feigenbaum, L., Ramakrishnan, K., Karwan, M., Shirota, H., Klinman, D. M., Dunleavy, K., Pittaluga, S., Anderson, S. K., Donnelly, R. P., Wilson, W. H. & Young, H. A. (2011). A novel role for IL-22R1 as a driver of inflammation. *Blood* Vol. 117, No. 2, pp. 575-584, ISSN. 1528-0020

Scarpa, R., Altomare, G., Marchesoni, A., Balato, N., Matucci Cerinic, M., Lotti, T., Olivieri, I., Vena, G. A., Salvarani, C., Valesini, G. & Giannetti, A. (2010). Psoriatic disease: concepts and implications. *J Eur Acad Dermatol Venereol* Vol. 24, No. 6, pp. 627-630, ISSN. 1468-3083

Schlaak, J. F., Buslau, M., Jochum, W., Hermann, E., Girndt, M., Gallati, H., Meyer zum Buschenfelde, K. H. & Fleischer, B. (1994). T cells involved in psoriasis vulgaris belong to the Th1 subset. *J Invest Dermatol* Vol. 102, No. 2, pp. 145-149, ISSN. 0022-202X

Schon, M. P. & Boehncke, W. H. (2005). Psoriasis. *N Engl J Med* Vol. 352, No. 18, pp. 1899-1912, ISSN. 1533-4406

Sewgobind, V. D., van der Laan, L. J., Kho, M. M., Kraaijeveld, R., Korevaar, S. S., Mol, W., Weimar, W. & Baan, C. C. (2010). The calcineurin inhibitor tacrolimus allows the induction of functional CD4CD25 regulatory T cells by rabbit anti-thymocyte globulins. *Clin Exp Immunol* Vol. 161, No. 2, pp. 364-377, ISSN. 1365-2249

Shear, N. H., Prinz, J., Papp, K., Langley, R. G. & Gulliver, W. P. (2008). Targeting the interleukin-12/23 cytokine family in the treatment of psoriatic disease. *J Cutan Med Surg* Vol. 12 Suppl 1, No., pp. S1-10, ISSN. 1203-4754

Shehata, I. H. & Elghandour, T. M. (2007). A possible pathogenic role of CD4+CD25+ T-regulatory cells in psoriasis. *Egypt J Immunol* Vol. 14, No. 1, pp. 21-31, ISSN. 1110-4902

Shevach, E. M., Thornton, A. & Suri-Payer, E. (1998). T lymphocyte-mediated control of autoimmunity. *Novartis Found Symp* Vol. 215, No., pp. 200-211; discussion 211-230, ISSN. 1528-2511

Shuster, S. (1971). Research into psoriasis--the last decade. *Br Med J* Vol. 3, No. 5768, pp. 236-239, ISSN. 0007-1447

Sobell, J. M., Kalb, R. E. & Weinberg, J. M. (2009). Management of moderate to severe plaque psoriasis (part 2): clinical update on T-cell modulators and investigational agents. *J Drugs Dermatol* Vol. 8, No. 3, pp. 230-238, ISSN. 1545-9616

Squire, B. (1873). The Etiology of Psoriasis. *Br Med J* Vol. 1, No. Feb, pp. 141, ISSN.

Stock, P., Akbari, O., DeKruyff, R. H. & Umetsu, D. T. (2005). Respiratory tolerance is inhibited by the administration of corticosteroids. *J Immunol* Vol. 175, No. 11, pp. 7380-7387, ISSN. 0022-1767

Sugiyama, H., Gyulai, R., Toichi, E., Garaczi, E., Shimada, S., Stevens, S. R., McCormick, T. S. & Cooper, K. D. (2005). Dysfunctional blood and target tissue CD4+CD25high regulatory T cells in psoriasis: mechanism underlying unrestrained pathogenic effector T cell proliferation. *J Immunol* Vol. 174, No. 1, pp. 164-173, ISSN. 0022-1767

Toichi, E., Torres, G., McCormick, T. S., Chang, T., Mascelli, M. A., Kauffman, C. L., Aria, N., Gottlieb, A. B., Everitt, D. E., Frederick, B., Pendley, C. E. & Cooper, K. D. (2006). An anti-IL-12p40 antibody down-regulates type 1 cytokines, chemokines, and IL-12/IL-23 in psoriasis. *J Immunol* Vol. 177, No. 7, pp. 4917-4926, ISSN. 0022-1767

Tonel, G., Conrad, C., Laggner, U., Di Meglio, P., Grys, K., McClanahan, T. K., Blumenschein, W. M., Qin, J. Z., Xin, H., Oldham, E., Kastelein, R., Nickoloff, B. J. & Nestle, F. O. (2010). Cutting edge: A critical functional role for IL-23 in psoriasis. *J Immunol* Vol. 185, No. 10, pp. 5688-5691, ISSN. 1550-6606

Trinchieri, G. (1998). Interleukin-12: a cytokine at the interface of inflammation and immunity. *Adv Immunol* Vol. 70, No., pp. 83-243, ISSN. 0065-2776

Trinchieri, G., Pflanz, S. & Kastelein, R. A. (2003). The IL-12 family of heterodimeric cytokines: new players in the regulation of T cell responses. *Immunity* Vol. 19, No. 5, pp. 641-644, ISSN. 1074-7613

Valdimarsson, H., Bake, B. S., Jónsdótdr, I. & Fry, L. (1986). Psoriasis: a disease of abnormal Keratinocyte proliferation induced by T lymphocytes. *Immunology Today* Vol. 7, No. 9, pp. 256-259, ISSN. 0167-5699

Vanaudenaerde, B. M., Verleden, S. E., Vos, R., De Vleeschauwer, S. I., Willems-Widyastuti, A., Geenens, R., Van Raemdonck, D. E., Dupont, L. J., Verbeken, E. K. & Meyts, I. (2010). Innate and Adaptive IL-17 Producing Lymphocytes in Chronic Inflammatory Lung Disorders. *Am J Respir Crit Care Med* Vol., No., pp., ISSN. 1535-4970

Vaz, N. M., Ramos, G. C., Pordeus, V. & Carvalho, C. R. (2006). The conservative physiology of the immune system. A non-metaphoric approach to immunological activity. *Clin Dev Immunol* Vol. 13, No. 2-4, pp. 133-142, ISSN. 1740-2522

Volpe, E., Servant, N., Zollinger, R., Bogiatzi, S. I., Hupe, P., Barillot, E. & Soumelis, V. (2008). A critical function for transforming growth factor-beta, interleukin 23 and proinflammatory cytokines in driving and modulating human T(H)-17 responses. *Nat Immunol* Vol. 9, No. 6, pp. 650-657, ISSN. 1529-2916

Vukmanovic-Stejic, M., McQuaid, A., Birch, K. E., Reed, J. R., Macgregor, C., Rustin, M. H. & Akbar, A. N. (2005). Relative impact of CD4+CD25+ regulatory T cells and tacrolimus on inhibition of T-cell proliferation in patients with atopic dermatitis. *Br J Dermatol* Vol. 153, No. 4, pp. 750-757, ISSN. 0007-0963

Watanabe, H., Kawaguchi, M., Fujishima, S., Ogura, M., Matsukura, S., Takeuchi, H., Ohba, M., Sueki, H., Kokubu, F., Hizawa, N., Adachi, M., Huang, S. K. & Iijima, M. (2009). Functional characterization of IL-17F as a selective neutrophil attractant in psoriasis. *J Invest Dermatol* Vol. 129, No. 3, pp. 650-656, ISSN. 1523-1747

Weiner, H. L., da Cunha, A. P., Quintana, F. & Wu, H. (2011). Oral tolerance. *Immunol Rev* Vol. 241, No. 1, pp. 241-259, ISSN. 1600-065X

Wilhelm, A. J., Zabalawi, M., Owen, J. S., Shah, D., Grayson, J. M., Major, A. S., Bhat, S., Gibbs, D. P., Jr., Thomas, M. J. & Sorci-Thomas, M. G. (2010). Apolipoprotein A-I modulates regulatory T cells in autoimmune LDLr-/-, ApoA-I-/- mice. *J Biol Chem* Vol. 285, No. 46, pp. 36158-36169, ISSN. 1083-351X

Wilson, N. J., Boniface, K., Chan, J. R., McKenzie, B. S., Blumenschein, W. M., Mattson, J. D., Basham, B., Smith, K., Chen, T., Morel, F., Lecron, J. C., Kastelein, R. A., Cua, D. J., McClanahan, T. K., Bowman, E. P. & de Waal Malefyt, R. (2007). Development, cytokine profile and function of human interleukin 17-producing helper T cells. *Nat Immunol* Vol. 8, No. 9, pp. 950-957, ISSN. 1529-2908

Wolk, K., Haugen, H. S., Xu, W., Witte, E., Waggie, K., Anderson, M., Vom Baur, E., Witte, K., Warszawska, K., Philipp, S., Johnson-Leger, C., Volk, H. D., Sterry, W. & Sabat, R. (2009a). IL-22 and IL-20 are key mediators of the epidermal alterations in psoriasis while IL-17 and IFN-gamma are not. *J Mol Med* Vol. 87, No. 5, pp. 523-536, ISSN. 1432-1440

Wolk, K., Kunz, S., Asadullah, K. & Sabat, R. (2002). Cutting edge: immune cells as sources and targets of the IL-10 family members? *J Immunol* Vol. 168, No. 11, pp. 5397-5402, ISSN. 0022-1767

Wolk, K., Kunz, S., Witte, E., Friedrich, M., Asadullah, K. & Sabat, R. (2004). IL-22 increases the innate immunity of tissues. *Immunity* Vol. 21, No. 2, pp. 241-254, ISSN. 1074-7613

Wolk, K., Witte, E., Wallace, E., Docke, W. D., Kunz, S., Asadullah, K., Volk, H. D., Sterry, W. & Sabat, R. (2006). IL-22 regulates the expression of genes responsible for antimicrobial defense, cellular differentiation, and mobility in keratinocytes: a potential role in psoriasis. *Eur J Immunol* Vol. 36, No. 5, pp. 1309-1323, ISSN. 0014-2980

Wolk, K., Witte, E., Warszawska, K., Schulze-Tanzil, G., Witte, K., Philipp, S., Kunz, S., Docke, W. D., Asadullah, K., Volk, H. D., Sterry, W. & Sabat, R. (2009b). The Th17 cytokine IL-22 induces IL-20 production in keratinocytes: A novel immunological cascade with potential relevance in psoriasis. *Eur J Immunol* Vol., No., pp., ISSN. 1521-4141

Yeilding, N., Szapary, P., Brodmerkel, C., Benson, J., Plotnick, M., Zhou, H., Goyal, K., Schenkel, B., Giles-Komar, J., Mascelli, M. A. & Guzzo, C. (2011). Development of the IL-12/23 antagonist ustekinumab in psoriasis: past, present, and future perspectives. *Ann N Y Acad Sci* Vol. 1222, No., pp. 30-39, ISSN. 1749-6632

Yu, P., Lee, Y., Liu, W., Krausz, T., Chong, A., Schreiber, H. & Fu, Y. X. (2005). Intratumor depletion of CD4+ cells unmasks tumor immunogenicity leading to the rejection of late-stage tumors. *J Exp Med* Vol. 201, No. 5, pp. 779-791, ISSN. 0022-1007

Zaba, L. C., Cardinale, I., Gilleaudeau, P., Sullivan-Whalen, M., Suarez-Farinas, M., Fuentes-Duculan, J., Novitskaya, I., Khatcherian, A., Bluth, M. J., Lowes, M. A. & Krueger, J. G. (2007). Amelioration of epidermal hyperplasia by TNF inhibition is associated with reduced Th17 responses. *J Exp Med* Vol. 204, No. 13, pp. 3183-3194, ISSN. 1540-9538

Zheng, Y., Danilenko, D. M., Valdez, P., Kasman, I., Eastham-Anderson, J., Wu, J. & Ouyang, W. (2007). Interleukin-22, a T(H)17 cytokine, mediates IL-23-induced dermal inflammation and acanthosis. *Nature* Vol. 445, No. 7128, pp. 648-651, ISSN. 1476-4687

8

Psoriasis

Adolfo Fernandez-Obregon
Hoboken
USA

1. Introduction

Psoriasis is a common, chronic inflammatory and proliferative condition of the skin, sometimes affecting joints, in which both genetic and environmental influences play a critical role. Most characteristically, it consists of scaly, sharply demarcated red and indurated plaques, present particularly over extensor surfaces sometimes overlying the joints, and occasionally involving the scalp.

2. Epidemiology

Psoriasis affects between 2% and 3% of people worldwide. [1] This varies from an incidence of 1.5% to 4.8% in Northern Europe [2] to China, where the lower prevalence of 0.3% has been observed. [3] Nearly one quarter of these have moderate to severe psoriasis consistent with involvement of >3% of body surface area. Women (OR = 1.37, 95% CI: 1.14–1.64) are slightly more likely than men and African Americans less likely than Caucasians (OR = 0.54; 95% CI: 0.34–0.85) to report a psoriasis diagnosis. [4]

Psoriasis can develop at any age, but symptoms typically first appear between ages 15 and 25 years. Approximately one half of patients diagnosed with psoriasis report suffering with pruritus. [5] In a large US survey, the average age of onset was 28 years, while in China it was 36. In other studies, both sexes appear to be equally affected. Table 1 shows world-wide studies on prevalence of psoriasis.

Looking at the white population in Rochester, MN, Bell *et al* reported an incidence of 60.4 per 100,000 adjusted for sex and age, during the 1980 Rochester Epidemiology Project. [6] From the same project Shbeeb *et al* looked at the population from 1982 and 1991 and reported a rising incidence to 107.7 per 100,000. [7] Those same increasing trends were confirmed by similar studies by Icen *et al* in the same population, and by Huerta *et al* looking at the population in the United Kingdom. [8] [9] The reasons for this increase cannot be explained alone on known genetic factors. Other environmental influences or unknown genetic factors may play a role in this observation. The lack of obvious family history in many cases of newly diagnosed disease underscores this concept.

3. Genetic & environmental causes

3.1 Genetic basis of psoriasis

A search for the genetic basis of psoriasis has been seriously undertaken by Gunnar Lomholt who studied heredity in residents of the Faroe Islands. Farber and Nall subsequently studied the concordance rates in monozygotic twins and documented kindreds having multiple family members afflicted with the diseases. [10] [11] Population studies revealed a higher incidence of psoriasis among first- and second-degree relatives than in the general population. However, just as the pathogenesis is complex, the mode of inheritance is also complex. Of nine distinct chromosomal loci, 7 of which have been clearly identified as being associated with psoriasis.

World Region & Reference	Prevalence (%)
Europe	
Norway	1.4-4.8
Sweden	2.3
Denmark 28	2;5-3.2
United Kingdom 28	1.5-2.8
Croatia 28	1.55
Italy	0.8-4.5
Germany	2.5-3.5
France	3.58-5.2
Spain	1.43
Czechoslovakia 28	1.2
Hungary 28	2.0
Netherlands 28	1.8
New World	
North America 28	0.5 – 4.7
African-Americans	1.3
Newfoundland, Canada	2-3
South America 28 28	0.2-4.2
Caribbean 28 28	1.3-6.0
Africa	
West Africa 28	0.05-0.9
East Africa 28	2.8-3.5
North Africa 28	3.0
South Africa 28	1.5
Oceania	
Australian Aborigines	0.47
Australian Caucasians	2.3-2.57
Samoa Islands 28	0
Asia	
China 28 28	0.05-1.23
Japan 28	0.29-1.18
India 28	0.5-2.3
Malaysia 28	1.1-5.5

Table 1. Worldwide Prevalence of Psoriasis

The most important genetic determinant of psoriasis is PSORS1 (psoriasis susceptibility locus), widely considered to be a susceptibility locus for the development of psoriasis accounting probably for 35 to 50% of the heritability of the disease. [12] PSORS1 is found within the major histocompatibility complex (MHC) on chromosome 6p. Identification of the specific gene has been difficult because of the extensive linkage disequilibrium observed within the MHC. There are 3 genes within this locus that are strongly associated with inheriting the disease. [13] [14] These genes code proteins that may be over-expressed in psoriasis.[15] Others are found are exclusively found in the granular and cornified layers of the epidermis. [16] Studies show variants of psoriasis may be genetically heterogeneous. Guttate psoriasis appears to be strongly associated with PSORS1, [17] as opposed to late onset cases of psoriasis, generally occurring in persons over 50 years of age. [18]

Genetic Marker	Chromosome Location	Function	Associated Diseases
PSOR 1 54, 55 [19]	6p	HLA-CW6 & corneodesmposin	?
PSOR 2 62	17q	Immune synapse	?
IL12B 63, 64 [20]	5q	T-cell differentiation	Crohn's Disease
IL23R 55, 68, 69, [21] [22]	1p	T-cell differentiation	Crohn's Disease, ankylosing spondylitis, psoriatic arthritis, type I diabetes, celiac disease
ZNF 313 (RNF114) 55 69	20q	Ubiquitin pathway	?
CDKAL1 [23] [24]	6p	?	Crohn's Disease, type 2 diabetes mellitus
PTPN22 75, [25] [26]	6p	T cell signaling	Type 1 diabetes mellitus, juvenile idiopathic arthritis, systemic lupus erythematosus, rheumatoid arthritis, autoimmune thyroid disease
IL-4 - IL-13 cytokine gene cluster 55 [27]	5q	T-cell differentiation	Crohn's Disease (variant)
LCE3B/3C 66 [28]	1q	Epidermal differentiation	

Table 2. Genetic Markers associated with Psoriasis

PSORS2 is the second gene locus found associated with psoriasis. [29] Two genes in this region, SLC9A3R1 and NAT9, reside in chromosome 17q24-q25. [30] They contribute to the immunopathogenesis of psoriasis through their role on immunological synapse. This refers to the signaling accomplished by multimolecular complex formation between the mature T cell through its receptor (TCR), and the antigen presenting cell (APC). Through a series of adhesion molecules, like LFA-1, T cells can bind to ICAM-1 expressed in an adjacent cell like a keratinocyte or APC. The LFA-1 component was found particularly useful in therapy. By blocking this adhesion interaction, efalizumab was used to treat psoriasis. [31] Other adhesion molecules exist, and have been evaluated for a possible role in defining hereditary patterns of psoriasis and targeting these processes for therapy. For instance, LFA-3 Ig fusion protein (alefacept) has been found to reduce psoriasis lesions.[32]

Additional findings suggest LCE3B/3C, located within the epidermal differentiation complex on chromosome 1, is also strongly associated with the development of psoriasis. [33] Deletion of these genes is associated with a significant fraction in individuals of European ancestry with psoriasis. [34] Other genes that have been linked to psoriasis include ZNF313 (allele RNF114), which plays a role in the ubiquitin pathway, and CDKAL1, the function of which is not known at this time. [35] PTPN22 plays a role in T cell signaling. Other associations involve variants of the gene encoding the IL-23 receptor (IL-23R) and a region of the IL-12B (p40) gene as being closely linked to risk for psoriasis. IL-23R also appears in association with psoriatic arthritis and ankylosing spondylitis. CDKAL1 shows association with psoriasis and Crohn's disease, and type 2 diabetes mellitus. [36] [37] Nearly all of the genes listed are associated with the immune response strongly implicating an immunologic basis for the pathogenesis of psoriasis.

3.2 Environmental causes of psoriasis

As with many other diseases, there are interactions between genetic factors and the environment. Psoriatic lesions appearing at the site of injury are a well known phenomenon (Koebner or isomorphic response). This injury can be a physical, chemical, electrical, infective, sun-burn or other inflammatory insult. The reverse Koebner phenomenon has also been observed to occur and refers to clearing of psoriasis after an injury or illness. [38]

Streptococcal infection has been shown to precede the onset of guttate psoriasis, especially in those with a family history of plaque psoriasis, and drugs have been implicated as an initial cause or exacerbating bouts of psoriasis. [39] Among these are lithium salts, antimalarials, beta-adrenergic blocking agents, non-steroidal anti-inflammatory drugs, angiotensin converting enzyme inhibitors, and the sudden withdrawal of corticosteroids. [40]

Other factors that may play a role include pregnancy, [41] alcohol, smoking, [42] psychogenic stress factors [43] and concomitant HIV disease and acquired immune deficiency. [44]

4. Psycho-social considerations

Many patients with psoriasis, particularly those with severe disease, are frustrated with the management of their disease and the ineffectiveness of their therapies. A National Psoriasis Foundation (NPF) survey looking at a large number of patients revealed individuals suffering with psoriasis want to communicate their frustrations about their disease, and the disappointment about their treatments.[45]

Other studies reported that psoriasis sufferers experience difficulties in the workplace and in socialization with family members and friends, exclusion from public facilities, difficulties obtaining a job, and even contemplation of suicide. Other opinions expressed included feeling embarrassed, unattractive and depressed. The disease process was often described as a large problem in everyday life, influencing the choice of clothing used to cover psoriasis. Many claimed psoriasis interfered with their ability to sleep, and interfered with their sexual activities. About one third of those evaluated claimed having problems using their hands, walking, sitting, or standing for prolonged periods. [46] Another study reported 48% of respondents were not working, 20% of whom attributed their unemployment to their psoriasis or psoriatic arthritis. [47]

5. Clinical presentation – Subtypes of psoriasis (adults & children)

Psoriasis most commonly presents as the chronic stable large plaque disorder commonly referred to as psoriasis vulgaris. The scales are silvery and have been described as "micaceous" on an underlying salmon pink in color. The thickened epidermis allows the cutaneous vessels to come very close to the scaly *stratum corneum*. Dislodging the scale in essence causes a tear in the epidermis resulting in bleeding, known as the Auspitz sign. Psoriasis plaques are characterized by thickened silvery white scales on a red base of skin. Lesions may occur as a few small plaques or become more widespread throughout the body. [48] In one survey, the most frequent symptoms experienced were scaling, itching, skin redness, lightness of the skin, bleeding at lesion sites, burning sensation, and fatigue. [49]

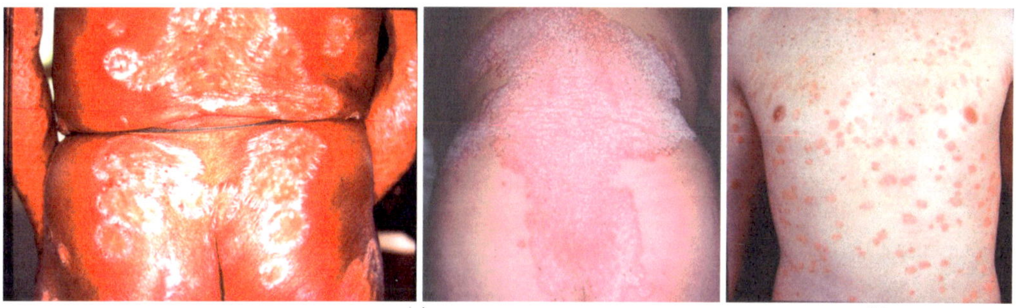

a) b)

Fig. 1. a) Large Chronic Plaque Psoriasis in an obese Caucasian and in a member of the Choclo natives of Southern Panama, with extensive plaques in spite of an outdoor life style while wearing minimal clothing. b) Guttate Psoriasis

A ring of hypopigmented normal skin often surrounds the psoriatic plaque, commonly referred o as the Woronoff ring. [50] Customarily it appears as the skin tries to repair itself, an has been used as an indication therapy is working. [51] [52]

Guttate psoriasis describes a "shower" of smaller less scaly and erythematous lesions appearing in a widespread to generalized distribution. They occur less commonly on the face. This variant occurs more commonly in children and young adults, often secondary to an acute infection, usually streptococcal.

Erythrodermic psoriasis results when chronic lesions evolve and coalesce into a generalized exfoliative phase. In this scenario it behaves either like an extensive form of large plaque psoriasis, which generally responds to therapy, or as the "unstable" form of psoriasis which can result from discontinuation of systemic corticosteroids, [53] Not commonly it can seen with joint involvement, or as the end result of a generalized pustular psoriasis. Individuals with this form tend to be febrile, highly resistant to tolerating any topical regimen, or phototherapy, and can present with metabolic complications related to sweating imbalance leading to abnormal thermoregulation, electrolyte abnormalities, intestinal absorption, and negative protein balance. [54] [55] [56]

Histological changes of psoriasis (hematoxylin and eosin), from a punch biopsy of a large plque, shows epidermal thickening with parakeratosis, and elongation of the rete ridges with mixed cellular infiltrate - T-cells an polymorphonuclear neutrophils (PMN). Vascular dilatation, and microabscesses (Munroe) with PMN form with disease progression.

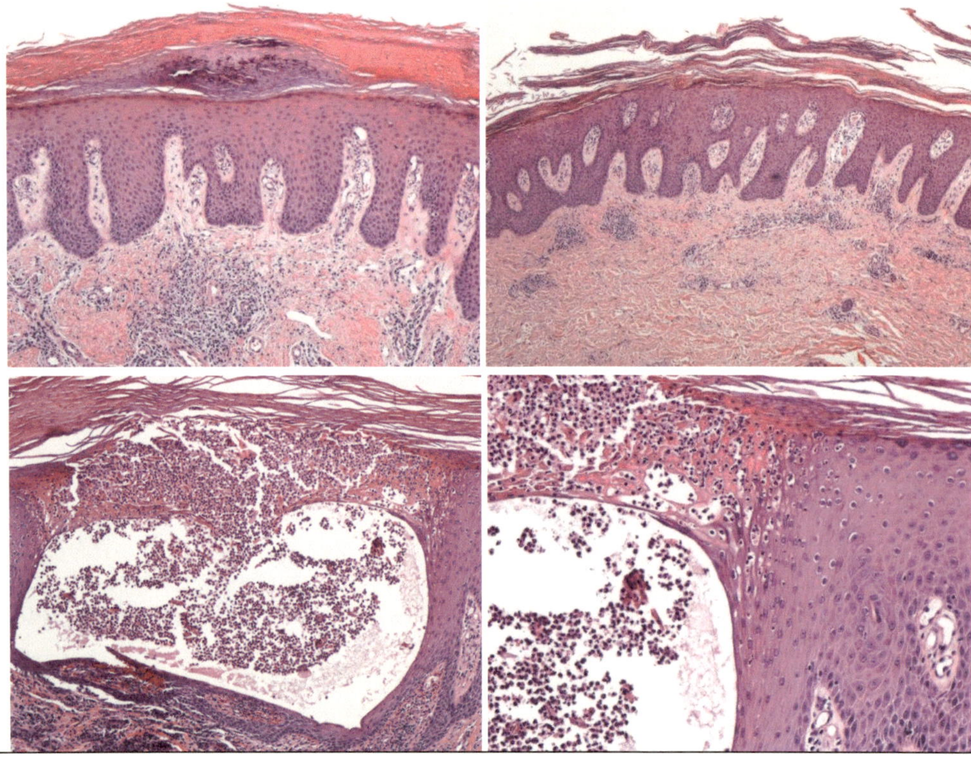

Fig. 2. Histologic Features of Psoriasis

Another manner to categorize psoriasis involves the anatomical distribution. Scalp psoriasis can be a part of large plaque psoriasis. Often it is seen as the sole anatomic area involved in the skin, presenting a therapeutic challenge due to the very thick nature of the plaques that form.

Genital involvement in males and females may occur as part of widespread disease or as a sole manifestation involving the glans mimicking erythroplasia or Zoon's balanitis. Sometimes, it can also occur on the flexural surface of the groins and vulva as part of inverse psoriasis, which can also exist on the axillas, submammary, gluteal cleft and other body folds. This is more common in older adults. Scaling is greatly reduced. Failure of these eruptions to respond to suspected fungal or yeast infections should raise suspicion.

Hands and feet may occur as well-defined plaques resembling hyperkeratotic eczema (palmo-plantar plaque psoriasis), or as a pustulosis, (palmo-plantar pustular psoriasis) or as a mixture of the two. It can be seen in connection with occupational use of irritants. [57]

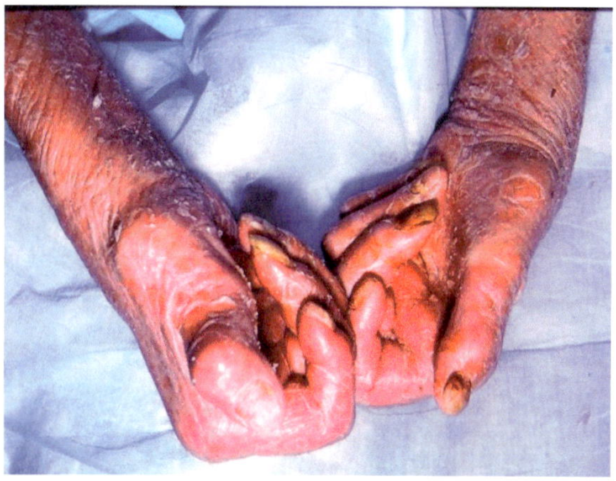

Fig. 3. Erythrodermic psoriasis & psoriatic arthritis with chronic joint deformity

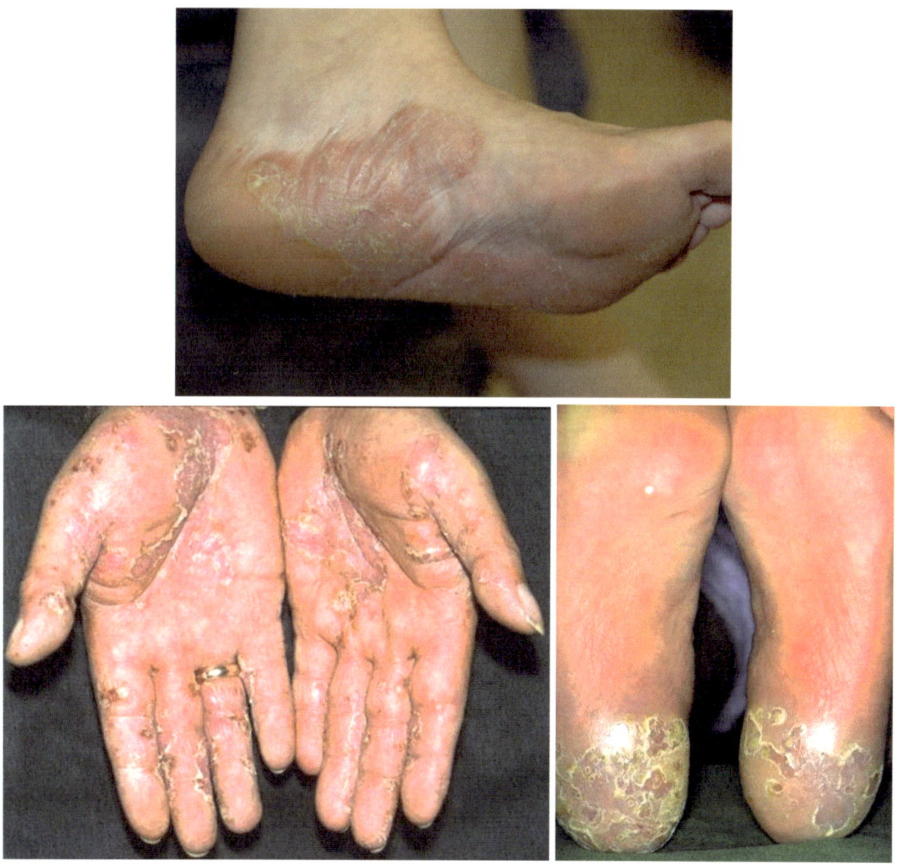

Fig. 4. Palmoplantar Plaque Psoriasis

Nail involvement can be seen in association with all types of psoriasis. It can be a predictor of psoriatic arthropathy, and as such is often seen in psoriatic patients with psoriatic arthritis. [58] Although pitting is the most frequent change seen, discoloration, subungual hyperkeratosis, and onycholysis are common. Splinter hemorrhages can occur. Nail disease is more severe in familial cases and when disease onset is early. Patients over 40 years of age are twice as affected as those under 20. [59] Longitudinal biopsy of the nail bed and matrix studies have shed some light on the cause of these changes. [60] Nail pits, ridges and grooves result from psoriasis of the nail matrix, whereas onycholysis, subungual hyperkeratosis, and splinter hemorrhages are attributable to disease of the nail bed or hyponychium. [61] Circular discoloration of the nail bed and hyponychium may resemble an "oil drop" below the nail. This observation represents histologically psoriatic change in the hyponychium. [62] Candidal onychomycosis is a common find in psoriatic nails, but dermatophytes are rare. [63]

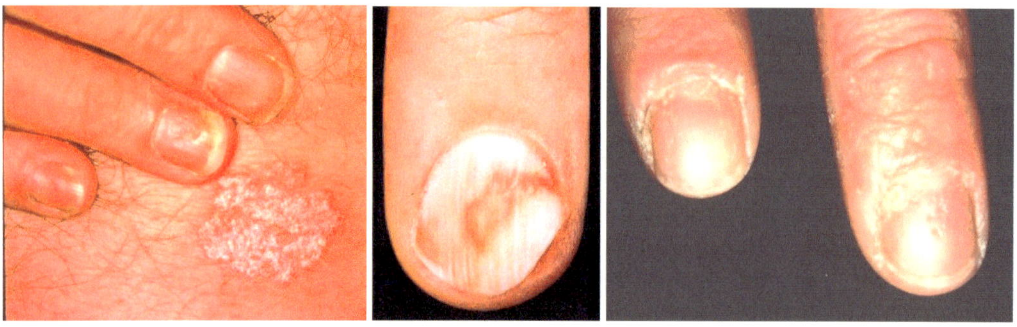

Fig. 5. Nail changes in Psoriasis

5.1 Psoriasis in children

Psoriasis occurs approximately 1/3 of the time during the first two decades of life, and is therefore quite common in children. [64] Guttate psoriasis is frequently seen in children. Inverse psoriasis can present in the form of a toe cleft intertrigo, a chronic blepharitis, or perleche on the angle of the mouth or a lateral eye lid. Psoriasis on the face occurs more often in children than in adults. Scalp involvement and a psoriatic rash in the napkin area are common.

5.2 Differential diagnosis

The rash of eczema, at times, can present with a psoriasiform appearance. As mentioned previously, psoriasis of the hands can appear indistinguishable from contact dermatitis, since irritants can often exacerbate or herald onset of activity. Lichen planus (LP) can at times have a dusky red presentation similar to early psoriasis. LP can also coexist with psoriasis. When involving skin close to the elbows, knees or shins, lichen simplex can mimic psoriasis. Pityriasis lichenoides chronica or Muccha-Habermann Disease, can appear like guttate psoriasis. Skin biopsy is sometimes necessary to differentiate these entities. Candidiasis, particularly in the flexural areas has been mistaken for psoriasis. Dermatophytosis is generally differentiated from psoriasis by the nature of the scale that spreads over the expanding margins. Pityriasis rubra pilaris and secondary syphilis can be confused with erythroderma. Lymphoma of the skin, and toxic erythema caused by drugs can present similarly with an erythrodermic presentation. Psoriasis cutaneous lymphoma, and leprosy are three clinical entities that can typically present with secondary lesions that have "skip areas." This refers to islands of normal skin appearing within the lesion.

5.3 Psoriatic arthritis

Psoriatic arthritis (PsA) is inflammatory in nature. These patients tend to present with pain, stiffness, and swelling of affected joints. [65] Up to 30% of psoriatic patients have PsA, a progressive and destructive disease. Psoriatic arthritis usually develops between 30-50 years of age. Generally, skin symptoms appear earlier than joint symptoms (70% of cases). Likelihood of developing PsA may also correlate with duration and severity of psoriasis. However, in 15 % of patients, the joint manifestations may appear before the skin changes by as many as 10-15 years. In the remaining 15% the skin and joint symptoms appear simultaneously. Sensitizing clinicians to the morbidity of these diseases may aid in optimizing psoriasis management and patient care. [66] [67] [68] [69] [70] Nail involvement is observed in 70-80% of these patients making this clinical observation a valuable predictive clinical sign for the development of PsA. 28 [71] Severity of nail disease correlates with severity of skin disease. As early as 2008, the American Academy of Dermatology (AAD) issued guidelines for the management of psoriasis and psoriatic arthritis. The most commonly affected joints were listed to be those in the wrist, knees, ankles, lower back, and neck. [72]

Prolonged morning stiffness, lasting longer than 60 minutes, is a common complaint, and results from inflammatory involvement of entheses, the point at which tendons or ligaments insert to bone. It tends to improve throughout the day. What begins as oligoarthritis (4 or less joints) may progress to polyarticular (more than 4 joints) over years, and may revert back to oligoarthritis with treatment. Though patterns of presentation are not helpful to identify PsA, the distal inter-phalangeal joint (DIP) may be the most readily recognizable because it is unique to PsA. It occurs in 5%-10% of patients and is seen predominantly in men. An asymmetric oligoarthritis occurs in 30% of cases, a large joint is generally involved like a knee, in association with a few small joints of the hands and feet, commonly with dactylitis. The polyarthritis pattern, practically as common, is seen more often in women, it involves fingers, wrists, toes and ankles. It involves DIP joints and is asymmetric. In comparison with RA, in PsA all joints of one digit tend to be involved while sparing other digits, whereas in RA the same joint is involved in all the digits. Whereas synovitis is the primary lesion of rheumatoid arthritis (RA), synovitis along with enthesitis characterizes PsA. [73] The most common sites of entheseal involvement in PsA include the attachment of the Achilles tendon or the plantar fascia to the calcaneus, as well as the ligaments around the rib cage, pelvis, vertebral bodies, posterior tibial tendon, quadriceps muscle, patellar tendon, and the elbow.

Arthritis mutilans of hands and feet occurs infrequently, about 5% of the times. Axial disease, when it occurs alone, is equally infrequent and is seen in 5% of cases. More commonly, it is seen in association with peripheral arthritis. About 40% of patients in general have some form of axial disease. The cervical pine is involved more frequently than the thoraco-lumbar. [74]

Constitutional symptoms associated with PsA are similar to those observed in other types of inflammatory arthritis, and include fatigue, anorexia, weight loss and general weakness. Conjunctivitis and or uveitis (pain, lacrimation and photophobia) may present in up to 1/3 of cases. It tends to be chronic and bilateral.

5.3.1 Physical examination

Proper evaluation requires an examination of all joints; this includes the feet, which often reveal significant pathology. Erythema overlying the joints, and often over the distal phalanges is often seen in hands as well as feet. Selling of the second and third metacarpo-phalangeal joint of the hands may be prominent. Swelling of the large joints like the knees may be noted as well. Dactylitis or fusiform swelling of the digits or toes is the result of inflammation of the phalangeal joints along with enthesitis. Mutilating psoriatic arthritis can result with shortening of the fingers opera (opera glass or telescoping effect).

5.3.2 Laboratory & imaging studies

There is no specific serologic marker for PsA. Though acute phase reactants like CRP, and ESR may be elevated, they are far from specific. HLAB27 is not much better in specificity. While it may appear in 50%-70% of sufferer with axial disease, and less than 15% of those with peripheral disease, it may appear in 7% of normal North American Caucasians, and its presence is independent of disease severity. [75]

Imaging findings center on visualizing radiographic evidence of new bone proliferation or periostitis observed adjacent to erosions, and at sites of entheseal attachments. Marginal erosions of bones may progress to involve the central articular surface resulting in the characteristic "pencil in cup" finding. This progressive loss of bone results in collapse of the phalanges and metacarpal bone resulting in the opera glass or telescoping deformity. MRI and ultrasound are of greater value than plain radiographic film when evaluating the presence of enthesitis. [76] Rheumatoid Factor (RF) may help confirm the diagnosis of RA (at least in 2/3 of the cases); however, RF is positive in 5% of adults, increasing in frequency with age, so that 20% of those over 65 years of age may have a positive RF. In patients with PsA, RF may be positive 5%-10% of the time. Even antibodies to citrullinated-containing proteins (AntiCCP) with improved sensitivity and specificity over RF for RA, are positive in PsA in less than 7%. [77]

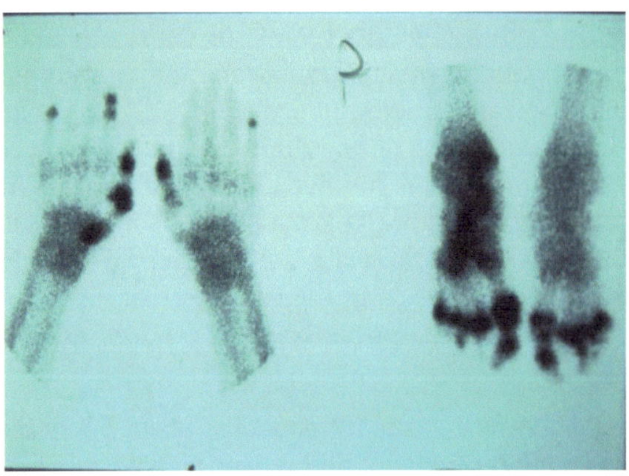

Fig. 6. Nuclear scan of hands and feet - in a psoriatic patient showing asymmetric uptake of radiolabeled Technitium-99 material taken up by inflamed joints

5.3.3 Classification of psoriatic arthritis

Two types of classification (Moll & Wright and CASPAR) are commonly used to categorize psoriatic arthritis. It is often helpful to use one of these when describing clinical severity.

This exercise is useful when seeking approval for systemic therapy from government or private insurance carriers. According to the AAD, the Moll and Wright criteria for classifying psoriatic arthritis, developed in 1973, are frequently used. The Moll & Wright Classification criteria have a specificity of 98% and a sensitivity of 91%.

To meet the Moll and Wright classification criteria, a patient must present with psoriasis, and seronegative inflammatory arthritis with one of several different criteria including:

- Polyarticular, symmetric arthritis (rheumatoid arthritis-like)
- Oligoarticular (< 5 joints), asymmetric arthritis
- Distal interphalangeal joint predominant
- Spondylitis predominant
- *Arthritis mutilans*

The CASPAR (classification criteria for psoriatic arthritis) criteria consist of established inflammatory arthritis defined by the presence of tender and swollen joints and prolonged morning- or immobility-induced stiffness with at least 3 points from the following features1,2:

- Current psoriasis (assigned a score of 2; all other features are assigned a score of 1)
- A personal history of psoriasis (unless current psoriasis is present)
- A family history of psoriasis (unless current psoriasis is present or there is a personal history of psoriasis)
- Current dactylitis or history of dactylitis recorded by a rheumatologist
- Juxtaarticular new bone formation
- Rheumatoid factor negativity
- Typical psoriasis nail dystrophy including onycholysis, pitting, and hyperkeratosis

The CASPAR criteria have a specificity of 99% and a sensitivity of 91%. 28 28

5.4 Psoriasis Area and Severity Index (PASI) & its role in clinical research

Psoriasis Area and Severity Index (PASI) score provides a means of assessing psoriasis that takes into account both the severity and extent of disease. The PASI score for an individual patient is calculated by adding the scores of the four body regions: the head, the trunk, the arms, and the legs. It ranges from 0 to 72. [78] The score for a single region is obtained by multiplying the percentage of surface area occupied by the region (e.g., 0.1 for the head) times the degree of involvement for that region, assessed on a scale of 0 to 6. The result is multiplied by the overall severity score for the region, defined as the sum of scores for redness, thickness, and scale, calculated on a scale of 0 to 4. The resultant scores are then added for each body region to yield the overall PASI score. The PASI has become a tool for measuring disease severity and evaluating how a therapeutic agent lowers the subject's score.

One problem with this index is that it presumes the area of involvement corresponds with severity of disease. It would be possible for a patient with thick plaques on the scalp, elbows and knees to have the same score as one having minimal plaques in the arms and trunk. The former would pose a therapeutic challenge in comparison with the latter, yet their index scores would fail to capture this discrepancy.

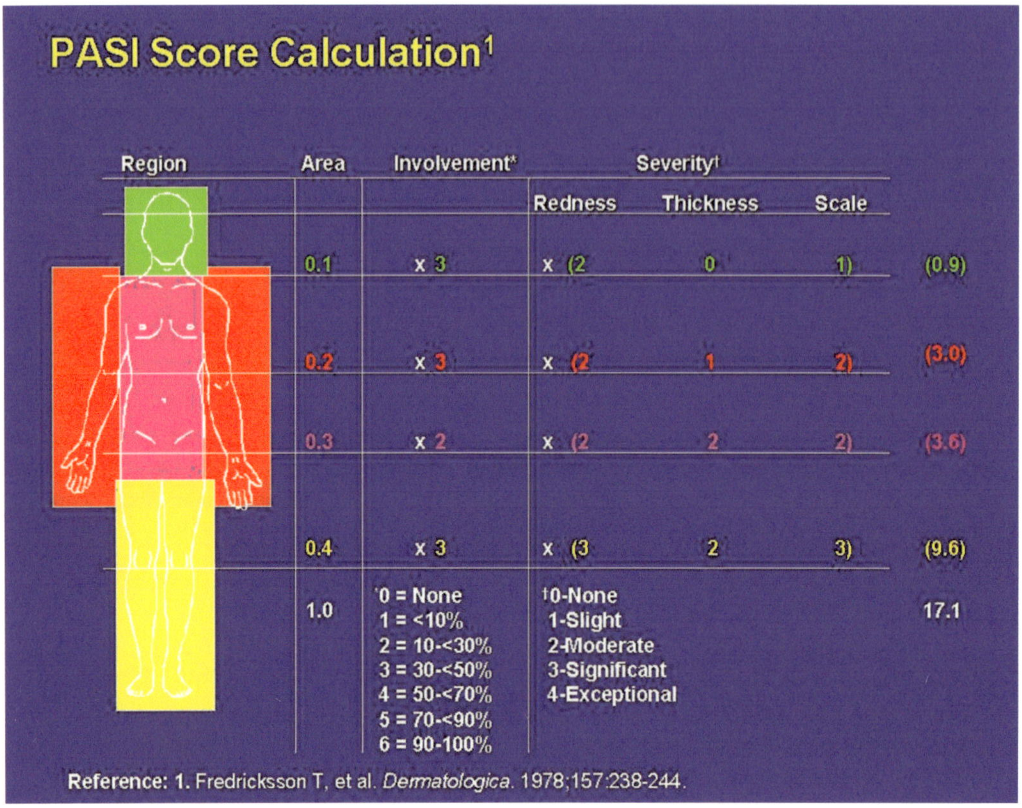

Fig. 7. PASI Score scale. In the example shown here, the score for the trunk is obtained by multiplying 0.3 x 2 x the sum of 2 + 2 + 2, to yield a score of 3.6. When the scores for the four regions are added, we get a PASI Score of 17.1.

Other indices used to categorize disease severity include body surface area (BSA), dermatology life quality index (DQLI), .[79] and the global physician assessment (GPA). [80]

Puzenat *et al* studies a group of indices used to evaluate psoriasis severity. Based on this systematic review, it appears that none of the severity scores used for psoriasis meets all of the validation criteria required for an ideal score. However, we can conclude that the PASI score is the most extensively studied psoriasis clinical severity score and the most thoroughly validated according to methodological validation criteria. Despite certain limitations, use of the PASI score can be recommended for scientific evaluation of the clinical severity of psoriasis. [81]

6. Immunopathophysiology

The cytokine networking theory for the cause of psoriasis was postulated 20 years ago. [82] Proponents maintain that cytokines rather than non-protein type mediators like eicosanoids, orchestrate the multicellular conspiracy among immunocytes such as dentritic cells and T-cells as well as the cross talk between immunocytes and epidermal keratinocytes that culminates in the formation of the psoriatic plaque. There is mounting evidence the innate immune system, by carrying out its intended role of providing an early response mechanism against harm to the host through its nonspecific effectors, may also help induce psoriasis. [83] Plasmacytoid dentritic cells, the foremost producers of interferon-α, a documented inducer of psoriasis,[84] are activated and increased in psoriatic lesions through complexes of the antimicrobial peptide LL37 (*cathelicidin*) and DNA in a toll-like receptor (TLR) 9 - dependent manner. [85] This provides a possible explanation of the mechanism by which host DNA is turned into a proinflammatory stimulus that breaks the immunologic tolerance in psoriasis.

Psoriatic keratinocytes are a rich source of antimicrobial peptides, including IL37, β-*defensins*, and S100A7 (*psoriasin*). These antimicrobial peptides also have strong chemotactic properties, and can help direct other cell functions in dendritic cells and T-cells. In addition, keratinocytes have a potential accessory role in skin immune response. They respond to cytokines derived from dendritic cells and T-cells including interferons, TNF, IL-17, & the IL-20 family of cytokines. They can also produce proinflammatory cytokines like IL-1, IL-6, TNF- α, and chemokines like IL-8 (CXCL*), CXCL10, and CCL20. (see Figure 1)

Dendritic cells bridge the gap between innate and adaptive immunity. Myeloid dermal dendritic cells are increased in psoriatic lesions and induce autoproliferation of T-cells and T_H1 cells. [86] A specialized subgroup (TIP dendritic cells) produce TNF- α, and inducible nitric oxide synthetase. [87] Targeted immunotherapy and psoralen and ultraviolet A (PUVA) therapy reduce the number of dendritic cells in psoriatic patients, adding validity to the role these cells play in the pathogenesis of psoriasis.[88] Clearly, it becomes evident the psoriatic inflammatory response is shaped by a complex interface between elements of the innate and the adaptive immune response. [89]

In two different studies, Zheng *et al* [90] and Chan [91] give IL-23 a potential role in the pathogenesis of psoriasis. Injecting IL-12 into mice skin leads to increased IFN-γ, whereas IL-23 injections increased production of other cytokines including IL-17 and IL-22, but not INF-γ. The traditional belief has been to categorize IL-12 and IFN-γ producing immunocytes as T_H1 type, promoting a cell-mediated immune response to intracellular pathogens. In contrast, T cells producing another collection of cytokines such as IL-4, IL-5, and IL-13 promote a humoral or antibody response to combat extracellular pathogens in a classical T_H2 type reaction. A new cytokine network has been identified belonging to the $CD4^+$ subset producing a different set of cytokines. This third effector cell is the T_H17, and it is directed by IL-23 with help from transforming growth factor (TGF-β) and IL-7 [92] It is apparent that through the promotion of T_H17 cells, IL-23 can play a role in the clearance of infections agents, but has the ability of mediating autoimmune inflammatory disease such as psoriasis and Crohn's Disease. These T_H17 cells produce IL-22, which is responsible for the epidermal thickening seen on psoriasis, and the production of antimicrobial peptides as well as chemokines (including Il-17, and Il-22). 28 It is believed this may be accomplished through the phosphorilation of Sta3, which has been found elevated in psoriatic plaques. [93] IL-22 also mediates the keratinocyte production of *defensins* & other molecules (antimicrobial cytokines) that help enhance the mobility and amplification of the inflammatory response leading to the phenotype of psoriasis [94] [95] With successful anti-TNF treatment, T_H17 cells are reduced, adding still further support to their functional role in psoriasis. [96] Figure 1 illustrates how targeting specific focal points responsible for the pathogenesis of psoriasis may lead to effective prevention of disease and its progression.

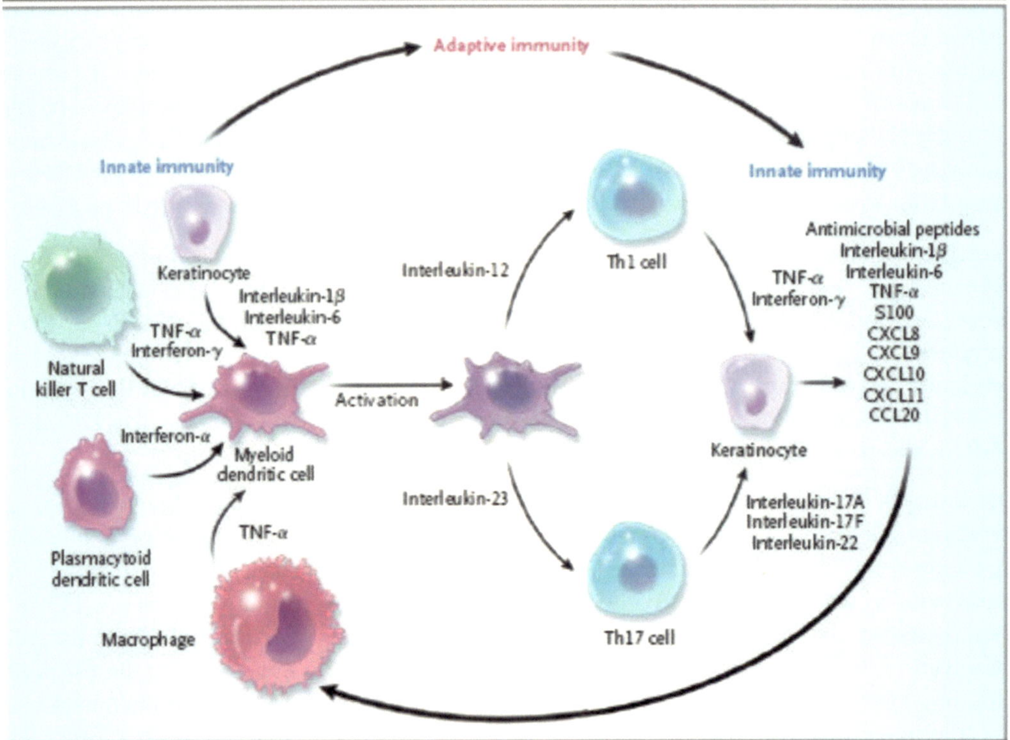

Fig. 8. Key Cells & Mediators in the transition from innate to adaptive immunity in the pathophysiology of psoriasis

Innate immature cells produce key cytokines (TNF-α, interferon- α, interferon-γ, interleukin-1β and interleukin 6) that activate myloid dendritic cells. Activated dendritic cells present antigens and secrete mediators such as interleukin-12 and interleukin-23, leading to the differentiation of type 17 and type 1 helper T cells (Th17 and Th1). T cells, in turn, secrete mediators (e.g. interleukin-17A, interleukin-17F, and interleukin-22) that activate keratinocytes and induce the production of antimicrobial peptides (e.g.LL-37 cathelicidin and β-defensins), proinflammatory cytokines (TNF-α, interleukin-1β, and interleukin 6), chemokines (CXCL8 through CXCL11 and CCL20) and S100 proteins. These soluble mediators feed back into the proinflammatory disease cycle and shape the inflammatory infiltrate.

It seems possessing the gene encoding the IL23 receptor (IL23R) confers strong protection against Crohn Disease [97] Chan et al showed other molecules cross talk between IL23 activated monocytes and the epidermal response including TNF-α and members of the IL19 mainly (IL19, IL20, IL24). IL23 induced epidermal response was depended on the presence of TNF-α as well as the IL20R receptor - which is shared by IL19 family members. There is observed reciprocal exchange of signals between epidermal keratinocytes and immunocytes.

An effort has been ongoing to search for that elusive high-affinity foreign antigen possibly derived from an infectious agent to drive the distinct cell clones in the clonal adaptive immune response. However, to date, no clonal T-cell expansion has been consistently indentified. Alternatively, investigators began to look at the innate immune system as the one responsible for contributing to an inappropriate local tissue inflammatory reaction in psoriasis. It has been noted that IL-23 has been implicated in local mucosal immunopathology by means of innate immune mechanisms. [98] Noting that dendritic cells serve as the bridge between the innate and the adaptive immune system, it may well be it is not an antigenic stimulus that sparks the process, but a genetically programmed hyperactivity of these cells through their altered mechanism of immunologic synapse.

As a final thought in this section, vitamin D and its analogs have been well established as therapeutic agents in the treatment of psoriasis. The mechanism of action by which these agents improve psoriasis is via the vitamin D receptor (VDR), which mediates its effects on the proliferation and differentiation of epidermal keratinocytes,[99] [100] and on the immunological features of psoriasis, including shifting the T_H 1 cytokine profile of plaques towards a T_H 2 cytokine profile. [101]

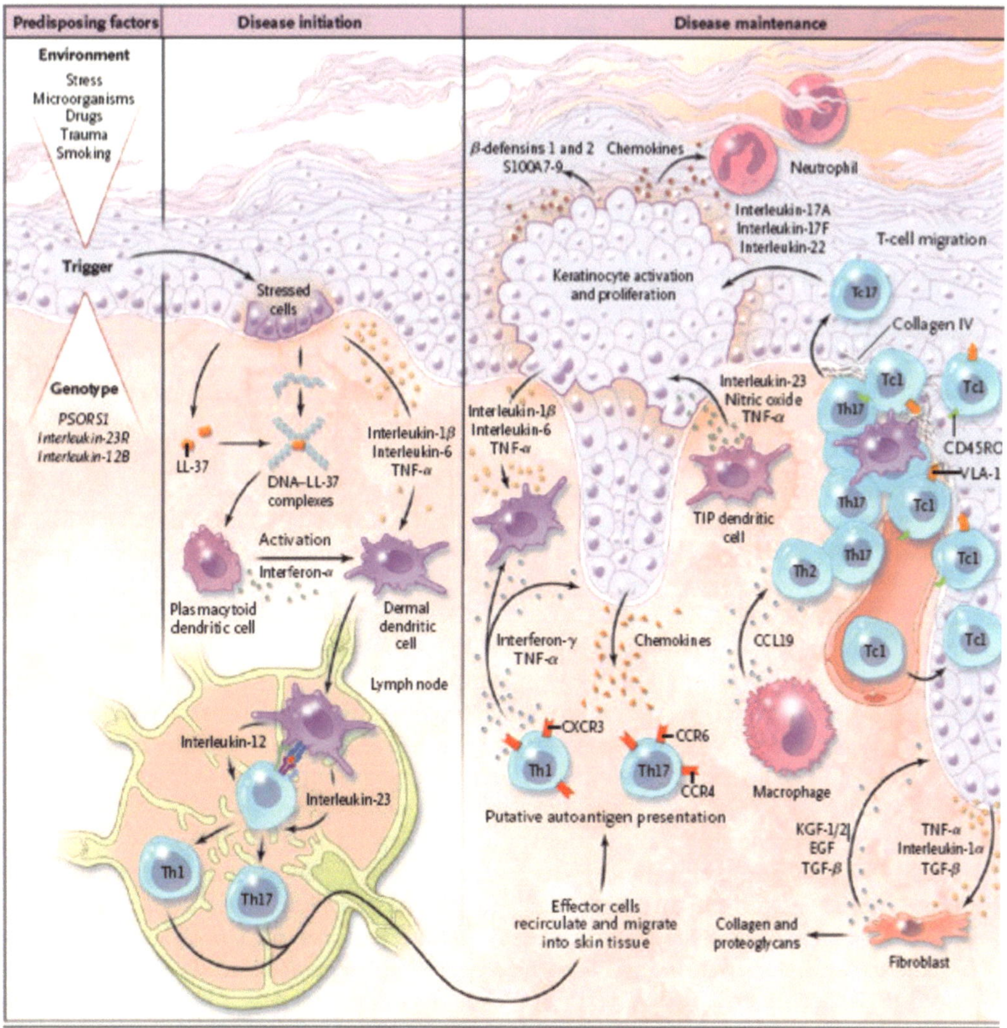

Fig. 9. Overview of the immunopathophysiology of Psoriasis

Vitamin D, through its action by interaction with the VDR offers a beneficial effect on reducing the psoriatic plaque. Keratinocyte differentiation is evident through observed increased levels of transglutaminase I and involucrin and enhanced cornified envelope formation of suprabasal cells [102] [103] , and down regulation of epidermal growth factor, keratin & other markers. The immunomodulatory activity of VDR includes a decrease in the expression or protein levels of IL-2, IL-6, IL-8, IFNγ and GM-CSF. These cytokines play a role in cutaneous inflammation and proliferation of T-lymphocytes and keratinocytes. The expression of IL-12 and GMCSF is negatively regulated through VDR by ligand-dependent inhibition of NF-AT-AP1 composite element activity. [104] [105] 1α,25-dihydroxyvitamin D3 and calcipotriol have also been shown to increase the expression of the receptor for the anti-inflammatory cytokine IL-10 in cultured keratinocytes. [106] [107]

The overall scheme illustrating the various players in the process that leads to the development of psoriasis is illustrated in Figure 2.

7. Comorbidities & other medical considerations

The basis for these observations began from noting psoriasis is characterized by increased T-cell activation leading to production of various cytokines leading to inflammation in the skin as well as other organ targets. 28 These next sections will look at recent data exploring the possibility of a link between psoriasis and cardiovascular disease, chronic obstructive pulmonary disease, metabolic syndrome and obesity, diabetes, pregnancy, celiac disease, and malignancies.

7.1 Cardiovascular disease

Psoriasis may be a risk factor for development of coronary artery calcification (CAC) according to a small study in which 32 patients with psoriasis and 32 matched controls were compared to assess their degree of CAC using non-contrast-enhanced, 16-row, spiral computed tomography. Patients and controls were matched for age, sex, race, cardiovascular risk factors with the exception of family history of cardiovascular diseases. CAC scores were determined for these various individuals and the scores were correlated with the likelihood of coronary artery disease (CAD). Nearly 72% of control patients were found to be free of evidence of CAC, as opposed to only 40.6% of psoriasis patients. In the category where stenosis was likely to be found (those with a CAC score 101-400), 9.4% of control subjects were found to have CAD in comparison with 18.8% in the psoriasis group. For those subjects with a CAC score above 400, no patient in the control group was found to have CAD; whereas 6.3% of the psoriasis group showed nearly certain evidence of CAD. [108] In one larger study investigators from the United Kingdom employed the General Practice Research Database (UKGPRD) to determine whether severe psoriasis is associated with an increases risk of cardiovascular mortality. They identified 3603 patients with severe psoriasis, and compared that to 14,330 who had no history of psoriasis. Severe psoriasis was defined as anyone given the diagnosis of severe psoriasis, and systemic therapy consistent with severe psoriasis. The unadjusted risk of mortality measures incidence per 1,000 person-years, due to cardiovascular disease, and was significantly increased in patients with severe psoriasis (8.75), compared with unexposed patients (6.19). Even as severe psoriasis was shown to be an independent risk factor for death due to cardiovascular disease, after adjusting for traditional cardiovascular risk factors (age, sex, hyperlipidemia, hypertension, smoking, diabetes), the relative risk (RR) of cardiovascular death associated with severe psoriasis was highest in younger individuals with a RR of cardiovascular death of 2.69 for a 40-year-old, as opposed to 1.92 for a 60-year old. [109]

Using the UKGPRD, Gelfand *et al* embarked in a more ambitious prospective, population-based cohort study. Patients with psoriasis (aged 20 to 90 years) were compared with a matched sample of persons without psoriasis from 1987 to 2002. There were 555,995 controls, 127,139 patients with mild psoriasis, and 3837 patients with severe psoriasis (defined like in the previous study). The rates of myocardial infarction (MI) were compared between controls and psoriasis patients after a mean follow-up time of 4-5 years. Out of the group of patients with mild disease the adjusted relative risk for MI was 1.54, while the rate in the group having severe psoriatic disease was 7.08. Separating the groups according to age showed similar results as the earlier study. The younger individuals displayed a greater risk for MI than older patients, and severity of disease was again proportionally more likely to confer a greater risk in the younger age group. Additional analysis suggested men and women with severe psoriasis died 3.5 and 4.4 years younger respectively than patients without psoriasis. The results persisted after adjustment for risk factors associated with mortality. [110] Further evaluation of this data in a recent publication concluded severe psoriasis confers an additional 6.2% absolute risk of 10-year rate of major adverse cardiac events compared to the general population. This has important therapeutic implications for cardiovascular risk stratification and prevention in patients with severe psoriasis. [111]

Very similar results were obtained in a study of two US health care databases analyzed adult patients at least 17 years old in 2001. The population examined totaled around 17 million. Cardiovascular disease (CVD) or CVD risk factors generally increased with disease severity. Severe disease was defined as disease requiring at least one systemic drug. In both databases, higher disease severity raised the risk for coronary heart failure, diabetes mellitus (type 2), hypertension, and ischemic heart disease. [112] An observational study analyzed computerized records of all outpatients who were diagnosed with psoriasis between January 1, 1985 and December 31, 2005 at the Miami VA Medical Center. A total of 3,236 patients with psoriasis and 2,500 controls were evaluated. An association was observed between psoriasis and coronary artery, cerebrovascular, and peripheral vascular diseases.[113]

Osteopontin is a phosphoprotein secreted by osteoblasts, lymphocytes, macrophages, epithelial cells, and smooth muscle cells. It is a byproduct of inflammation, and has been known to be elevated in patients with atherosclerotic heart disease. Chen *et al* have noted increased levels of *osteopontin* in patients with psoriasis, and have suggested it be a cardiovascular risk factor for patients suffering with psoriasis, further validating the notion inflammatory factors may coexist in both heart disease and psoriasis. [114]

Anti-TNF therapy may reduce risk for MI in patients with psoriasis. A retrospective cohort group study at Kaiser Permanente in Southern California looked at 30,467 patients from January 2004 to December 2008 The average age was 50.2 years, with 48.4% being males. Severe psoriasis was defined as anyone getting systemic therapy including phototherapy. There were 5,392 (18%) patients in this group. The TNF-α inhibitor cohort had 2,064 (7%) patients. The overall MI rate was 0.42 per 100 patient years for all patients, while the cohort that had mild psoriasis had an MI rate of 0.43 per 100 patient year, and the severe psoriasis group had a rate of 0.44 per 100 patient years. Patients treated with a TNFα antagonist showed a rate of 0.34 per 100 patient years. This data suggest that effective therapy with a

TNF-α antagonist should reverse the cardiovascular risk profile for patients that respond to this therapy. Further research is needed before this claim can be verified. [115]

7.2 Metabolic syndrome & obesity

Metabolic syndrome is a cluster of risk factors that often accompany obesity, and is associated with increased risk for atherosclerotic cardiovascular disease and type 2 diabetes. The 5 components of metabolic syndrome, as defined by the United States National Cholesterol Education Program, are abdominal obesity (measured by waist circumference), elevated fasting glucose (suggestive of insulin resistance), hypertension, hypertriglyceridemia and, reduced high-density lipoprotein cholesterol (HDL-C). Persons meeting any 3 or more of these 5 criteria are now considered to have metabolic syndrome. The metabolic syndrome is a cluster of risk factors that often accompany obesity and are associated with increased risk for cardiovascular disease and type 2 diabetes. Certain adjustments to waist circumference measurement should be made for persons of Asian origin (cut point ≥ 90 cm in men and ≥ 80 cm in women). The prevalence of metabolic syndrome in the US is estimated to be 22.8% among men and 22.6% among women. It is highest among those of Mexican-American heritage and lowest in blacks. [116] [117] [118]

It has been suggested that there may be a relationship between the risk of psoriasis, and obesity. Both conditions result in a state of chronic systemic inflammation that can have deleterious effects on cardiovascular health, glucose, and lipid metabolism. Obesity is associated with a state of chronic low-level inflammation and the presence of inflammatory cytokines, particularly tumor necrosis factor alpha (TNF-α), which are presumed to derive from macrophages into adipose tissue or activated adipocytes themselves. [119] [120] [121] [122] [123]

Adipocytes (fat cells) store lipids and regulate metabolic homeostasis under normal conditions, while macrophages play a key role in the inflammatory response.

However, each has the ability to perform both functions if necessary. Both types of cells share certain common features, including production of inflammatory cytokines and fatty acid binding proteins. In obese persons, infiltration of macrophages into adipose tissue and release of inflammatory cytokines by adipocytes results in adipocytes becoming inflamed. Several of the cytokines released by adipocytes affect the immune stress response, and many more are key to inflammation (TNF-α, interleukin-6).[124] [125] [126]

In a recent survey conducted by the National Psoriasis Foundation, many psoriasis and psoriatic arthritis patients surveyed reported having at least one other critical health condition. Of those surveyed, almost 70% were overweight or obese; 28% had another chronic inflammatory disease such as lupus, Crohn's disease, or multiple sclerosis; while 24% of patients had hypercholesterolemia. Survey responses were obtained between 2004 and 2009 from telephone and internet surveys. Survey respondents were screened so that 75% had moderate to severe psoriasis, based on expected body surface area (BSA) coverage of 3% or greater without medication, while the remaining 25% had mild disease, or BSA coverage of less than 3%. Among respondents, 62% had psoriasis alone, while 38% also had psoriatic arthritis. [127]

Using the WHO definition of metabolic syndrome, a retrospective study compared records of 581 adults hospitalized with chronic moderate to severe plaque psoriasis with those of

1,044 hospitalized controls without psoriasis. The patients with psoriasis had chronic plaque disease requiring hospitalization because of the severity of their disease or treatment resistance. The median duration of psoriasis was 13 years for men and 16 years for women. Metabolic syndrome was found in 4.3% of the chronic plaque psoriasis patients and only 1.1% in the control group. These psoriasis patients were at significantly increased risk for type 2 diabetes, hypertension, dyslipidemia, and coronary heart disease, and were also more likely to consume alcohol and to be smokers than controls. [128]

Another case-controlled study compared 338 adult patients with psoriasis and psoriatic arthritis and 334 patients with non-psoriatic skin diseases to see if metabolic syndrome was more common among the former. In this study, the mean age of patients was 62.1 years in the control group and 63.8 years in the psoriasis group, and more persons in the psoriatic diseases group were smokers. Fifty five percent of psoriasis patients had BSA ≥ 10%, 43% had PASI scores ≥ 10. [129] In a retrospective case-control study, information from the database of a large managed care organization, with approximately 3.8 million members, was used to assess the potential association between metabolic syndrome and psoriasis. In total, nearly 17,000 patients with psoriasis and 49,000 controls were included; about half were women. The proportion of patients with conditions associated with metabolic syndrome, such as diabetes mellitus, hypertension, and obesity, were increased in those with psoriasis versus controls. Triglyceride and total cholesterol levels were also higher in the psoriasis group by a small but significant amount. [130]

7.3 Diabetes

The association of psoriasis with obesity and diabetes is implicitly evident with the data presented under metabolic syndrome. In a population-based observational study using the UKGPRD, the electronic records of about 73,000 patients were examined between 1994 and 2005. The group was matched between those with a first-time diagnosis of psoriasis and those without. Analysis showed that, as compared to those without psoriasis, the odds ratio (OR) of developing diabetes mellitus in those with psoriasis was 1.31. This odds ratio was corrected for smoking status, body mass index (BMI), hyperlipidemia, infections, and systemic steroid use. Among overweight patients (BMI=25), the OR of developing diabetes mellitus, as compared to normal weight patients, was 7.04 among overweight patients without psoriasis, but this OR was elevated to 8.27 among overweight patients with psoriasis. The risk of developing diabetes mellitus in the psoriasis cohort appeared independent of BMI. Specifically, the risk for developing diabetes mellitus in psoriatic patients of normal weight, or BMI less than 25, increased twofold, 2.02, compared with normal weight patients without psoriasis. [131]

To evaluate further the potential relationship between obesity and psoriasis, Setty and colleagues conducted a prospective, 16-year longitudinal study that evaluated the relationship between adiposity and incidence of psoriasis in a prospective cohort of nearly 117,000 female registered nurses who were between the ages of 25 and 42 years and who had no previously diagnosed psoriasis. The study investigators measured body mass index (BMI), weight change, waist circumference, hip circumference, waist-hip ratio, and incident psoriasis. Data were collected in 78,626 women and in the study time period, 892 newly diagnosed cases of psoriasis were identified. Using a BMI of 21.0 to 22.9 as the reference, the relative risk of psoriasis increased significantly as the BMI increased in all three evaluations: updated, baseline, and after18 years. In the baseline evaluation, the relative risk for the 30.0-34.9 BMI range was 1.73, rising to 2.23 when the BMI was greater than or equal to 35. For the updated evaluation, which was updated every 2 years during follow-up, the relative risk was 1.48 in the 30-34.9 BMI range, and 2.69 when the BMI was over 35. Additionally, a BMI value under 21 was associated with a lower psoriasis risk. Taken together, these data show that multiple measures of adiposity, such as BMI, weight gain since the age of 18, and waist and hip circumference, are substantial risk factors for the development of psoriasis. [132]

Using the same study that began in 1989, Qureshi and colleagues published data on the risk of diabetes and hypertension in female patients with psoriasis. Out of 84,039 women who responded to a questionnaire in 2005 regarding psoriasis, 5,978 women were excluded due to reporting diabetes or hypertension at baseline. Out of the remaining 78,061 women, 1,813 reported a lifetime history of physician-diagnosed psoriasis. During the 14-year follow up from 1991 to 2005, 1500 incident cases of diabetes occurred in the group without psoriasis and 60 incident cases of diabetes occurred in the group with psoriasis. Of those that did not have psoriasis, there were 15,338 incident cases of hypertension and 386 incident cases of hypertension in the group that reported psoriasis (excluding any individuals with concomitant diabetes and hypertension). Mean BMI, alcohol intake, and proportions of current and past smokers were higher in the psoriasis group. There was no difference in mean age between the groups with and without psoriasis. Concomitant psoriasis therapies were unknown. [133]

7.4 Chronic Obstructive Pulmonary Disease (COPD)

More recently Chiang & Lin looked at the National Health Insurance database in Taiwan from 2004 to 2006. The risk of COPD was compared between patients with psoriasis and a matched reference cohort. Their study included 2096 patients with psoriasis and 8384 randomly selected subjects. After adjusting for sociodemographic characteristics and selected co-morbid medical disorders, results showed a hazards ratio (HR) of COPD for mild psoriasis (defined as those just getting topical therapy) to be 2.22. Patients in the comparison cohort with severe psoriasis (defined as those under phototherapy or systemic medication) had an HR of COPD of 2.81. Analysis stratified by patient age and gender showed an adjusted HR for COPD occurring during the 18-month follow-up period to be 2.19 times higher for patients with psoriasis who were > 50 years old than for the same age group of the comparison cohort. There was no significant difference in patients ≤ 50 years old. In male subjects, the adjusted HR of COPD during the follow-up period was 2.38 times greater for those with psoriasis than those without; however, there was no significant difference in the female group. This study places a distinct association among male patients with severe psoriasis, especially those over 50 years of age and psoriasis.[134]

7.5 Venous thromboembolism

Using the multivariate Poisson regression model controlling for age, gender, comorbidity, concomitant medication, socio-economic data and calendar year, Ahlehoff *et al* looked at data from a Danish nationwide cohort derived from records of hospitalization, drugs dispensing from pharmacies, socio-economic data, and listed causes of death. The intent was to look at the risk of venous thromboembolism (VTE) in patients with psoriasis. A total of 35,138 patients with mild psoriasis and 3,526 patients with severe psoriasis were identified, and compared with 4,126,075 controls. The rate ratio (RR) for VTE was elevated in all patients with psoriasis, with RR 1.35 for mild psoriasis, and RR 2.06 for more severe disease. Excluding patients with malignancies and undergoing surgery did not alter results. There was a highest risk noted in young patients with severe psoriasis.[135]

7.6 Pregnancy

Pregnant women with psoriasis (n = 47) and non-pregnant controls (n = 27) were assessed 5 times over 1 year at approximately 10, 20, and 30 weeks of pregnancy and 6 and more than 24 weeks postpartum. A change of more than 3% body surface area defined "Improvement" and "Worsening"; no change was defined as a change in body surface area between 3% and -3%. Most pregnant women with psoriasis experienced improvement in psoriasis or no change during their pregnancies. Psoriasis worsened in fewer than one-fourth of the patients. Conversely, nearly two-thirds of the patients experienced worsening of their psoriasis postpartum. [136] Retrospective examination of psoriasis data from 358 women with psoriasis and 131,424 without psoriasis indicates that psoriasis may be associated with poor pregnancy outcomes, including: spontaneous abortion risk ratio (RR) 3.90; preterm birth RR 2.92; severe pre-eclampsia and eclampsia RR 4.92; *placenta previa* with/without hemorrhage RR 3.49; and ectopic pregnancy RR 4.56. [137] Many of the treatments to be discussed later need to be avoided in the pregnancy state.

7.7 Celiac disease

The association between psoriasis and celiac disease has already been mentioned. Patients with psoriasis often have increased serum levels of IgA antibodies to gliadin. Out of 302 patients with psoriasis, 16% (18 females and 31 males) showed serum IgA

Anti-Gliadin A (AGA) levels above the 90th percentile value (51 u/ml) of the reference group. Palmoplantar pustulosis was found more often than other types of psoriasis. Some patients had signs of gluten sensitive enteropathy. It is noteworthy that 10% of patients with celiac disease fail to show AGA. [138] Out of 33 AGA-positive patients with psoriasis patients, 15 had an increased number of lymphocytes in the duodenal epithelium, and two had IgA antibodies to endomysium (EmA). Thirty of the 33 patients with AGA completed a gluten-free diet for a trial period, after which they showed a highly significant decrease in mean PASI. Resumption of a regular diet resulted in a return of pre-study psoriasis. [139]

7.8 Malignancies

Using the UKGPRD populations of 153,197 from 1988 ton 2002, patients with psoriasis (including 3994 with severe psoriasis) and 765,950 matched controls were identified for a retrospective cohort analysis. Psoriasis patients were classified as severe if they received a systemic treatment. It is important to note that the disease severity classification was based on the treatment the patient had received. The potential causal relationship between therapy and risk of malignancy was not addressed in this study. Highest risk was noted on the occurrence of T-cell lymphoma among the severe psoriasis population. [140]

Adjusted Relative Risk (RR, 95% CI)*	Mild Psoriasis	Severe Psoriasis
All lymphoma	1.34 (1.16, 1.54)†	1.59 (0.88, 2.89)‡
Non-Hodgkin's lymphoma £	1.15 (0.97, 1.37)‡	0.73 (0.28, 1.96)§
Hodgkin's lymphoma	1.42 (1.00, 2.02)**	3.18 (1.01, 9.97)**
T-cell lymphoma	4.10 (2.70, 6.23)†	10.75 (3.89, 29.76)†
*RR = relative risk(confidence interval), adjusted for gender and age † P <0.001 ‡ P <0.1 § P = 0.5 ** P = 0.05 £ Excludes cutaneous T-cell lymphoma		
(Gelfand JM, Shin DB, Neimann AL, Wang X, Margolis DJ, Troxel AB. The risk of lymphoma in patients with psoriasis. *J Invest Dermatol*. 2006;126:2194-2201.)		

Table 3. Risk of Lymphoma in Psoriasis (UK General Practice Research Database) 28

A study in Sweden examined records of patients with a hospital discharge diagnosis of psoriasis between the years of 1965 and 1983, and identified 9,773 patients who were alive and free of cancer one year after admission. Relative rates of cancer were compared to the Swedish national population by computing the standardized incidence ratios (SIR). The table gives the SIR for different cancer types. The most commonly seen cancers were prostate in men (77 cases) and breast in women (78 cases). Other common cancers were lung (65 cases in men, 25 in women), colon (26 cases each in men and women), and squamous cell cancer of the skin (35 cases in men,10 in women). An increased risk of squamous cell cancer was seen in all anatomic regions except the head and neck. However, no increased risk of melanoma was seen with psoriasis. [141]

SIR (95% CI)	Male	Female	Both Genders
Oral/Pharyngeal	2.60 (1.68-3.84)	3.37 (1.68-6.04)	2.80 1.96-3.87)
Esophagus	3.00 (1.59-5.13)	3.03 (082-7.76)	3.01-1.75-4.81)
Liver	2.52 (1.49-3.98)	1.36 (0.68-2.44)	1.91 (1.28-2.74)
Pancreas	1.34 (0.73-2.24)	1.82 (0.99-3.05)	1.56 (1.02-2.23)
Lung	1.91 (1.48-2.44)	3.00 (1.94-4.43)	2.13 (1.71-2.61)
Skin, Squamous Cell Carcinoma	2.75 (1.92-3.83)	1.92 (1.02-3.28)	2.46 (1.82-3.27
Genital organs	2.69 (1.16-5.30)	2.47 (0.90-5.37)	
Kidney, pelvis	1.10 (0.58-1.88)	2.45 (1.37-4.04)	1.56 (1.04-2.25)
Mycosis fungoides	26.7 (8.60-62.3)	0.07 (0.51.3)	19.3 (6.22-45.1)
Non-lymphocytic leukemia	1.74 (0.64-3.79)	2.18 (0.70-5.09)	1.92 (0.96-3.43)
* Incidence ratio of select neoplasms among patients hospitalized for psoriasis			
Boffetta P, Gridley G, Lindelof B. Cancer risk in a population-based cohort of patients hospitalized for psoriasis in Sweden. *J Invest Dermatol*. 2001;117:1531-1537.			

Table 4. Prevalence of Malignancies in Psoriasis * (Swedish Hospital Study) 28

A cohort US study assessing incidence of cancer in 1,105 patients with severe psoriasis and 16,519 patients with less severe psoriasis looked at patients in the government public assistance program of three states from July 1992 to March 1996. One state was located in the mid-Atlantic region, one in the midwest, and one in the southern region of the US The states were not identified. The incidence of cancer in the psoriasis population was compared with the general population (N=259,808). Margolis *et al* designed a 4-year retrospective cohort study using Medicaid data from three large states to compare the risk of malignancy among adult patients ≥ 20 years with severe psoriasis treated with ≥ 1 systemic agents and less severe psoriasis not treated with a systemic agent. Comparison groups included patients with hypertension, patients with severe eczema, and organ transplant recipients. The hypertension group was selected as the reference group because the cancer risk among hypertensive persons is not expected to be substantially different from the risk in the general population.

Patients with severe psoriasis were more likely to develop a malignancy than those patients in the hypertension, severe eczema, and less severe psoriasis groups.

Patients with less severe psoriasis may have had a slightly increased risk of developing cancer compared with the hypertension group. A limitation of this study is that it did not differentiate between potential causes for increased risk of cancer: psoriasis severity and systemic agent use. [142]

Relative Rate Ratio (RR, 95% CI)*	Less Severe Psoriasis	Severe Psoriasis †
All malignancies	1.13 (1.03-1.25)	1.78 (1.32-2.40)
Lymphoproliferative malignancies	2.11 (1.63-2.74)	7.95 (4.94-12.79)
Skin malignancies (non-melanoma & unknown behavior	2.35 (1.96-2.82)	4.15 (2.52-6.84)
Malignancies(excluding non-melanoma skin and lymphoproliferative malignancies	1.00 (0.90-1.12)	1.46 (1.04-2-05)

* Poisson regression used to estimate relative rate ratio compared with hypertensive population adjusted for age, patioent's state of origin, and sex.
† Psoriasis patients were classified as severe if they received treatment with systemic medications.

Margolis D, et al. *Arch Dermatol.* 2001;137:778-783.

Table 5. Prevalence of Malignancies in Psoriasis (US Study)

7.9 Management of psoriasis & psoriatic arthritis

Studies looking at cognitive behavior therapy as an adjunct to pharmaceutical therapies in patients with psoriasis showed clinical improvement in comparison to patients receiving pharmacological therapy alone. [143] High levels of worry and stress have been found to aggravate disease activity, and aggravate the therapeutic benefit of Psoralen and UVA therapy (PUVA). [144] Attempts to look at diet including diets rich in zinc, [145] and turkey meat, [146] diets low in tryptophan, [147] protein, [148] or calories [149] seem to have little impact. As mentioned before, in patients with both celiac disease and psoriasis, diets low in gluten have been shown to be useful in improving both conditions. 28

It is well documented sunlight exposure (heliotherapy), and spa treatments such as those in the Israeli Dead Sea can be beneficial. [150]

Traditionally, pharmacological therapy has been divided into topical therapy, systemic therapy and photo-pharmacological therapy (PUVA). Some include all forms of phototherapy in systemic therapy. Before steroids were introduced, topical therapy was limited to tar, anthralin and keratolytics like urea and salicylic acid. The impossibility to standardize biological activity on tar products, and arrive at a consensus on measuring disease severity to gauge therapeutic success has hindered the ability to define and compare various reported efficacies of these topical regimens.

7.10 Tar with & without UV therapy

Tar had been used as topical monotherapy for a century before it was combined with Ultraviolet B (UV-B at 290-320 nm) in the Goeckerman regimen. [151] Crude coal tar (2.5-5%) was applied daily in combination with a tar bath and UV therapy, usually as an inpatient facility. It became clear UVB was more valuable than UVA. [152] In addition, tar could sensitize the skin to UVA, but not UVB. It is believed UVB erythema thresholds prevent UVA exposure sufficient to cause photosensitization in the Goeckerman regimen. [153] The risk from therapeutic tar is small. [154] [155] It may be wise to avoid prolonged application to the anogenital areas including the scrotum, and avoid prolonged UV exposure. [156] [157] [158] [159]

7.11 Anthralin (dithranol)

Chrysarobin, from the bark of a tree, was found to be useful in the treatment of psoriasis. Dithranol, a synthetic derivative, was found to be unstable, but salicylic acid was found to stabilize it and lead to the development of the Ingram regimen. [160] After a tar bath, followed by UVB, the lesions were covered with dithranol paste in increasing concentrations seeking a maximum response while avoiding irritation. The regimen became popular in Europe. It was later found use of dithranol in Lassar's paste was equally effective. Short contact dithranol therapy - twice daily and in high concentration regimes, was also effective. [161] Newer formulations have been developed to limit staining and reduce irritation. In some parts of the world, anthralin is available as a combination preparation with potent topical steroids, and effective results have been seen. [162]

7.12 Topical corticosteroids

Held by many as the topical treatment of choice, several preparations are widely available worldwide. The more potent forms of topical corticosteroids, are needed to treat hyperkeratotic plaques, and difficult to treat areas like the scalp, hands and feet. Besides their direct effect in limiting psoriasis, these agents are helpful in reducing symptoms like pruritus, and limiting irritation caused by other therapies. Better results are often obtained using occlusive dressings; a recent study found even better effectiveness when occluded with a hydrocolloid dressing. [163] Cutaneous side effects include telangiestasias, atrophy and striae. [164] Besides cutaneous adverse events adrenal suppression leading to lowering plasma cortisol levels can be observed with the most-potent preparations. [165] As little as 7 g/day of 0.05% clobetasol propionate or 0.05% betamethasone dipropionate was sufficient to suppress morning plasma cortisol levels in 20% of patients. [166] Tolerance or tachyphylaxis is not uncommon. To avoid this, as well as other adverse side effects, sequential therapy incorporating other topical agents, and pulse therapy rotating the various agents, have been implemented limiting total contact with skin, and any significant absorption.[167 168 169]

7.13 Intralesional corticosteroids

Resistant and thick plaques in awkward anatomical areas, like the knuckles, where it is difficult to keep topical preparations during daily living activities, often respond to intralesional injections with triamcinolone acetonide with remarkable success.

7.14 Vitamin D analogs

Naturally occurring and synthetic vitamin D analogues have been found to be effective in the topical treatment of psoriasis. Vitamin D_3 and its active metabolite, 1,25 dihydroxyvitamin D_3, (calcitriol), as well as the three synthetic analogues - calcipotriol (known in the US as calcipotriene), 1-24-dihydroxyvitamin D_3 (tacalcitol), and 1,25-dihydroxyvitamin D_3 (maxacalcitol). Calcipotriol ointment is the most widely prescribed vitamin D analog. The mechanism by which these molecules affect their therapeutic benefit has already been described in a previous section. Current concern on their use includes irritation, and the potential for hypercalcemia, which has not been observed with the use or recommended maximum topical dosing of up to 100 g/week.[170] Ointment preparations appear to be more effective than the others available. A combination stable formulation using calcipotriol 50 µg/g and betamethasone diproprionate 0.5%mg/g, applied once daily shows better results than either product alone.[171] Calcitriol ointment 3 µg/g has shown long term effectiveness in the treatment of chronic large plaque psoriasis. Comparison between this agent, calcipotriol and other topical agents used to treat psoriasis show unclear results except for the superiority of calcitriol in the treatment of face and flexural regions, and a lower relapse rate following withdrawal compared with topical steroids.[172 173] Tacalcitol 4 µg/g ointment is effective in the treatment of chronic plaque psoriasis, but does not appear to show superiority to calcipotriol 50 µg/g.[174] Preliminary studies indicate maxacalcitol applied once daily may be more effective in short-term studies than calcipotriol 50 µg/g.[175]

It is important to note salient interesting interactive relations when considering use of vitamin D analogues. Use of calcipotriol 50 µg/g used in combination with methotrexate allows the use of lower doses of methotrexate.[176] Clinical and *in vitro* studies have been performed analyzing the compatibility of using clobetasol propionate spray or lotion together with calcitriol ointment 3 µg/g. Results suggest calcitriol remains stable in the presence of each of the other compounds. The sequence used was not relevant to their continued efficacy.[177 178]

Calcipotriol ointment enhances the efficacy of PUVA and UVB therapy, Howeverr, UVA partly inactivates calcipotriol, while UVB serves to absorb calcipotriol. When used with phototherapy, these products should be applied after the UV therapy session. 28 Tacalcitols ointment when combined with PUVA is UVA sparing,[179] while calcitriol is UVB sparing when used in combination.[180]

When used in combination with topical steroids, vitamin D analogs offer the advantage of sustained efficacy while offering a desirable steroid sparing effect.[181] This has lead to a wide range of pulsing and sequential therapy regimens with anecdotal reports attesting to their efficacy. Controlled corroborating studies are lacking.

7.15 Vitamin A analogs

Retinoids have been suspected to be a successful alternative to the treatment of psoriasis. With their direct effect on cellular proliferation and subsequent differentiation, it would be expected they would be the ideal preparation. Initial trials revealed efficacy, but significant irritation. [182] The development of the products that selectively used the retinoid acid receptor ushered in tazarotene, a synthetic retinoid, whose main metabolite binds the RARs β and γ. [183] Applied as its 0.05% or 0.1% gel once daily for three months, showed significant improvement over its gel vehicle in the treatment of chronic plaque psoriasis. [184] Irritation was its principal drawback, which was reduced when the 0.05% and 0.1% creams were introduced. [185] Reports using a topical steroid helped maintain a longer standing remission, while reducing some of the irritation. [186]

7.16 Topical calcineurin inhibitors

The two products in this category currently available are tacrolimus and pimecrolimus. Developed initially for the treatment of childhood atopic dermatitis, both preparations have been found effective for the management of psoriasis involving the face, neck, flexular areas, the genitals and mucosal surfaces. They have a safer profile than topical steroids, and do not produce skin atrophy where used. [187]

7.17 Phototherapy

7.17.1 UVB

The Goeckerman regimen, which used UVB was already described [188] Subsequent to the time this treatment was being offered, it was learned that broad band UVB at 290-320 nm (BBUVB) alone was effective in clearing psoriasis [189] [190] [191] [192] and even as effective as PUVA [193] While some studies have not shown an increased rate of skin cancer risk in UVB treated psoriasis patients [194] [195] [196], suspicion still exists that long term exposure may contribute to total risk. One study does suggest an added risk for genital tumors in men treated with BBUVB, [197] making it prudent to protect that area during treatment. More recently, a narrow-band source of UVB at 311nm, (NBUVB) has offered longer remissions, and suggested a lower incidence of burning. [198] [199] [200] Studies comparing a higher intensity (100W) NBUVB have suggested better results still. However, when compared to PUVA several studies provide conflicting results suggesting patient selection, level of disease activity, and need for larger population studies are needed before reliable results can be compared. [201] [202] [203] Data showing a lower risk for UV carcinogenesis is limited to one study, which failed to reveal significant association between NBUVB and squamous cell carcinoma, malignant melanoma and basal cell carcinoma. [204] One observation peculiar to NBUVB, which has not been observed in BBUVB, is the occurrence of painful blisters at the site of psoriatic lesions appearing in the middle of the treatment course. They are self limiting, but can be painful and require a brief interruption in the regimen. [205] Both NBUVB and BBUVB units are commercially available for home therapy.

In addition, end results can often be improved by supplementing phototherapy with topical dithranol, and oral retinoids, Heliotherapy, described previously, enjoys the therapeutic benefit of the full-range light spectrum of the sun. A retrospective study looked at 1488 psoriasis patients treated at a Dead Sea Clinic from 1983 to 1986. Patients were treated by sun exposure and bathing in the mineral-rich sea. Nearly three quarters improved by 90% or more. [206]

UVB can be used effectively for the treatment of guttate psoriasis, as well as those relatively rare forms of head and neck or "seborrheic" psoriasis. It is also helpful in patients who live in colder climates and experience seasonal exacerbation during winter months. UVB can also be used as adjunct therapy for a temporary period for patients who have responded to systemic therapy, but experience an unexpected setback in disease activity. Skin types should always be considered, especially if long-term care is a reasonable expectation, due to the potential for UV related carcinogenesis. This risk would be theoretically greater on individuals of Fitzpatrick skin types I-III.

7.18 Psoralen photochemotherapy (PUVA)

Success with the Goeckerman regimen, and use of psoralen photochemotherapy lead to thinking it might help psoriasis. [207] [208] By the early 1970's, there was ample evidence 8-methoxypsoralen (8-MOP) and UVA would treat psoriasis effectively, and thus lead to the treatment definition of photochemotherapy. [209] PUVA soon became its modified acronym. Other forms of psoralen like 5-methoxypsoralen (5-MOP) and trimethylpsoralen have been used with similar results as 8-MOP. [210] [211]

The treatment essentially involves the ingestion of one of several preparations of 8-MOP available at the recommended calculated dose. Bioavailability varies from various preparations, and from patient to patient. Intestinal absorption is affected by fat content. It is customary to use one preparation, take it on an empty stomach and insist on a constant time interval from ingestion to UVA exposure. Dose calculation based on weight is 0.6mg/kg given 2 hours before irradiation. Patients must wear appropriate eye protection for a period of 24 hours from the time the psoralen is ingested to prevent sun-induced cataracts. Treatment is given 2-4 times weekly. Initial UVA dose is based on skin type and is incrementally increased with each treatment by 0.5-1.5 J/cm^2 each time. [212] Once remission is achieved the frequency of treatment is gradually reduced and given every 1-4 weeks. Patient selection is important. Individuals must have physical stamina to stand for prolonged periods of time during the irradiation sessions. Previous exposure to arsenic, prior radiation therapy, pregnancy, and ingestion of medication that is photosensitizing are all contraindicated. Persons less than 18 years of age should not receive PUVA. Persons with any medical condition that can be exacerbated by UV exposure including patients with collagen vascular disease should be identified.

Clearance rates topping 90% have been reported, with substantial clearance being achieved with 15-25 treatments. [213] [214] [215] [216] [217] PUVA can be helpful in erythrodermic psoriasis, psoriasis involving palms and soles, pustular psoriasis, and psoriasis involving the nails. Results in these resistant forms of disease vary, and are not as successful. PUVA can be combined with dithronol, [218] methotrexate, [219] and calcipotriol.[220] Risk of cancer is increased further with concomitant methotrexate use. [221] Calcipotriol use reduces the required the UVA exposure, and as mentioned previously, should be used after irradiation to prevent its inactivation. PUVA and UVB have been used effectively in patients who fail to response to PUVA or UVB alone. [222] Topical PUVA offers similar therapeutic advantage with fewer side effects. It is not generally available to the individual patient requiring in-patient administration, and thus too costly for practical use.

Early reports raised the concern that PUVA treated patients would experience an increased rate of developing tumors in patients with xeroderma pigmentosa. [223] PUVA appeared to have a promoter effect on patients previously exposed to X-irradiation, arsenic, and several cytotoxic drugs. [224] Subsequent studies have corroborated the same association with patients receiving PUVA. The risk is most profound on patients of fair skin. [225] [226] Stern et al reported an increase rate of squamous cell carcinoma among patients that received PUVA for a prolonged period of time. No association was found with malignant melanoma or basal cell carcinoma. [227] In a further follow-up study, the same group identified a risk for melanoma in association with long-term exposure to PUVA. [228] Subsequent Swedish study found a similar association with squamous cell carcinoma but no association with malignant melanoma or basal cell carcinoma. [229] Until more definitive studies define the proper course, current prudence suggests to avoid using PUVA on patients with family or past medical history of malignant melanoma, and to those that have already received 200 treatments. [230]

8. Systemic therapy

Systemic therapy is reversed for the more severe forms of psoriasis and the treatment of psoriatic arthritis. For the latter a Disease Modifying Anti Rheumatic Drug (DMARD) is generally used with the double aim of arresting inflammation, and halting disease progression. Some systemic agents can treat PsA while others do not.

8.1 Methotrexate (MTX)

An initial observation in 1951 demonstrated that aminopterin was beneficial in the treatment of psoriasis, and led to exploring use of its more stable analogue methotrexate, which can be administered orally, intramuscularly, subcutaneously and intravenously.[231] Its oral absorption may be impeded in psoriatic patients. [232] Twenty to 70% of methotrexate is bound to plasma albumin, [233] [234] [235] and excretion is largely by the kidney, but there is extensive entero-hepatic cycling. [236] [237] [238] Initially its mechanism was felt to be its anti-metabolite effect on keratinocyte proliferation through competitive inhibition of dihydrofolate reductase in DNA synthesis, [239] More recently, it has been learned that at low doses (0.1 to 0.3 mg/kg weekly), a dose too low to affect keratinocytes, methotrexate is 10-100 times more effective in inhibiting proliferation of lymphoid cells through its inhibition of 5-aminoimidazole-4-carboxamide ribonucleotide transformylase leading to accumulation of extracellular adenosine, which has anti-inflammatory activities including slowing chemotaxis of polymorphonuclear leukocytes. [240] [241] [242] These latter two mechanisms may have a greater effect on its ability to treat psoriasis. Addition of folic acid supplementation (1-5 mg/day) reduces the side effects of nausea, oral ulcers, and megaloblastic anemia.

Controlled trials attest to the effectiveness of methotrexate for the treatment of psoriasis. [243] [244] Initially 5-10 mg is given orally once a week to avoid early toxicity (the elderly can be started often with 2.5 mg). Doses can be increased by 2.5 mg/week to achieve a maximum of 25 mg/week. [245] Clinical response is generally noted within 2 weeks. Pustular psoriasis and psoriatic erythroderma tend to respond to this regimen. Transient anorexia, nausea, and other upper gastrointestinal symptoms are the most common symptoms.

Before treatment, baseline renal, hepatic, and marrow function should be obtained. The presence of chronic hepatitis (B and C) should be ruled out. Due to methotrexate's direct effect on the immune system, latent tuberculosis, [246] and, where geographically appropriate, chronic fungal and other parasitic infection should be ruled out as well. [247]Since standard serum liver function tests cannot evaluate hepatic damage reliably, current guidelines suggest a liver biopsy be performed when a cumulative dose of 1.5 g is achieved, and repeated every 1.0-2.0 g thereafter. A liver biopsy has been the preferred method of monitoring the damaging effect of methotrexate, since serological liver function studies have been known to conceal evolving harm, and reveal significant hepatic scarring only too late in the course of therapy.[248] Hepatotoxicity is a well established effect of methotrexate. [249] [250] Renal impairment, previous intake of hepatotoxins, and alcohol use can increase this risk [251] In some parts of the world monitoring amino terminal type III procollagen peptide (PIIINP) assay every three months is being done in lieu of liver biopsy. In the US, the FDA has not approved the use of this assay yet. [252]

Myelosuppression is a serious issue with the use methotrexate. It can occur 7-10 days after an initial dose is given. It can also be seen in the setting of folate deficiency, as an initial response in the beginning of therapy, due to toxicity, or quite innocently when the patient receives sulfonamides or other drug (usually a sulfa based agent) interfering with dihydrofolate reductase activity. This is a potentially fatal reaction, and must be identified and treated with folinic acid given at a dose 20 mg. parenterally or orally, and repeated every 6 hours. [253]

There is no evidence that splitting the dose in three parts, and giving it every 12 hours, a practice that was common to synchronize the therapy to the keratinocyte cell cycle when it was believed the treatment was all about epidermal cell turnover, offers any advantage over single weekly dose, except when it comes to reducing nausea. Pharmacokinetic studies indicate the bioavailability of MTX after oral ingestion is highly variable and unreliable.[254] Subcutaneous administration offers the same advantage as intramuscular. Compared with the highly variable and unpredictable bioavailability following oral administration (25–80%), parenteral dosing achieves more consistent and complete absorption. [255] Intramuscular or subcutaneous administrations achieve equivalent pharmacokinetic profiles with a bioavailability of 87% of that following intravenous dosing.

Concern exists over the possible development of malignancies while on long-term therapy with methotrexate. Evidence supports an increase risk for developing cutaneous squamous cell carcinoma in those with cumulative doses in excess of 3 g over 4 years. Thus risk was independent of PUVA. Pneumonitis, oligospermia, and osteopathy can occur. The latter can be confused with psoriatic arthritis [256] Methotrexate is teratogenic, and an abortifacient in early pregnancy. [257] Conception is regarded safe 3 months after discontinuation of therapy. [258]

Methotrexate has been used in combination with UVB, PUVA, [259] and systemic retinoids.[260] Use with the latter must be done with caution due to greater risk of hepatitis. Methotrexate and cyclosporine helps patients with psoriatic arthritis [261], while combining methotrexate with colchicine has been used in generalized pustular psoriasis. [262]

8.2 Cyclosporine

Used principally as an immune-suppressant in organ-transplant recipients, cyclosporine is a cyclic undecapeptide derived from the fungus *Tolypocladium inflatum gams*. It was found to clear psoriasis in 1979. [263] Its mechanism of action is presumed to be related to its inhibitory effect on T-cell activation. [264] Because of it toxic effects, and its potential to cause malignancies, its use is generally limited to patients that have failed other systemic alternatives. Exclusion criteria for its use include renal dysfunction, uncontrolled hypertension, past or present malignancy, epilepsy, acute infections, other immunosuppressive therapy, concomitant therapy with neurotoxins, previous serious side effects from prior use, or known hypersensitivity. Candidates for using cyclosporine must be reliable to undergo proper frequent monitoring. As a highly lipophilic agent metabolized in the liver by means of the cytochrome P-450, there are many drugs that could interact with cyclosporine such as anticonvulsants, which can prevent therapeutic levels of cyclosporine. NSAIDs (non-steroidal anti-inflammatory drugs) may enhance nephrotoxicity. [265] The recommended initial daily oral regimen is 2.5 mg/kg divided in two doses. Improvement often starts in days, and failure to see any benefit in two weeks should warrant a dose escalation to a maximum of 5 mg/kg/day.[266] Sudden withdrawal may lead to relapse, but nothing like the flares seen with systemic steroid withdrawal.[267] [268] Ideally, this should be limited to 3-4 months.[269] [270] In the US, the FDA recommends cyclosporine should be used for less than one year. One study compared intermittent cyclosporine with continuous use for psoriasis, and found an intermittent regimen was probably safer. [271]

Dose-related hypertension and nephrotoxicity are the most serious side effects associated with cyclosporine use. Blood pressure can increase sharply weeks after beginning therapy. Glomerular filtration rate may decrease while plasma creatinine levels may rise. Serum uric acid may rise prior to elevation in creatinine or blood urea nitrogen. Other side effects include gum hyperplasia, hypertrichosis, elevated sebum production, mild anemia, and paraesthesias. [272] The mechanism by which cyclosporine reverses the clinical signs of psoriasis is by blocking transcription and synthesis of lymphokines such as interleukin-2 (IL-2) and interferon-y (IFN-y). [273] [274] This product inhibits the accessory cell function of Langerhans cells, [275] decreases the capacity of dendritic cells to enhance mitogenic stimulation of lymphocytes, and induces secretion of thymic hormone. Thus, cyclosporine could inhibit cytokine-mediated cellular activation that may contribute to the pathogenesis and progression of this disease. [276] [277]

Immunosuppression with long term use of cyclosporine may be associated with an increased risk for cutaneous malignancies, lymphomas. This is seen especially in patients with previous history of getting UV irradiation in any therapeutic regimen, or arsenic and methotrexate. 28 Females observed to develop cervical intraepithelial neoplasia, and males with HPV-associated penile carcinoma suggests the need for frequent cervical smears for females and examination for males especially when there is prior history of HPV infection. [278] [279]

8.3 Oral retinoids

Retinoids refer to a family of natural and synthetic derivatives of vitamin A. Their role in skin physiology has been long established enhancing epithelial differentiation. Deficiency causes squamous metaplasia and cutaneous hyperkeratosis, while their presence in excess can lead to xerosis with cutaneous exfoliation, hair loss, bony abnormalities, liver toxicity, and abnormalities in serum lipids. Oral retinoids are also well known for their teratogenic effect. They have been found to have a protective effect in slowing down or preventing the progression and development of cutaneous neoplasms arising out of chronic sun exposure. [280] [281] [282] While isotretinoin is the most widely known retinoid, used principally in the treatment of nodular acne and other forms of severe acne, and its successful use in the treatment of psoriasis has been documented, [283] other retinoids have been found more effective in the management of psoriasis. Because serum lipids are often elevated and hepatotoxic effects can occur with their use, proper monitoring is recommended.

8.4 Etretinate

First reported in 1975 to be useful in the treatment of psoriasis, [284] it was found effective for the treatment of psoriasis vulgaris, pustular psoriasis, [285] and erythrodermic psoriasis. [286] Its use has been replaced by acitretin in most countries.

8.5 Acitretin

This retinoid is the main active metabolite of etretinate. It has decreased lipophilicity resulting from being a free acid as opposed to an ester as in the case of etretinate. Its half life is 50 hours compared to 80 days for etretinate, making it a more desirable drug. Several clinical trials confer on acitretin the same profile of efficacy as etretinate. [287] [288] [289] [290] However, acitretin has been found to convert to etretinate in an unpredictable number of patients, requiring female patients of child-bearing age who use to refrain from pregnancy for 2 years after discontinuation of the drug. Retinoids should not be used in children except for exceptional circumstances, nor in anyone with pre-existing hyperlipidemia or liver disease. In the US, general practice is not to use an oral retinoid for psoriasis on any female of child-bearing age. Though a very small percentage of patients on acitretin may acquire a toxic hepatitis (1.5%), histological sign of hepatic damage is not found. Oral dosing can begin at 10 mg daily and increment to an optimum dose of 50 mg/day. Lipids should be monitored, and patients cautioned about photosensitivity. [291] The combination of acitretin with PUVA appears superior to PUVA alone. [292] Similarly acitretin improves the efficacy of UVB. [293]

Acitretin may help reduce the risk of cutaneous neoplasia brought on by chronic phototherapy. For this reason, its use has been advocated on patients with other risk factors for skin cancer who have received extensive phototherapy. 28 [294]

8.6 Systemic corticosteroids

Despite the fact that the use of systemic corticosteroids has not been advocated for the treatment of psoriasis, the practice of intramuscular injections with triamcinolone acetonide, commonly used for reduction of itching, inflammation, arthralgias and related symptoms associated with psoriasis, eczema, and other dermatoses is recognized as an effective clinical practice by many clinicians. However, in the case of psoriasis, there is often a break through of symptoms with repeated treatments. Rebound can also result. This phenomenon occurs often when patients with psoriasis undergo surgery. Current practice among anesthesiologists is to administer a stress dose of corticosteroid prior to surgery, leading to an observed marked improvement of the psoriasis while in the hospital and following the immediate post-operative period. A rebound is generally noted a few weeks afterwards prompting a visit to the dermatologist's office. In spite of it all, systemic corticosteroids can be helpful in cooling down the skin during the erythrodermic phase of disease, especially if the treatment is supplemented with another systemic agent that can assist in bringing a remission. Systemic corticosteroids also have a place in the treatment of the von Zumbush reaction, [295] and the hyperacute polyarthritis with potential for joint damage. Lability of disease with steroids is common, and often difficult to dispel. [296] Systemic corticosteroids have been helpful with concomitant use of methotrexate in the management of rebound or acute flares associated with the use of efalizumab. [297]

8.7 Other systemic agents used for the treatment of psoriasis

8.7.1 Hydroxyurea

Hydroxyurea is an antimetabolite used mainly for the treatment of chronic myeloid leukemia among other malignancies. It is converted to its active metabolite which blocks the conversion of ribonucleotides to deoxyribonucleotides by blocking the action of ribonucleoside diphosphate reductase, and thus inhibiting DNA synthesis in proliferating cells. [298]

It was first conceived to be used on psoriasis in 1969.[299] Oral regimens are generally up to 0.5 g three times daily for a minimum of 2 months before considering the treatment suboptimal. Principal side effects include bone marrow suppression, profound anemia, and thrombocytopenia. Macrocytosis and leucopenia are practically universal. It is teratogenic, making it essential to be avoided during pregnancy. However, it is less hepatotoxic than methotrexate with less gastrointestinal side effects, and also less effective with a satisfactory response rate of 45-80%. [300] [301] [302] It is generally used when other systemic agents have failed, especially methotrexate. Besides, it can be used in combination with methotrexate, [303] cyclosporine, [304] and acitretin. [305] A drug related cutaneous vasculitis has been reported. 28 [306] Leg ulcers can occur, and are often difficult to manage. [307]

8.8 6-Thioguanine

Closely related to 6-mercaptopurine, 6-thioguanine was shown to be effective in the treatment of psoriasis. [308] [309] Its mechanism of action, as an antimetabolite, appers to be depletion of T-cells in the skin. The studies show remarkable efficacy in patients that had failed other systemic therapies. Oral regimens ranged in dose from 20 mg twice weekly to 120 mg/day, and the duration averaged 15 months. [310] [311] In one study 14 out of 18 patients experienced greater than 90% improvement. Increased liver enzymes and veno-occlusive disease of the liver may be seen. [312]

8.9 Fumaric acid

German speaking countries in Europe enjoy the most experience with the use of this family of compounds for the treatment of psoriasis. The mechanism of action seems to suggest the ability of fumarates to inhibit nuclear binding of nuclear Kappa B and promoting the secretion of Th2 cytokines such as IL-10, found to be beneficial in treating psoriasis. [313] [314]

Preparations commercially available incorporate several salts. Fumaderm is one such preparation with a mixture of dimethylfumarate, and the calcium, magnesium and zinc salts of monoethylfumaric acid. These compounds are not yet approved for use in the US. After ingestion, dimethylfumarate is hydrolysed to monomethylfumarate - the main active metabolite. Clinical trials show efficacy. [315] [316] [317] Regimen includes starting at 30 mg/day orally building up over several weeks to a maximum dosage of 240 mg three times daily. Dyspepsia and diarrhea are common appearing in about two thirds of patients, and one third develop flushing. Lymphocyte counts fall in nearly all, and can drop to 50%. Though it is prudent to monitor renal and liver function, it is rarely impaired.

9. Biologics – The latest modality

The mechanisms by which biologic agents exert their therapeutic benefit have been reviewed in the immunopathophysiology section of this chapter, and illustrated in Figure 1. In the US as in Europe and most parts of the world, their use is relegated generally to the patients suffering with moderate to severe disease, with or without psoriatic arthritis.

The Food & Drug Administration (FDA) approved the use of efalizumab in November 2003, and the European Medicines Agency (EMEA) in September 2004. This was one of several biologics approved for the treatment of psoriasis on the basis of favorable findings obtained from well-designed clinical trials. [318] Ongoing monitoring of sustained efficacy, tolerability, and possible side effects lead to the discovery of 3 newly diagnosed cases of progressive multifocal leukoencephalopathy. [319] In 2009, efalizumab was voluntarily withdrawn from the market by Genentech, its manufacturer. This unexpected experience underscores the importance of vigilance and careful monitoring when treating a medical condition with any immunosuppressant - biologics being no exception.

Another issue that relates to the use of biologics is the emergence of loss of therapeutic response. This may occur as a temporary minor flare of disease activity in spite of continuing use. It may also appear as a nearly total loss of therapeutic activity. Though this can occur with any biologic currently being used to treat psoriasis, it has been shown to occur more often with the monoclonal antibodies. It has been postulated this is due to the development of neutralizing antibodies, as in the case of infliximab and adalimumab, which generally follows with a subsequent drop in therapeutic serum level of the biologic being used.[320] Concomitant use of methotrexate at low doses has been shown to diminish chances of developing neutralizing antibodies. [321] Anti-adalimumab antibodies in rheumatoid arthritis patients have been recently reported to be associated with interleukin-10 gene polymorphism. [322] IL 10 is a key cytokine in antibody formation, and its role has been implicated in other autoimmune diseases. Neutralizing antibodies have not been detected to etanercept to date. Loss of response to the TNFα antagonists may also occur independent of adequate serum levels and lack of detectable antibodies. One thing is clear, the mechanism of loss of response is not as simple as one is lead to belief by reviewing current literature. One observation held by canvassing opinion from multiple thought leaders is resistance to therapy tends to arise early in therapy, and rarely after a patient shows adequate response to an agent for several years (personal communication). Further studies, especially comparative studies are needed to clarify the pathogenesis of this phenomenon, and learn which treatment is most appropriate to any given patient.

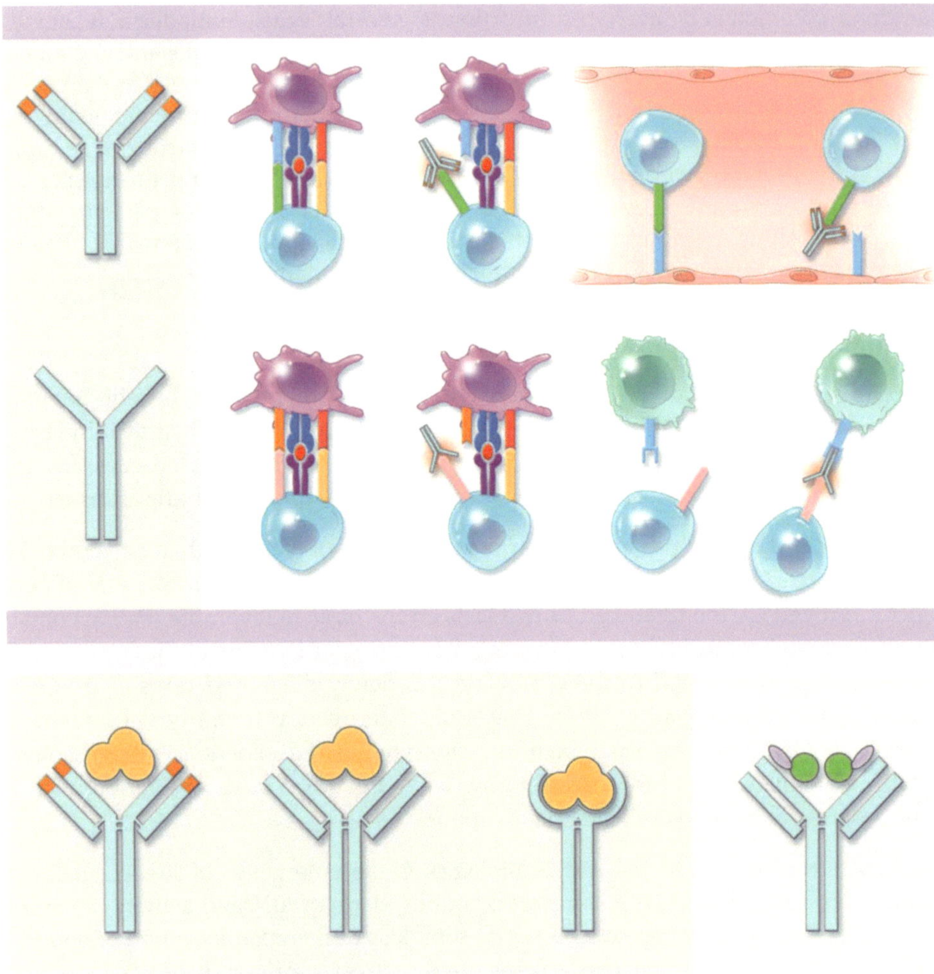

Fig. 10. Immunopathogenesis & Target Therapy (Legend)
New approaches to the treatment of psoriasis include targeted biologic therapies. Of those that been approved for marketing, the two major therapeutic classes are T-cell–targeted therapies (alefacept and efalizumab) and anticytokine therapies (anti–tumor necrosis factor [TNF] therapies): infliximab, adalimumab, etanercept, and a monoclonal antibody against interleukin-12 and interleukin-23 (ustekinumab). Efalizumab (which has been withdrawn from the market) is a chimeric monoclonal anti-CD11a antibody. It blocks the interaction of CD11a (lymphocyte-function–associated antigen -1 (LFA- 1) with intercellular adhesion molecule 1 (ICAM-1), leading to a disruption of the interaction between dendritic cells and T cells at tissue sites and in lymph nodes as well as blocking of immune cell binding to blood vessels. Alefacept is a human LFA-3 Fc fusion protein that blocks the interaction between CD2 on T cells and LFA-3 on antigen-presenting cells. It also induces antibody-dependent cytotoxicity in T cells bound to alefacept. At this point, anti-TNF strategies have three targeted therapies: a humanized chimeric anti–TNF-α monoclonal antibody (infliximab), a fully human monocolonal anti–TNF-α antibody (adalimumab), and a human p75 TNF-receptor Fc fusion protein (etanercept). Blocking of Il-12 and Il13 is achieved by means of antibodies targeting the common p40 chain of these cytokines. (CD=cluster designaton; FcR=Fc receptor)

Agent	Efficacy	Side effects
Sulfasalazine [323 324] (anti-inflammatory)	57% of assessed patients in treated group showed marked improvement. Effective in psoriatic arthritis	25% patients get Headches, nausea, vomiting oligospermia, prutitis, anemia 1-2
Azathioprine [325 326] (purine analog antimetabolite)	No conclusive studies	Bone marrow suppression
Mycophenolate mofetil (purine antimetbolite)[327 328 329]	Effective but with limited experience	GI and bone marrow
Cytokines IL-10 [330 331] IL-4 [332]	 50% reduction in severity Short trials- 10 patients & 28 patients More than 68% improvement in 20 patients	 Mild anemia, decrease response in delayed-type hypersensitivity reaction
Zidovudine [333]	Improvement noted in AIDS-associated psoriasis - Of 19 evaluable patients, 90% had partial (58%) or complete (32%) improvement	Failed to improve associated arthritis, and long term relapses were common
Somatostatin [334] Liarozole (retinoic acid metabolism blockers) [335 336]	Small series of patients, Similar to other systemic retinoids, but rapid clearance from blood once discontinued	Blood levels of somatostatin are inversely proportional to clinical response Teratogenicity, hyperlipidemias, and other muco-cutaneous symptoms
Photodynamic therapy (5-aminolevulinic acid followed by UVB irradiation) [337 338]	Small series of patients - not all sites respond to treatment	Local pain at siote of therapy
Lasers Carbon dioxide and pulsed dye laser Excimer laser (308 nm UVB) [339 340]	 Insufficient data Effective especially when using high dose therapy with long remissions	 Potential for burning as with phototherapy

Oral calcineurin antagonists Oral tacrolimus [341] [342] Oral Pimecrolimus [343]	Oral tacrolimus can improve severe psoriasis in short term (10 weeks) Oral Pimecrolimus showed similar results	Paraesthesias, headache, elevation in serum creatinine, and blood pressure

Table 6. List of Other Systemic Agents Less Commonly Used for Treating Psoriasis

Biologic	Alefacept [344]	Etanercept [345] [346]	Infliximab [347] [348]	Adalimumab [349] [350] [351] [352]	Ustekinumab [353] [354]
Dose & Route & duration	15 mg. im weekely for 12 weeks	50 mg. sub cut 2x/wk for 12 weeks then once per week thereafter	3-10 mg/kg IV infusion over 2 hrs. at week 0, 2, 6, and every 8 weeks thereafter *	80 mg. given sub cut on week 0, 40 mg. given week one, then every other week *	For under 100 kg. body weight: 45 mg. sub cut week 0 week 4 then q 3 months. (over 90 kg body weight- 90 mg.)
Type of Rx course	Pulse of 12 weeks	Continuous	Continuous	Continuous	Continuous
Pre-Rx w/u	Baseline PPD	Baseline PPD US: Viral Hepatitis screen Monitor Deep Fungal where geographicallya ppropriate †	Baseline PPD US: Viral Hepatitis screen Monitor Deep Fungal where geographicallya ppropriate †	Baseline PPD US: Viral Hepatitis screen Monitor Deep Fungal where geographicallya ppropriate †	Baseline PPD US: Viral Hepatitis screen Monitor Deep Fungal where geographicallya ppropriate
Efficacy	28% achieved a PASI 75 at 12 weeks. After 2 courses the PASI-75 goes to 40%	49% achieved PASI 75% after 12 weeks (50 mg biw) vs. 59% at 24 weeks.	For 3 mg/kg body weight: PASI 75 was 72% at 10 weeks, and 88% for 5 mg/kg body wegight	At week 12, 53% achieved PASI 75 or >	PASI 75 ay week 12 was 66.7% for those taking the 45 mg dose; 75.7% who received one 90 mg dose.
Concurrent use of live vaccines	Not studied	Not recommended	Not recommended	Not recommended	Not recommended
Efficacious for treationg PsA	-	+	+	+	-/+

Safety	Lympho-penia, malignancy, serious infections (Contraindicated on HIV +)	Serious infections, exacerbation of demyelinating diseases like (MS & optic neuritis), pancytopenia malignancy, worsening of CHF, lupus like symptoms, +ANA, Improves glucose tolerance for diabetics lowering insulin needs	Infusion-related reactions, Serious infections, exacerbation of demyelinating diseases like (MS & optic neuritis), malignancy, or lymphoprilifera-tive disorders, worsening of CHF, lupus like symptoms, +ANA	Injection site reactions, exacerbation of demyelinating diseases like (MS & optic neuritis), cytopenias, malignancy, worsening of CHF, lupus like symptoms, +ANA	Clinical experience is short to compare with other biologics- serious infections, malignmancy, Reversible posrerior leukoencepha-lopathy syndrome, and cardiovascular events
Monitoring	CD4+ T-cell counts every 2 weeks,	Annual PPD	Annual PPD	Annual PPD	Annual PPD
Long Term Data	Data on small number of patients	PASI response continues to improve to week 24. Restarting therapy after prolonged absence restores previous response. Long term safety profile established	Gradual loss of response is observed over time, especially in patients using the lower range	Loss of response was observed in 33 weeks if treatment was discontinued. Recent data shows efficacy with retreatment can restore initial gains	Not enough time has elapsed since its introduction for long term data
Pregnancy Category	B	B	B	B	B

* Low dose methotrexate (5-15 mg/week) often used to prevent antibody formation.

† Persons inhabiting or traveling through Ohio River Valley should be monitored for Histoplasmosis. Thoe inhabiting or traveling through San Joaquin Valley should be monitored for Coccidiodomycosis.

Table 7. Currently available Biologics to treat Psoriasis & Psoriatic Arthritis

9.1 Mortality in psoriasis

Mortality when it comes to psoriasis tends to occur in 3 major settings. The first tends to occur as a result of the specific co-morbidities commonly associated with severe psoriasis. Abuakara *et al* looked at a population-based cohort in the UK and found cardiovascular death as the major cause of mortality among patients with severe psoriasis. [355] Roth *et al* looked retrospectively over a 20 year period from 1965 to 1985 in France. Though the total number of patients documented to die from lethal psoriasis over a century reported in this review was 72, this number may be suspect since other causes may have lead to fatality. This study found patients whose cause of death was also related to co-morbidities including the metabolic syndrome, and visceral amyloidosis. Another group was identified with the most severe forms of psoriasis such as erythrodermic psoriasis, pustular psoriasis and psoriasis with polyarthritis. The third group was identified in which the cause of death was medication given to treat psoriasis. The largest number in this category was patients taking methotrexate. [356] Methotrexate should be used cautiously. Evidence is mounting that severe psoriasis along with the co-morbidities seen in this disease category may represent a risk factor for mortality. Well-controlled long term studies are needed to address this vital aspect.

9.2 Final comments

Certain intriguing aspects of psoriasis continue to haunt us as Nickoloff has stated on so many occasions. Psoriatic lesions in human skin have distinct clinical, histological and immunopathological features, of which not all can be reproduced in other experimental models such as mouse skin. Psoriatic skin can be restored grossly to clinical normal appearance, in spite of the fact that there may still be histological vestiges of disease activity found in clinically normal appearing skin. [357] In spite of the persistence, and often quite prominent inflammatory milieu, only rarely does one need to treat infection in psoriatic skin. Cellulitis, impetigo, viral or fungal and other parasitic infections are more commonly sequelae of atopic dermatitis, and are not generally seen in patients suffering with chronic psoriasis. Innate immunity as well as adaptive immunity are likely to play the role in maintaining the contrasting difference between these two disorders. [358] It is even rarer to record a progression to malignancy in specifically involved psoriatic skin. The interactions between the T_H1 and T_H17 networks needs further elucidation *vis a vis* the role IL-23 and IL-22 may play in this relation and its implication in the pathogenesis of psoriasis. As IL-23 has been found to promote tumor incidence and growth, this paradox needs to be resolved. A search for that elusive antigen which may be responsible to initiate and maintain the cascade of events that activates the cytokine network and leads to psoriasis continues. As more is learned about the intricacies of this pathogenesis process, it may become clear, that the sensitivity of the intercellular and intracellular interactions observed in this complicated web of events may be the result of overactive cellular forces, which may not require a specific antigenic trigger. Newer therapies are entering the arena.

10. Acknowledgements

The author wishes to recognize the invaluable assistance from Dr. Kenneth Shulman, and Dr. Jason Cohen for their contribution to the histopathology sections included in this chapter. David Pompei was instrumental in reviewing material and offering suggestions for the preparation of the manuscript. Special recognition goes to Ioanna Agams for her library services throughout this project. Lastly, I wish to thank William Jochimsen for proofreading the completed manuscript, and Gabriel Fernandez-Obregon for the illustrations.

11. References

[1] Christophers E. Psoriasis – epidemiology and clinical spectrum. *Clin Exp Dermatol* 2001;26:314.
[2] Farber EM, Nall ML. The natural history of psoriasis in 5600 patients. *Dermatologica*.1974;148:1-18.
[3] Yui YS. The prevalence of psoriasis in the mongoloid race. J *Am Acad Dermatol*.1984;10:965-8.
[4] Stern RS, Nijsten T, Feldman SR, Margolis DJ, Rolstad T. Psoriasis is common, carries a substantial burden even when not extensive, and is associated with widespread treatment dissatisfaction. *J Investig Dermatol Symp Proc.* 2004;9:136-139.
[5] Pariser DM, Bagel J, Gelfand JM, *et al.* National Psoriasis Foundation clinical consensus on disease severity. *Arch Dermatol.*2007;143:239-242.
[6] Bell LM, Sedlack R, Beard CM, Perry HO, Michet CJ, Kurland LT. Incidence of psoriasis in Rochester, Minn, 1980-1983. *Arch Dermatol* 1991;127:1184-7.
[7] Shbeeb M, Sunku J, Hunder G, Gibson L, O'Fallon W, Gabriel S. Incidence of psoriasis and psoriatic arthritis, a populationbased study. *Arthritis Rheum* 1995;38:S379.
[8] Icen M, Crowson CS, McEvoy MT, Dann FJ, Gabriel SE, Maradit Kremers H. Trends in incidence of adult-onset psoriasis over three decades: a populationbased study. *J Am Acad Dermatol* 2009;60:394-401.
[9] Huerta C, Rivero E, Rodriguez LA. Incidence and risk factors for psoriasis in the general population. *Arch Dermatol* 2007;143: 1559-65.
[10] Lomholt G. Psoriasis, Prevalence, Spontaneous Course and Genetics: a census study on the prevalence of skin diseases on the Faroe Islands. Copenhagen. *Denmark GEC Gad*, 1963: 54-6.
[11] Farber EM, Nall ML.The natural history of psoriasis in 5600 patients. *Dermatologica.* 1974;148:1-18.
[12] Trembath RC, Clough RL, Rosbotham JL, *et al.* Identification of a major susceptibility locus on chromosome 6p and evidence for further disease loci revealed by a two stage genome-wide search in psoriasis. *Hum Mol Genet* 1997;6:813-20.
[13] Nair RP, Duffin KC, Helms C, *et al.* Genome-wide scan reveals association of psoriasis with IL-23 and NF-kappaβ pathways. *Nat Genet* 2009;41:199-204.
[14] Nair RP, Stuart PE, Nistor I, *et al.* Sequence and haplotype analysis supports HLA-C as the psoriasis susceptibility 1gene. *Am J Hum Genet* 2006;78:827-51.
[15] Asumalahti K, Laitinen T, Itkonen-Vatjus R, *et al.* A candidate gene for psoriasis near HLA-C, HCR (pg8) is highly polymorphic with a disease-associated susceptibility allele. *Hum Mol Genet.* 2000;9;1533-42. Erratum, Hum Mol Genet. 2001;10:301.)
[16] Allen MH, Veal C,Faassen A. *et al.* A non-HLA gene within the MHC in psoriasis. *Lancet*.1999;353:1589-90.
[17] Asumalahti K, Ameen M, Suomela S, *et al.* Genetic analysis of PSORS1 distinguishes guttate psoriasis and palmoplantar pustulosis. *J Invest Dermatol.* 2003;120:627-32.
[18] Allen MH, Ameen H, Veal C, et al. The major psoriasis susceptibility locus PSORS1 is not a risk factor for late-onset psoriasis. *J Invest Dermatol* 2005;124:103-6.

[19] Duffin KC, Woodcock J, Krugger GG. Genetic Variations associated with psoriasis and psoriatic arthritis found by genome-wide associaton. *Dermatol Ther* 2010 Mar;23(2):101-13.
[20] Tsunemi Y, Saeki H, Nakamura K, Sekiya et al. Interleukin-12 p40 gene (IL12B) 3'-untranslated region an polymorphism is associated with susceptibility to atopic dermatitis and psoriasis vulgaris. *J Dermatol Sci* 2002;30:161-6.
[21] Duerr RH, Taylor KD, Brant SR, Rioux JD, *et al.* A genome-wide association study identifies IL23R as inflammatory bowel disease gene. *Science* 2006;314(5804):1461-1463.
[22] Barton A, Eyre S, Ke X, Hinks A, *et al.* Identification of AF4/FMR2 family, member 3 (AFF3) as a novel rheumatoid arthritis susceptibility locus and confirmation of two further pan-autoimmune susceptibility genes. *Hum Mol Genet* 2009;18(13):2518-2522.
[23] Wolf N, Quaranta M, Prescott NJ, Allen M *et al.* Psoriasis is associated with pleiotropic susceptibility loci identified in type II diabetes and Crohn disease. J *Med Genet* 2008;45:114-6.
[24] Li Y, Liao W, Chang M, Schrodi SJ *et al.* Further genetic evidence for three psoriasis-risk genes: ADAM33, CDKAL1, and PTPN22. *J Invest Dermatol* 2009;129:629-34.
[25] Huffmeier U, Steffens M, Burkhardt H, Lascorz J *et al.* Evidence for susceptibility determinant(s) to psoriasis vulgaris in or near PTPN22 in German patients. *J Med Genet* 2006;43:517-22.
[26] Smith RL, Warren RB, Eyre S, Ke X *et al.* Polymorphisms in the PTPN22 region are associated with psoriasis of early onset. *Br J Dermatol* 2008;158:962-8.
[27] Chang M, Li Y, Yan C, Callis-Duffin KP *et al.* Variants in the 5q31 cytokine gene cluster are associated with psoriasis. *Genes Immun* 2008;9:176-81.
[28] Zhang XJ, Huang W, Yang S, Sun LD *et al.* Psoriasis genome-wide association study identifies susceptibility variants within LCE gene cluster at 1q2. *Nat Genet* 2009;41:205-10.
[29] Tomfohrde J, Silverman A, Barnes R, Fernandez-Vina MA, *et al.* Gene for familial psoriasis susceptibility mapped to the distal end of human chromosome 17q. *Science*. 1994.;264:1141-45.
[30] Helms C, Caol L, Krueger JG, Wijsman EM. *et al.* A putative RUNX1 binding site variant between SLC9A3R1 and NAT9 is associated with susceptibility to psoriasis. *Nat Genet*. 2003;349-56.
[31] Bromley SK, Burack WR, Johnson KG, Somersalo K. *et al.* The immunological synapse. *Ann Rev Immunol* .2001;19:375-96.
[32] Ellis CN, Krueger GG. Treatment of chronic plaque psoriasis by selective targeting of memory effector T lymphocytes. *N Eng J Med*;345:248-55.
[33] Jackson B, Tilli CM, Hardman MJ, *et al.* Late cornified envelope family in differentiating epithelia--response to calcium and ultraviolet irradiation. *J Invest Dermatol.* 2005;124:1062-1070.
[34] de Cid R, Riveira-Munoz E, Zeeuwen PL, *et a*l. Deletion of the late cornified envelope LCE3B and LCE3C genes as a susceptibility factor for psoriasis. *Nat Genet.* 2009;41:211-215.
[35] Nestle FO, Kaplan DH, Barker J. Psoriasis. *N Engl J Med.* 2009;361:496-509.

[36] Cargill M, Schrodi SJ, Chang M, *et al.* A large-scale genetic association study confirms IL12B and leads to the identification of IL23R as psoriasis-risk genes. *Am J Hum Genet.* 2007;80:273-90.
[37] Capon F, Di Meglio P, Szaub J, *et al.* Sequence variants in the genes for the interleukin-23 receptor (IL23R) and its ligan (IL12B) confer protection against psoriasis. *Hum Genet.* 2007;122:201-6.
[38] Eyre RW. Krueger GG. The Koebner response in psoriasis. In Roenig HH,Maibach HI eds. Psoriasis. New York Marcel Decker; 1984:105-16.
[39] Telfer NR, Chalmers RJ,Whale K, Colman G. The role of streptococcal infection in the initiation of guttate psoriasis. *Arch Dermatol.*1992;128:39-42.
[40] Abel EA, DiCicco LM, Orenberg EK *et al.* Drugs in exacerbation of psoriasis. *J Am Acad Dermatol.* 1986; 15:1007-22.
[41] Ben-David G, Sheiner E, Hallak M, Levy A. Pregnancy outcome in women with psoriasis. *J Reprod Med* 2008; 53: 183–7.
[42] Higgins E. Alcohol, smoking and psoriasis. *Clin Exp Dermatol* 2000; 25: 107–10.
[43] Seville RH. Psoriasis and stress. *Br J Dermatol.* 1977; 97: 279–302.
[44] Lazar AP, Roenigk HH. Acquired immunodeficiency syndrome (AIDS) can exacerbate psoriasis. *J Am Acad Dermatol* 1988; 18: 144.
[45] Krueger G, Koo J, Lebwohl M, *et al.* The impact of psoriasis on quality of life: results of a 1988 National Psoriasis Foundation patient-membership survey. *Arch Dermatol.* 2001; 137:280-84. *Arch Dermatol.* 2001; 137:280-84.
[46] National Psoriasis Foundation. Spring 2005 Survey Panel Snapshot. Available at: http://www.psoriasis.org/files/pdfs/research/2005_spring_survey_panel.pdf. Accessed October 30, 2007.
[47] NSF Fall 2004 Survey Panel Snapshot.Available at: www.psoriasis.org/files/pdfs/research/2004_fall_survey_panel.pdf. Accessed October 30, 2007.
[48] Pardasani AG, Feldman SR, Clark AR Treatment of psoriasis:an algorithm-based approach for primary care physicians. *Am Fam Phys.* 2000;61:725-33.
[49] NPF. Available at www.psoraisis.org/about/stats. Accessed March 2006
[50] Ingram JT, The significance and management of psoriasis. BMJ.1954; ii:823-8.
[51] Griffiths CE, Christopher E, Barker JN, Chalmers RJ *et al.* A classification of psoriasis according to phenotype. *Br J Dermatol.* 2007;156: 258-62.
[52] Rakkit T, Panko JM, Christensen TE, Wong B *et al.* Plaque thickness and morphology in psoriasis vulgaris associated with therapeutic response. *Br J. Dermatol* 2009; 160:1083-9.
[53] Baker H. Corticosteroids and pustular psoriasis. *Br J Dermatol.* 1976; 94 (Suppl.12):83-8.
[54] Grice K, Blendis LM, Keir MI, Harvey RF. Accidental hypothermia in erythroderma from generalized psoriasis. *Arch Dermatol* 1968; 98:263-7.
[55] Johnson C. Shuster S. Eccrine sweating in psoriasis. *Br. J. Dermatol.* 1969; 81: 119-24.
[56] Preger L, Maibach HI, Osborne RB, Shapiro HA *et al.* On the question of psoriatic enteropathy. *Arch Dermatol.* 1970; 102:151-3.
[57] Samitz MH. Albom JJ. Palmar Psoriasis. *Arch Dermatol.* 1951;64:199-204.
[58] Baker H, Golding DN, Thompson N. The nails in psoriatic arthritis. *Br J Dermatol.* 1964;76:549-54.

[59] Stuart P, Malick F, Nair RP, Henseler T *et al.* Analysis of phenotypic variation in psoriasis as a function of age at onset, and family history. *Arch Dermatol.* 2002;294:207-13.

[60] Zaias N. Psoriasis of the nail. Arch *Dermatol.* 1969;99:567-79.

[61] Robbins TO, Kouskoukis CE, Ackerman AB. Onycholysis in psoriatic nails. *Am J. Dermatopathol.* 1983;5:39-41.

[62] Kouskoukis CE. Scher RK. Ackerman AB. The "oil drop" sign of psoriatic nails: a clinical finding specific for psoriasis. *Am J Dermatopathol.*1983;5:259-62.

[63] Ganor S. Diseases sometimes associated with psoriasis. *Dermatologica.* 1977;154:268-72.

[64] Nyfors A. Psoriasis in children. *Acta Derm Venereol (Stockh)* 1981;61 (Suppl. 95);47-53.

[65] Gladman DD. Psoriatic arthritis. *Rheum Dis Clin North Am.* 1998;24:829-844.

[66] Fisher VS. Clinical monograph for drug formulary review: systemic agents for psoriasis/psoriatic arthritis. *J Manag Care Pharm.* 2005;11:33-55.

[67] Gladman DD, Antoni C, Mease P, Clegg DO *et al.* Psoriatic arthritis: epidemiology, clinical features, course, and outcome. *Ann Rheum Dis.* 2005;64(suppl 2):ii14-7.

[68] Reich K. Approach to managing patients with nail psoriasis. *J Eur Acad Dermatol Venereol.* 2009;23(suppl 1):15-21.

[69] Williamson L, Dalbeth N, Dockerty JL, Gee BC *et al.* Extended report: nail disease in psoriatic arthritis—clinically important, potentially treatable and often overlooked. *Rheumatology.* 2004;43:790-794.

[70] Leung YY, Tam LS, Kun EW, Li EK. *et al.* Psoriatic arthritis as a distinct disease entity. *J Postgrad Med.* 2007;53:63-71.

[71] Pariser DM, Bagel J, Gelfand JM, Korman NJ *et al;* for the National Psoriasis Foundation. National Psoriasis Foundation clinical consensus on disease severity. *Arch Dermatol.* 2007;143:239-242.

[72] Gottlieb A, Korman NJ, Gordon KB, Feldman SR *et al.* Guidelines of care for the management of psoriasis and psoriatic arthritis, section 2, psoriatic arthritis: Overview and guidelines of care for treatment with an emphasis on the biologics. *J Am Acad Dermatol.* 2008;58:851-64.

[73] Fernández-Sueiro JL, Willisch A, Pértega-Díaz S, Tasende JA *et al.* Evaluation of ankylosing spondylitis spinal mobility measurements in the assessment of spinal involvement in psoriatic arthtitis. *Arthritis Rheum* 2009;61:386-92.

[74] Veale D, Rogers S, Fitzgerald O. Classification of clinical subsets in psoriatic arthritis. Br J Rheumatol 1994;33:133-8.

[75] Chandran V. Epidemiology of psoriatic arthritis. J Rheumatol 2009;36:213-15.

[76] Gisondi P, Tinazzi I, El-Dalati G, Gallo M *et al.* Lower limb enthesopathy in patients with psoriasis without clinical signs of arthropathy: a hospital-based case control study. *AnnRheum Dis* 2008;67:26-30.

[77] Taylor W, Gladman D, Helliwell P, Marchesoni A *et al.* Classification criteria for psoriatic arthritis: development of new criteria from a large international study. *Arthritis Rheum.* 2006;54:2665-2673.

[78] Fredriksson T, Pettersson U. Severe psoriasis—oral therapy with a new retinoid. *Dermatologica.* 1978;157:238-244.

[79] Finlay AY, Khan GK. Dermatology Life Quality Index (DLQI) - a simple practical measure for routine clinical use. *Clin Exp Dermatol.* 1994; 19: 210–216.

[80] Langley RG, Ellis CN. Evaluating psoriasis with psoriasis area and severity index, psoriasis global assessment, and lattice system physician's global assessment. *J Am Acad Dermatol* 2004;51:563–569.
[81] Puzenat E, Bronsard V, Prey S, Gourraud PA *et al.* What are the best outcome measures for assessing plaque psoriasis severity? A systematic review of the literature. J Eur Acad Dermatol Venereol. 2010 Apr;24 Suppl 2:10-6.
[82] Nickoloff, BJ. The cytokine network in psoriasis. *Arch Dermatol.* 1991;127(6):871-84.
[83] Nickoloff BJ. Skin innate immune system in psoriasis: friend or foe? *J Clin Invest.*1999;104:1161-4.
[84] Funk J, Langeland T, Schrumpf E, Hanssen LE. Psoriasis induced by interferon-alpha. *Br J Dermatol* 1991;125:463-5.
[85] Lande R, Gregorio J, Facchinetti V, Chatterjee B *et al.* Plasmacytoid dendritic cells sense self-DNA coupled with antimicrobial peptide. *Nature* 2007;449:564-9.
[86] Nestle FO, Turka LA, Nickoloff BJ. Characterization of dermal dendritic cells in psoriasis: autostimulation of T lymphocytes and induction of Th1 type cytokines. *J Clin Invest.* 1994;94:202-9.
[87] Lowes MA, Chamian F, Abello MV, Fuentes-Duculan J *et al.* Increase in TNF-alpha and inducible nitric oxide synthase-expressing dendritic cells in psoriasis and reduction with efalizumab (anti-CD11a*). Proc Natl Acad Sci U S A.* 2005;102:19057-62.
[88] Chamian F, Lowes MA, Lin SL, Lee E *et al.* Alefacept reduces infiltrating T cells, activated dendritic cells, and inflammatory genes in psoriasis vulgaris. *Proc Natl Acad Sci U S A.* 2005;102:2075-80.
[89] Buchau AS, Gallo RL. Innate immunity and antimicrobial defense systems in psoriasis. *Clin Dermatol.* 2007;25:616-24.
[90] Zheng Y, Danilenko DM, Valdez P, Kasman I *et al.* Interleukin-22 a T(H)17 cytokine, mediates IL-23-induced dermal inflammationm an acanthosis. Nature 2007; 445:648-51.
[91] Chan JR, Blumenschein W, Murphy E, Diveu C. *et. al.* IL-23 stimulated epidermal hyperplasioa via TNF and IL-20R2-dependent mechanisms with implications for psoriasis pathogenesis. *J Exp Med* 2006;203 (12): 2577-87.
[92] Iwakura Y, Ishigame H. The IL-23/IL-17 axis in inflammation. *J Clin Invest* 2006; 116: 1218-22.
[93] Sano S, Chan KS, Carbajal S, Clifford J *et al.* Stat3 links activated keratinocytes and immunocytes required for development of psoriasis in a novel transgenic mouse model. *Nat Med* 2005; 43-49.
[94] Boniface K, Bernard FX, Garcia M, Gurney AL, *et al.* IL-22 inhibits epidermal differentiation and induces proinflammatory gene expression and migration of human keratinocytes. *J Immunol* 2005;174 (6): 3695-702.
[95] Wolk K, Witte E, Wallace E, Döcke WD *et al.* IL-22regulated the expression of genes responsible for antimicrobial defense, cellular differentiation and mobility in keratinocytes: a potential role in psoriasis. *Eur J. Immunol* 2006;36(5):1309-23.
[96] Zaba LC, Cardinale I, Gilleaudeau P, Sullivan-Whalen M *et al.* Amelioration of epidermal hyperplasia by TNF inhibition is associated with reduced Th17 responses. *J Exp Med.* 2007; 204:3183-94. [Erratum, *J Exp Med.* 2008; 205:1941.])
[97] Duerr RH, Taylor KD, Brant SR, Rioux JD. *et al.* A genome\-wide association study indentifies IL23R as an inflammatory bowel disease gene. *Science.* 2006;314:1461-3.

[98] Uhlig HH, McKenzie BS, Hue S, Thompson C *et al.* Differential activity of IL12 and IL-23 in mucosal and systemic innate immune pathology. *Immunity* 2006;25; 309-18.
[99] Langner A, Ashton P, Van De Kerkhof PC, Verjans H *et al.* A long-term multicentre assessment of the safety and tolerability of calcitriol ointment in the treatment of chronic plaque psoriasis. *Br J Dermatol.* 1996; 135: 385–9.
[100] Binderup L, Bramm E. Effects of a novel vitamin D analogue MC903 on cell proliferation and differentiation *in vitro* and on calcium metabolism *in vivo. Biochem Biopharmacol.* 1998; 37: 889–95.
[101] Kang S, Yi S, Griffiths CE, Fancher L *et al.* Calcipotriene-induced improvement in psoriasis is associated with reduced interleukin-8 and increased interleukin-10 levels within lesions. *Br J Dermatol.* 1998; 138: 77–83.
[102] Bikle DD. 1,25(OH)2D3-modulated calcium induced keratinocyte differentiation. *J Invest Dermatol* ;1996:1:22-7.
[103] Su MJ, Bikle DD, Mancianti ML, Pillai S. 1,25-Dihydroxyvitamin D3 potentiates the keratinocyte response to calcium. *J Biol Chem.* 1994;269:14723-9.
[104] Takeuchi A, Reddy GS, Kobayashi T, Okano *T et al.* Nuclear factor of activated T cells (NFAT) as a molecular target for 1alpha,25dihydroxyvitaminD3-mediated effects. .*J Imunnol.* 1998;160; 209-18.
[105] Towers TL, Staeva TP, Freedman LP. A two-hit mechanism for vitamin D3-mediated transcriptional repression of the granulocyte-macrophage colony-stimulating factor gene: vitamin D receptor competes for DNA binding with NFAT1 and stabilizes c-Jun. *Mol Cell Biol.* 1999;19:4191-9.
[106] Michel G, Gailis A, Jarzebska-Deussen B, Muschen A. *et al.* 1,25-(OH)2-vitamin D3 and calcipotriol induce IL-10 receptor gene expression in human epidermal cells. *Inflamm Res.* 1997;46:32-4..
[107] Nagpal S, Lu J, Boehm MF. Vitamin D Analogs: Mechanism, of Action and Therapeutic Applications. *Cur Med Chem.*2001;8(13):1661-79.
[108] Ludwig RJ, Herzog C, Rostock A, Ochesendorf FR *et al.* Psoriasis: a possible risk factor for development of coronary artery calcification. *Br J Dermatol.* 2007;156:271-276.
[109] Mehta NN, Azfar RS, Shin DB, Neiman AL *et al.* Patients with severe psoriasis are at increased risk of cardiovascular mortality: cohort study using the General Practice Research Database. *Eur Heart J.* 2010;31:1000-1006.
[110] Gelfand JM, Niemann AL, Shin DB, Wang X, Margolis DJ, Troxel AB. Risk of myocardial infarction in patients with psoriasis. *JAMA.* 2006;296:1735-1741.
[111] Mehta NN, Yu Y, Pinnelas R, Krishnamoorthy P, Shin DB et al.Attributable risk estimate of severe psoriasis on major cardiovascular event. *Am J Med.* 2011 Aug;124(8):775.e1-6.
[112] Kimball AB, Robinson D Jr. Wu Y, Guzzo C *et al.* Cardiovascular disease and rik factors among psoriasis patients in two US healthcare databases, 2001-2002. *Dermatology.* 2008;217:27-7
[113] Prodanovich S, Kirsner RS, Kravetz JD Ma F *et.al.* Association of psoriasis with coronary artery, cerebrovascular, and peripheral vascular diseases and mortality. Arch Dermatol. 2009;145(6):700-3.
[114] Y-J Chen, J-L Shen, C-Y Wu, Y-T Chang. Elevated plasma *osteopontin* level is associated with occurrence of psoriasis and is an unfavorable cardiovascular risk factor in patients with psoriasis. *J Am Acad Dermatol.* 2009;60:225-30.

[115] Jashin Wu , Albert Yuh-Jer (Kaiser Permanente- Southern CA). *The effect of tumor necrosis factor alpha inhibitors on the risk of myocardial infarction in patients with psoriasis.* American Academy of Dermatology (AAD) 69th Annual Meeting. Abstract P400. Presented February 6, 2011.

[116] Grundy SM. Metabolic syndrome: connecting and reconciling cardiovascular and diabetes worlds. *J Am Coll Cardiol.* 2006;47:1093-1100.

[117] Park Y-W, Zhu S, Palaniappan L, Heshka S, Carnethon MR, Heymsfield SB. The metabolic syndrome. Prevalence and associated risk factor findings in the US population from the Third National Health and Nutrition Examination Survey, 1988-1994. *Arch Intern Med.* 2003;163:427-436.

[118] National Cholesterol Education Program. *Third Report of the National Cholesterol Education Program (NCEP) Expert Panel on Detection, Evaluation, and Treatment of High Blood Cholesterol in Adults (Adult Treatment Panel [ATP] III. Final Report.* Bethesda, Md: National Heart, Lung, and Blood Institute; 2002. NIH Publication No. 02-5215.

[119] Hamminga EA, van der Lely AJ, Neumann HAM, Thio Hb. Chronic inflammation in psoriasis and obesity: implications for therapy. *Med Hypotheses.* 2006;67:768-773.

[120] Wellen KE, Hotamisligil GS. Inflammation, stress, and diabetes. *J Clin Invest.* 2005;115:1111-1119.

[121] Wakkee M, Thio HB, Prens EP, Sijbrands EJG, Neumann HAM. Unfavorable cardiovascular risk profiles in untreated and treated psoriasis patients. *Atherosclerosis.* 2007;190:1-9.

[122] Mussi A, Bonifati C, Carducci M, D'Agosto G *et al.* Serum TNF-alpha levels correlate with disease severity and are reduced by effective therapy in plaque-type psoriasis. *J Biol Regul Homeost Agents.* 1997;11:115-18.

[123] Wakkee M, Thio HB, Prens EP, Sijbrands EJG, Neumann HAM. Unfavorable cardiovascular risk profiles in untreated and treated psoriasis patients. *Atherosclerosis.* 2007:190:1-9

[124] Wellen KE, Hotamisligil GS. Inflammation, stress, and diabetes. *J Clin Invest.* 2005;115:1111-1119.

[125] Ronti T, Lupattelli G, Mannarino E. The endocrine function of adipose tissue: an update. *Clin Endocrinol.* 2006;64:355-365.

[126] Wisse BE. The inflammatory syndrome: the role of adipose tissue cytokines in metabolic disorders lined to obesity. *J Am Soc Nephrol.* 2004;15:2792-2800.

[127] National Psoriasis Foundation. *Report on the Psycho-Social Impacts of Psoriasis.* 2009. Available at: http://www.psoriasis.org/NetCommunity/Document.Doc?id=619. Accessed June 6, 2010.

[128] Sommer DM, Jenisch S, Suchan M, Christophers E, Weichenthal M. Increased prevalence of the metabolic syndrome in patients with moderate to severe psoriasis. *Arch Dermatol Res.* 2006;298:321-328.

[129] Gisondi P, Tessari G, Conti A, Piaserico S et al. Prevalence of metabolic syndrome in patients with psoriasis: a hospital-based case-control study. *Br J Dermatol.* 2007;157:68-73.

[130] Cohen AD, Sherf M, Vidavsky L, Vardy DA, Shapiro J, Meyerovitch J. Association between psoriasis and the metabolic syndrome: a cross-sectional study. *Dermatology.* 2008;216:152-155.

[131] Brauchli YB, Jick SS, Meier CR. Psoriasis and the risk of incident diabetes mellitus: a population-based study. *Br J Dermatol.*2008;159:1331-37.

[132] Setty AR, Curhan G, Choi HK. Obesity, waist circumference, weight change, and the risk of psoriasis in women: Nurses' Health Study II. *Arch Intern Med.* 2007;167:1670-1675.

[133] Qureshi AA, Choi HK, Setty AR, Curhan GC. Psoriasis and the risk of diabetes and hypertension: a prospective study of US female nurses. *Arch Dermatol.*2009;145:379-382.

[134] Chiang YY, Lin H-W. Association between psoriasis and chronic obstructive pulmonary disease: a population based study in Taiwan. *J Eur Acad Dermatol Venereol.* 2011 Mar 9. doi: 10.1111/j.1468-3083.2011.04009.x. [Epub ahead of print]

[135] Ahlehoff O, Gislason GH, Lindhardsen J, Charlot MG. et al. Psoriasis carries an increased risk of venous thromboembolism: a Danish nationwide cohort study. *Plos One* 2011 Mar25;6(3)e18125.

[136] Murase JE, Chan KK, Garite TJ, Cooper DM *et al.* Hormonal effect on psoriasis in pregnancy and post partum. *Arch Dermatol.* 2005;141:601-6.

[137] Lima XT, Abuabara K, Kimball AB. Pregnancy outcomes in psoriasis: a retrospective analysis. Presented at: American Academy of Dermatology 68th Annual Meeting; March 5-9, 2010; Miami, FL. Presentation No. P3308.

[138] Michaëlsson G, Gerdén B, Ottosson M, Parra A *et al.* Patients with psoriasis often have increased serum levels of IgA antibodies to gliadin. *Br J Dermatol.* 1993 Dec;129(6):667-73.

[139] Michaëlsson G, Gerdén B, Hagforsen E, Nilsson B. *et al.* Psoriasis patients with antibodies to gliadin can be improved by a gluten-free diet. *Br J Dermatol.* 2000 Jan;142(1):44-51.

[140] Gelfand JM, Shin DB, Neimann AL, Wang X, Margolis DJ, Troxel AB. The risk of lymphoma in patients with psoriasis. *J Invest Dermatol.* 2006;126:2194-2201.

[141] Boffetta P, Gridley G, Lindelof B. Cancer risk in a population-based cohort of patients hospitalized for psoriasis in Sweden. *J Invest Dermatol.* 2001;117:1531-7.

[142] Margolis D, Bilker W, Hennessy S,Vittorio C *et al.* The risk of malignancy associated with psoriasis. *Arch Dermatol.* 2001;137:778-83.

[143] Fortune DG, Richards HL, Kirby B, Bowcock S *et al.* A cognitive-behavioral symptom management programme as an adjunct in psoriasis therapy. *Br J Dermatol* 2002;146: 458–65.

[144] Fortune DG, Richards HL, Kirby B. McElhone K *et al.* Psychological distress impairs clearance of psoriasis in patients treated with photochemotherapy. *Arch Dermatol* 2003;139: 752–6.

[145] Voorhees JJ, Chakrabarti SG, Botero F,Miedler L *et al.* Zinc therapy and distribution in psoriasis. *Arch Dermatol* 1969; 100: 669–73.

[146] Ellis JP, Sanderson KV, Savin JA. The turkey diet in psoriasis (Letter). *Lancet* 1968; i: 1429–30.

[147] Farber EM, Zackheim H. Turkey, tryptophan, and psoriasis (Letter). *Lancet* 1967; ii: 944.

[148] Zackheim HS, Farber EM. Low-protein diet and psoriasis. *Arch Dermatol* 1969;99: 580–6.

[149] Zackheim HS, Farber EM. Rapid weight reduction and psoriasis. *Arch Dermatol* 1971; 103: 136–40.
[150] Even-Pas Z, Gumon R, Hipnis V. Dead Sea sun vs. Dead Sea water in the treatment of psoriasis. *J Dermatol Treat* 1996; 7: 83–6.
[151] Goeckerman WH. Treatment of psoriasis. *Arch Dermatol Syphilol* 1931; 24: 446–50.
[152] .Petrozzi JW, Barton JO, Kaidbey K, Kligman AM *et al.* Updating the Goeckerman regimen for psoriasis. *Br J Dermatol* 1978; 98: 437–44.
[153] Parrish JA, Morison WL, Gonzalez E, Krop TM *et al.* Therapy of psoriasis by tar photosensitization. *J Invest Dermatol* 1978; 70: 111-2.
[154] Bickers DR. The carcinogenicity and mutagenicity of therapeutic coal tar: a perspective. *J Invest Dermatol* 1981; 77: 173–4.
[155] Henry SA. Occupational cutaneous cancer attributable to certain chemicals in industry. *Br Med Bull* 1946–47; 4: 389–401.
[156] Götz H, Deichmann B, Zobel M. Zur Frage der iatrogenen Karzinomprovokation durch teeranwendung in der Dermatologie. *Z Hautkr* 1978; 53: 751-5.
[157] Pittelkow MR, Perry HO, Muller SA, Maughan WZ *et al.* Skin cancer in patients with psoriasis treated with coal tar: A 25-year follow up study. *Arch Dermatol* 1981;117: 465–8.
[158] McGarry GW, Robertson JR. Scrotal carcinoma following prolonged use of crude coal tar ointment. *Br J Urol* 1989;63:211.
[159] Jones SK, Mackie RM, Hole DJ, Gillis CR. Further evidence of the safety of tar in the management of psoriasis. *Br J Dermatol* 1985; 113: 97–101.
[160] Ingram JT. The approach to psoriasis. *BMJ* 1953; ii: 591–4.
[161] Statham BN, Rowell NR. Short contact dithranoltherapy-twice daily and high concentration regimes. *Br J Dermatol* 1985; 113: 245–6.
[162] Monk BE, Hehir ME, Clement MI, Pembroke AC *et al.* Anthralin-corticosteroid combination therapy in the treatment of chronic plaque psoriasis. *Arch Dermatol* 1988; 124: 548–50.
[163] David M, Lowe NJ. Psoriasis therapy: comparative studies with a hydrocolloid dressing, plastic film occlusion, and triamcinolone acetonide cream. *J Am Acad Dermatol* 1989; 21: 511–4.
[164] Lebwohl M, Ali S. Treatment of psoriasis. I. Topical therapy and phototherapy. *J Am Acad Dermatol* 2001; 45: 487–98.
[165] Nilsson JE, Gip LJ. Systemic effects of local treatment with high doses of potent corticosteroids in psoriatics. *Acta Derm Venereol (Stockh)* 1979; 59: 245–8.
[166] Katz HI, Hien NT, Prawer SE, Mastbaum LI *et al.* Superpotent topical steroid treatment of psoriasis vulgaris: clinical efficacy and adrenal function. *J Am Acad Dermatol* 1987; 16: 804–11.
[167] Du Vivier A, Stoughton RB. Tachyphylaxis to the action of topically applied corticosteroid. *Arch Dermatol* 1975; 111: 581-3.
[168] Hradil E, Lindström C, Möller H. Intermittent treatment of psoriasis with clobetasol propionate. *Acta Derm Venereol (Stockh)* 1978; 58: 375–7.
[169] Katz HI, Prawer SE, Medansky RS, Krueger GG *et al.* Intermittent corticosteroid maintenance treatment of psoriasis: a double-blind, multicenter trial of augmented betamethasone dipropionate ointment in a pulse dose treatment regimen. *Dermatologica* 1991; 183: 269–74.

[170] Mortensen L, Kragballe K, Wegmann E, Schiffer S *et al.* Treatment of psoriasis vulgaris with topical calcipotriol has no short-term effects on calcium or bone metabolism. *Acta Derm Venereol (Stockh)* 1993; 73: 300–4.

[171] Guenther L, Van De Kerkhof PCM, Snellman E, Kragballe K *et al.* Efficacy and safety of a new combination of calcipotriol and betamethasone dipropionate (one or twice daily) compared to calcipotriol (twice daily) in the treatment of psoriasis vulgaris: a randomized, double-blind, vehicle-controlled clinical trial. *Br J Dermatol* 2002; 147: 316–23.

[172] Zhu X, Wang B, Zhao G, Gu J *et al.* An investigator-masked comparison of the efficacy and safety of twice daily applications of calcitriol 3μg/g ointment versus calcipotriol 50 μg/g ointment in subjects with moderate chronic plaque type psoriasis *J Eur Acad Dermatol Venereol* 2007; 21: 466–72.

[173] Langer A, Ashton P, Van De Kerkhof PC, Verjans H *et al.* A long-term multicentre assessment of the safety and tolerability of calcitriol ointment in the treatment of chronic plaque psoriasis. *Br J Dermatol* 1996; 135: 385–9.

[174] Mason J, Mason AR, Cork MJ. Topical preparations for the treatment of psoriasis: a systematic review. *Br J Dermatol* 2002; 146: 351–64.

[175] Barker JN, Ashton RE, Marks R, Harris RI *et al.* Topical maxacalcitol for the treatment of psoriasis vulgaris: a placebo-controlled, double-blind, dose-finding study with active comparator. *Br J Dermatol* 1999; 141: 274–8.

[176] de Jong EM, Mørk NJ, Seijger MM, De La Brassine M *et al.* The combination of calcipotriol and methotrexate coupled with methotrexate and vehicle in psoriasis: results of a multicentre, placebo-controlled, randomized trial. *Br J Dermatol* 2003; 148: 318–25.

[177] Galderma - personal communication and data on file.

[178] Henry M, Frankel A, Emer J, Lebwohl M. Bilateral Comparison Study on the Order of Application of Combination Clobetasol Propionate Spray and Calcitriol Ointment in the Treatment of Plaque Psoriasis. Poster Presentation.

[179] Tzaneva S, Honingsmann H, Tanew A, Seeber A. A comparison of psoralen plus ultraviolet A (PUVA) monotherapy, tacalcitol plus PUVA and tazarotene plus PUVA in patients with chronic plaque type psoriasis. *Br J Dermatol* 2002; 147: 748–53.

[180] Ring J, Kowalzick L, Christophers E, Schill WB *et al.* Calcitriol 3 μg/g ointment in combination with UVB phototherapy for the treatment of plaque psoriasis: results of a comparative study. *Br J Dermatol* 2001; 144: 495–9.

[181] Lebwohl M, Siskin SB, Epinette W, Breneman D *et al.* A multicenter trial of calcipotriene ointment and halobetasol ointment compared to either agent alone for the treatment of psoriasis. *J Am Acad Dermatol* 1996; 35: 268–9.

[182] Macdonald A, McMinn RM, Fry L. Retinoic acid in the treatment of psoriasis. *Br J Dermatol* 1972; 86: 524-7.

[183] Chandraratna RAS. Tazarotene: first of a new generation of receptor-selective retinoids. *Br J Dermatol* 1996; 135 (Suppl. 49): 18–25.

[184] Krueger GG, Drake LA, Elias PM, Lowe NJ *et al.* The safety and efficacy of tazarotene gel, a topical acetylenic retinoid, in the treatment of psoriasis. *Arch Dermatol* 1998; 134: 57–60.

[185] Weinsten GD, Koo JYM, Krueger GG, Lebwohl MG *et al.* Tazarotene cream in the treatment of psoriasis: two multicenter, double-blind, randomized, vehicle-controlled studies of the safety and efficacy of tazarotene creams 0.05% and 0.1% applied once daily for 12 weeks. *J Am Acad Dermatol* 2003; 48: 760–7.

[186] Lebwohl M. Strategies to optimize efficacy, duration of remission and safety in the treatment of plaque psoriasis by using tazarotene in combination with a corticosteroid. *J Am Acad Dermatol* 2000; 43 (Suppl.): S43–6.

[187] Menter A, Korman NJ, Elmetts CA, Feldman SR *et al.* Guidelines of care for the management of psoriasis and psoriatic arthritis. Section 3, Guidelines of care for the management and treatment of psoriasis with topical therapies. *J Am Acad Dermatol* 2009; 60: 643–59.

[188] Goeckerman WH. Treatment of psoriasis. *Arch Dermatol Syphilol* 1931; 24: 446–50.

[189] Adrian RM, Parrish JA, Momtaz TK *et al.* Outpatient phototherapy for psoriasis. *Arch Dermatol* 1981; 117: 623–6.

[190] Larkö O, Swanbeck G. Home solarium treatment of psoriasis. *Br J Dermatol* 1979; 101: 13–6.

[191] LeVine MJ, White HAD, Parrish JA. Components of the Goeckerman regimen. *J Invest Dermatol* 1979; 73: 170–3.

[192] LeVine MJ, Parrish JA. Outpatient phototherapy of psoriasis. *Arch Dermatol* 1980; 116: 552–4.

[193] Van Weelden H, Young E, van Der Leun JC. Therapy of psoriasis: comparison of photo-chemotherapy and several variants of phototherapy. *Br J Dermatol* 1980; 103: 1–9.

[194] Larkö O, Swanbeck G. Is UVB therapy of psoriasis safe? *Acta Derm Venereol (Stockh)* 1982; 62: 507–12.

[195] Lynfield Y, O'Donohue MN. Tar, UVL, PUVA and cancer (Letter). *J Am Acad Dermatol* 1981; 4: 612–3.

[196] Stern RS, Laird N. The carcinogenic risk of treatments for severe psoriasis. *Cancer* 1994; 73: 2759–64.

[197] Stern RS. Members of the Photochemotherapy Follow-up Study. Genital tumors among men with psoriasis exposed to psoralens and ultraviolet A radiation (PUVA) and ultraviolet B radiation. *N Engl J Med* 1990; 322: 1093–7.

[198] van Weelden H, Baart de la Faille H, Young E, van der Leun JC. A new development in UVB phototherapy of psoriasis. *Br J Dermatol* 1988; 119: 11–9.

[199] Green C, Ferguson J, Lakshmipathi T, Johnson BE. 311 nm UVB phototherapy: an effective treatment for psoriasis. *Br J Dermatol* 1988; 119: 691–6.

[200] Man I, Crombie IK, Dawe RS, Ibbotson SH, Ferguson J. The photocarcinogenic risk of narrowband UVB (TL-01) phototherapy: early follow-up data. *Br J Dermatol* 2005; 152: 755–7.

[201] Storbeck K, Hölzle E, Schürer N, Lehmann P *et al.* Narrow-band UVB (311 nm) versus conventional broad-band UVB with and without dithranol in phototherapy for psoriasis. *J Am Acad Dermatol* 1993; 28: 227–31.

[202] Gordon PM, Diffey BL, Matthews JNS, Farr PM. A randomized comparison of narrow-band TL-01 phototherapy and PUVA photochemotherapy for psoriasis. *J Am Acad Dermatol* 1999; 41: 728–32.

[203] Tanew A, Radakovic-Fijan S, Schemper M, Honigsmann H. Narrow-band UVB phototherapy versus photochemotherapy in the treatment of chronic plaque type psoriasis: a paired comparison study. *Arch Dermatol* 1999; 135: 519–24.

[204] Hearn RM, Kerr AC, Rahim KF, Ferguson J *et al.* Incidence of skin cancers in 3867 patients treated with narrow-band ultrraviolet B phototherapy. Br J. Dermatol 2008 Sep;159(4):931-5.

[205] George SA, Ferguson J. Lesional blistering following narrow-band (TL-01) UVB phototherapy for psoriasis: a report of four cases (Letter). *Br J Dermatol* 1992; 127: 445–6.

[206] Abel EA, Barnes S, Le Vine MJ, Seidman DR *et al.* Psoriasis treatment at the Dead Sea: second international study tour (Letter). *J Am Acad Dermatol* 1988; 19: 362–4.

[207] Lerner AB, Denton CR, Fitzpatrick TB. Clinical and experimental studies with 8-methoxypsoralen in vitiligo. *J Invest Dermatol* 1953; 20: 299–314.

[208] Anderson TF, Voorhees JJ. Psoralen photochemotherapy of cutaneous disorders. *Ann Rev Pharmacol Toxicol* 1980; 20: 235–57.

[209] Parrish JA, Fitzpatrick TB, Tanenbaum L, Pathak MA *et al.* Photochemotherapy of psoriasis with oral methoxsalen and long-wave ultraviolet light. *N Engl J Med* 1974; 291: 1207–11.

[210] Langner A, Wolska H, Kowalski J, Duralska H *et al.* Photochemotherapy (PUVA) and psoriasis: comparison of 8-MOP and 8-MOP/5-MOP. *Int J Dermatol* 1976; 15: 688–9.

[211] Dubertret L, Averbeck D, Zajdela F, Bisagni E *et al.* Photochemotherapy (PUVA) of psoriasis using 3-carbethoxypsoralen, a non-carcinogenic compound in mice. *Br J Dermatol* 1979; 101: 379–89.

[212] Parrish JA, LeVine MJ, Fitzpatrick TB. Oral methoxsalen photochemotherapy of psoriasis and mycosis fungoides. *Int J Dermatol* 1980; 19: 379–86.

[213] Wolff KW, Fitzpatrick TB, Parrish JA, Gschnait F *et al.* Photochemotherapy for psoriasis with orally administered methoxsalen. *Arch Dermatol* 1976; 112: 943–50.

[214] Melski JW, Tanenbaum L, Parrish JA, Fitzpatrick TB *et al.* Oral methoxsalen photochemotherapy for the treatment of psoriasis: a cooperative clinical trial. *J Invest Dermatol* 1977; 68: 328–35.

[215] Roenigk HH, Farber EM, Storrs F *et al.* Photochemotherapy for psoriasis. A clinical cooperative study of PUVA-48 and PUVA-64. *Arch Dermatol* 1979; 115: 576–9.

[216] Siddiqui AH, Cormane RH. Initial photochemotherapy of psoriasis with orally administered 8-methoxypsoralen and long-wave ultraviolet light (PUVA). *Br J Dermatol* 1979; 100: 247–50.

[217] Henseler T, Wolff K, Hönigsman H, Christophers E. Oral 8-methoxypsoralen photochemotherapy of psoriasis. *Lancet* 1981;1(8225): 853–7.

[218] Marx JL, Scher RK. Response of psoriatic nails to oral photochemotherapy. *Arch Dermatol* 1980; 116: 1023–4.

[219] Morison WL, Momtaz K, Parrish JA, Fitzpatrick TB. Combined methotrexate-PUVA therapy in the treatment of psoriasis. *J Am Acad Dermatol* 1982; 6:46–51.

[220] Speight EL, Farr PM. Calcipotriol improves the response of psoriasis to PUVA. *Br J Dermatol* 1994; 130: 79–82.

[221] Stern RS, Laird N. The carcinogenic risk of treatment for severe psoriasis: photochemotherapy follow-up study. *Cancer* 1994; 73: 2759–64.

[222] Momtaz K, Parrish JA. Combination of psoralens and ultraviolet A and ultraviolet B in the treatment of psoriasis vulgaris: a bilaterial comparison study. *J Am Acad Dermatol* 1984; 10: 481–6.
[223] Reed WB. Treatment of psoriasis with oral psoralens and long-wave ultraviolet light (Letter). *Acta Derm Venereol (Stockh)* 1976; 56: 315.
[224] Baker H, Darley CR, Johnson-Smith J *et al.* Skin neoplasia associated with PUVA therapy. *Br J Dermatol* 1981; 105 (Suppl. 19): 65–6.
[225] Stern RS, Laird N. The carcinogenic risk of treatments for severe psoriasis. *Cancer* 1994; 73: 2759–64.
[226] Paul CF, Ho VC, McGeown C, Christophers E *et al.* Risk of malignancies in psoriasis patients treated with cysclosporine: a 5 year cohort study. *J Invest Dermatol* 2003; 120: 211–6.
[227] Stern RS, Liebman EJ.Väkevä L. Oral Psoralenand Ultraviolet-A Light (PUVA) Treatment of Psoriasis and Persistent Risk of Non-melanoma Skin Cancer. *J Natl Cancer Inst* 1998;90:1278-84.
[228] Stern RS. The risk of melanoma in association with long term exposure to PUVA. *J Am Acad Dermatol* 2001 May;44 (5):755-61.
[229] Lindelöf B, Siqurgeirsson B, Tegner E, Larkö O *et al.* PUVA and Cancer risk: the Sweedish follow-up study. *Br J Dermatol* 1999 Jul;14(1):108-12.
[230] Lindelof B. Risk of melanoma with psoralen/ultraviolet A therapy for psoriasis. Do the known risks outweigh the benefits? *Drug Saf* 1999 Apr;20(4):289-97.
[231] Weinstein GD. Commentary: three decades of folic acid antagonist in dermatology. *Arch Dermatol* 1983; 119: 525–7.
[232] Hendel L, Hendel J, Johnsen A, Gudmand-Høver E.. Intestinal functional and methotrexate absorption in psoriatic patients. *Clin Exp Dermatol* 1982; 7: 491–8.
[233] Bannwarth B, Pehourcq F, Schaever-Beke T, Dehais J. Clinical Pharmacokinetics of low-dose pulse methotrexate in rheumatoid arthritis. *Clin Pharmacokinet.* 996;30:194-210.
[234] Furst DE, Herman RA, Koehnker R, Ericksen N *et al.* Effect of aspirin and sulindac on methotrexate clearance. *J Pharm Sci.* 1990;79:782-6.
[235] Edno L, Bressolle F, Gomeni R, Bologna C *et al.* Total and free methotrexate pharmacokinetics in rheumatoid arthritis patients. *Ther Drug Monit.* 1996;18:128-34.
[236] Wan SH, Huffman DH, Azarnoff DL, Stephens R *et al.* Effect of route of administration and effusions on methotrexate pharmacokinetics. *Cancer Res* 1974; 34: 3487–91.
[237] Calvert AH, Bondy PK, Harrap KR. Some observations on the human pharmacology of methotrexate. *Cancer Treat Rep* 1977; 61: 1647–56.
[238] Taylor JR, Halprin KM. Effect of sodium salicylate and indomethacin on methotrexate-serum albumin binding. *Arch Dermatol* 1977; 113: 588–91.
[239] Taylor JR, Halprin KM, Levine V, Woodyard C *et al.* Effects of methotrexate *in vitro* on epidermal cell proliferation. *Br J Dermatol* 1983; 108: 45–61.
[240] Jeffes EWB, McCullough JL, Pittelkow MR, McCormick A *et al.* Methotrexate therapy of psoriasis: differential sensitivity of proliferating lymphoid and epithelial cells to the cytotoxic and growth-inhibitory effects of methotrexate. *J Invest Dermatol* 1995; 104: 183–8.
[241] Cronstein BN, Naime D, Ostad E. The antiinflammatory effects of methotrexate are mediated by adenosine. *Adv Exp Med Biol* 1994; 370:411.

[242] Walsdorfer U, Christophers E, Schröder J-M. Methotrexate inhibits polymorphonuclear leukocyte chemotaxis in psoriasis. *Br J Dermatol* 1983; 108: 451–6.

[243] Comaish S, Juhlin L. Site of action of methotrexate in psoriasis. *Arch Dermatol* 1969; 100: 99–105.

[244] Steward WD, Wallace SM, Runikis JO. Absorption and local action of methotrexate in human and mouse skin. *Arch Dermatol* 1972; 106: 357–61.

[245] Montaudié H, Sbidian E, Paul C, Maza A, Gallini A, *et al.* Methotrexate in psoriasis: a systematic review of treatment modalities, incidence, risk factors and monitoring of liver toxicity. J Eur Acad Dermatol Venereol. 2011(May); 25(Suppl)2:12-8.

[246] Smith JD, Knox JM. Psoriasis, methotrexate and tuberculosis. *Br J Dermatol* 1971; 84: 590–3.

[247] Verdich J, Christensen AL. Pulmonary disease complicating intermittent methotrexate therapy of psoriasis. *Acta Derm Venereol (Stockh)* 1979; 59: 471–3.

[248] Roenigk HH Jr, AuerbachR, Maibach HI, Weinstein GD. Methotrexate in psoriasis: revised guidelines. *J Am Acad Dermatol* : 1988;19:145-56.

[249] Zachariae H. Psoriasis and the liver. In: Roenigk HH, Maibach HI, eds. Psoriasis. New York: Marcel Dekker, 1985: 47–64.

[250] Zachariae H, Kragballe K, Sogaard H. Methotrexate-induced liver cirrhosis. *Br J Dermatol* 1980; 102: 407–12.

[251] van de Kerkhof PC, Hoefnagels WH, van Haelst UJ, Mali JW. Methotrexate maintenance therapy and liver damage. *Clin Exp Dermatol* 1985; 10: 194–200.

[252] Chalmers RJ, Kirby B, Smith A, Burrows B *et al.* Replacement of routine liver biopsy by procollagen III aminopeptide for monitoring patients with psoriasis receiving long-term methotrexate: A multicentre audit and health economic analysis. *Br J Dermatol* 152:444, 2005.

[253] Orion E, Matz H, Wolf R: The life-threatening complications of dermatologic therapies. *Clin Dermatol* 23:182, 2005.

[254] Fraser AG. MTX: first-line or second-line immunomodulator? Eur. J. Gastroenterol. Hepatol. 2003; 15: 225–31.

[255] Stern RS, Laird N. The carcinogenic risk of treatments for severe psoriasis. *Cancer* 1994; 73: 2759–64.

[256] Zonneveld IM, Bakker WK, Dijkstra PF, Bos JD *et al.* Methotrexate osteopathy in long-term, low-dose methotrexate treatment for psoriasis and rheumatoid arthritis. *Arch Dermatol* 1996; 132: 184–7.

[257] Milunsky A, Graef JW, Gaynor MF. Methotrexate-induced congenital malformations. *J Pediatr* 1968; 72: 790–5.

[258] Baker H. Methotrexate: the conservative treatment for psoriasis. In: Farber EM, Cox AJ, eds. Psoriasis. Proceedings of the 2nd International Symposium. New York:Yorke Medical, 1977: 235–42.

[259] Paul BS, Momtaz K, Stern RS *et al.* Combined methotrexate: ultraviolet B therapy in the treatment of psoriasis. *J Am Acad Dermatol* 1982; 7: 758–62.

[260] Vanderveen EE, Ellis CN, Campbell JP, Case PC *et al.* Methotrexate and etretinate as concurrent therapies in severe psoriasis. *Arch Dermatol* 1982; 118: 660–2.

[261] Clark CM, Kirby B, Morris AD, Davison S *et al.* Combination treatment with methotrexate and cyclosporin for severe recalcitrant psoriasis. *Br J Dermatol* 1999; 141:279–82.

[262] Horiguchi M, Takigawa M, Imamura S. Treatment of generalized pustular psoriasis with methotrexate and colchicine (Letter). *Arch Dermatol* 1981; 117:760.

[263] Mueller W, Herrman B. Cyclosporin A for psoriasis (Letter). *N Engl J Med* 1979; 301: 555.

[264] Bos JD, Meinardi MM, van Joost T, Heule F *et al.* Use of cyclosporin in psoriasis. *Lancet* 1989;2:1500–2.

[265] Schofi eld OMV, Camp RDR, Levene GM. Cyclosporin A in psoriasis: interaction with carbamazepine (Letter). *Br J Dermatol* 1990; 122: 425–6.

[266] Mihatsch MJ, Wolff K. Consensus conference on cyclosporin A for psoriasis. *Br J Dermatol* 1992; 126: 621–3.

[267] Berth-Jones J, Voorhees JJ. Consensus conference on cyclosporin A microemulsion for psoriasis. *Br J Dermatol* 1996; 135: 775–7.

[268] Griffiths CE Dubertret L, Ellis CN, Finlay AY *et al.* Ciclosporin in psoriasis clinical practice: an international consensus statement. *Br J Dermatol* 2004; 150: 11–23.

[269] Berth-Jones J, Henderson CA, Munro CS, Rogers S *et al.* Treatment of psoriasis with intermittent short course cyclosporin (Neoral): a multicentre study. *Br J Dermatol* 1997; 136: 527–30.

[270] Ho VC, Griffiths CE, Berth-Jones J, Papp KA *et al.* Intermittent short courses of cyclosporine microemulsion for long-term management of psoriasis: a 2 year cohort study. *J Am Acad Dermatol* 2001; 44: 643–51.

[271] Ohtsuki M, Nakagawa H, Sugai J, Ozawa A *et al.* Long-term continuous versus intermittent cyclosporin: therapy for psoriasis. *J Dermatol* 2003; 30: 290–8.

[272] Bos JD, Meinardi MM, van Joost T, Heule F *et al.* Use of cyclosporin in psoriasis. *Lancet* 1989; 2: 1500–2.

[273] Shevach E: The effects of cyclosporin A on the immune system. *Am Rev Immunol.*1985:397.

[274] Bennett W, Norman D: Action and toxicity of cyclosporin. *Am Rev Med.* 1986;37:215.

[275] Fureu M, Katz S: The effect of cyclosporin on epidermal cells. Cyclosporine inhibits accessory cell functions of epidermal Langerhans cells in vitro. *J Immunol.* 1988;l40:4139.

[276] Palay D, Cliff C, Wentworth P, Ziegler H: Cyclosporin inhibits macrophage-mediated antigen presentation. *J Immunol.* 1986;136:4348.

[277] Knight SC, Balfour B, O'Brien J, Buttifant L Sensitivity of veiled (dendritic) cells to cyclosporin. *Transplantation.* 1986;41:96.

[278] Grossman RM, Maugée E, Dubertrel L. Cervical intraepithelial neoplasia in a patient receiving long-term cyclosporin for the treatment of severe plaque psoriasis (Letter). *Br J Dermatol* 1996; 135: 147–8.

[279] Noel JC, de Dobbeleer G. Development of human papillomavirus-associated Buschke-Löwenstein penile carcinoma during cyclosporine therapy for generalized pustular psoriasis. *J Am Acad Dermatol* 1994; 31: 299–300.

[280] Bollag W. From vitamin A to retinoids: chemical and pharmacological aspects. In: Orfanos CE, Braun Falco O, Farber EM *et al.*, eds. Retinoids: Advances in Basic Research and Therapy. Berlin: Springer-Verlag, 1981: 5–11.

[281] Fisher GJ, Talwar HS, Lin J, Lin P *et al.* Retinoic acid inhibits induction of c-Jun protein by ultraviolet radiation that occurs subsequent to activation of mitogen-activated protein kinase pathways in human skin *in vivo. J Clin Invest* 1998; 101:1432–40.
[282] Bavinck JN, Teiben LM, Van der Woude FJ *et al.* Prevention of skin cancer and reduction of keratotic skin lesions during acitretin therapy in renal transplant recipients: a double-blind, placebo controlled study. *J Clin Oncol* 1995; 13:1933–8.
[283] Gollnick HPM. Oral retinoids: efficacy and toxicity in psoriasis. *Br J Dermatol.* 1996; 135 (Suppl. 49): 6–17.
[284] Lassus A, Geiger J-M, Nyblom M, Virrankoski T *et al.* Treatment of severe psoriasis with etretin (RO 10-1670). *Br J Dermatol* 1987; 117: 333–41.
[285] Gupta AK, Goldfarb MT, Ellis CN, Voorhees JJ. Side-effect profile of acitretin therapy in psoriasis. *J Am Acad Dermatol* 1989; 20: 1088–93.
[286] Bleiker TO, Bourke JF, Graham-Brown RAC, Hutchinson PE. Etretinate may work where acitretin fails. *Br J Dermatol* 1997; 136: 368–70.
[287] Pilkington T, Brogden RN. Acitretin: a review of its pharmacological properties and therapeutic use. *Drugs* 1992; 43: 597–627.
[288] Gollnick H, Bauer R, Brindley C, Orfanos CE *et al.* Acitretin versus etretinate in psoriasis. *J Am Acad Dermatol* 1988; 19: 458–69.
[289] Ledo A, Martin M, Geiger J-M, Marrón JM. Acitretin (RO 10-1670) in the treatment of severe psoriasis: a randomized double-blind parallel study comparing acitretin and etretinate. *Int J Dermatol* 1988; 27: 656–60.
[290] Kingston TP, Matt LH, Lowe NJ. Etretin therapy for severe psoriasis: evaluation of clinical responses. *Arch Dermatol* 1987; 123: 55–8.
[291] Roenigk HH Jr, Callen JP, Guzzo CA *et al.* Effects of acitretin on the liver. *J Am Acad Dermatol* 1999; 41: 584–8.
[292] Tanew A, Guggenbichler A, Honigsmann H *et al.* Photochemotherapy for severe psoriasis without or in combination with acitretin: a randomized, double-blind comparison study. *J Am Acad Dermatol* 1991; 25: 682–4.
[293] Lowe N, Prystowsky JH, Bourget T, Edelstein J *et al.* Acitretin plus UVB therapy for psoriasis: comparisons with placebo plus UVB and acitretin alone. *J Am Acad Dermatol* 1991; 24: 591–4.
[294] Bavinck JN, Tieben LM, Van der Woude FJ, Tegzess AM *et al.* Prevention of skin cancer and reduction of keratotic skin lesions during acitretin therapy in renal transplant recipients: a double-blind, placebo controlled study. *J Clin Oncol* 1995; 13: 1933–8.
[295] Ryan TJ, Baker H. Systemic corticosteroids and folic antagonists in the treatment of generalized pustular psoriasis. *Br J Dermatol* 1969; 81: 134–45.
[296] Champion RH. Treatment of psoriasis. *BMJ* 1966; 2: 993–6.
[297] Fernandez-Obregon AC. Clinical management of a patient with psoriasis and comorbid vitiligo. *J Drugs Dermatol.* 2008 Jul;7(7):679-81.
[298] Smith CH. Use of hydroxyurea in psoriasis. *Clin Exp Dermatol* 1999; 24: 2–6. 846–7.
[299] Yarbro JW. Hydroxyurea in the treatment of refractory psoriasis. *Lancet* 1969; 2:846-7.:
[300] Layton AM, Sheehan-Dare RA, Goodfi eld MJD *et al.* Hydroxyurea in the management of therapy-resistant psoriasis. *Br J Dermatol* 1989; 121: 647–53.
[301] Moschella SL, Greenwald MA. Psoriasis with hydroxyurea. *Arch Dermatol* 1973 107: 363–8.

[302] Baker H. Antimitotic drugs in psoriasis. In: Farber EM, Cox AJ, eds. Psoriasis. Proceedings of the 3rd International Symposium. New York: Marcel Dekker, 1985:451-5.

[303] Sauer GC. Combined methotrexate and hydroxyurea therapy for psoriasis. *Arch Dermatol* 1973; 107: 369–70.

[304] Kirby B, Harrison PV. Combination low-dose cyclosporin (Neoral) and hydroxyurea for severe recalcitrant psoriasis. *Br J Dermatol* 1999; 140: 186–7.

[305] Choo D, McHenry P. Combination therapy with acitretin and hydroxyurea for severe psoriasis. *J Dermatolog Treat* 1999; 10: 71–2.

[306] Roe LD, Wilson JW. Hydroxyurea therapy (Letter). *Arch Dermatol* 1973; 108:426–7.

[307] Kirby B et al: Dermatomyositis-like eruption and leg ulceration caused by hydroxyurea in a patient with psoriasis. *Clin Exp Dermatol*. 2000;25:256.

[308] Zackheim HS, Maibach HI, Grekin DA. Thioguanine for psoriasis. In: Farber EM, Cox AJ, Nall L, eds. *Psoriasis. Proceedings of the 3rd International Symposium*. New York: Grune & Stratton, 1982: 405.

[309] Molin L, Thomsen K. Thioguanine treatment in psoriasis. *Acta Derm Venereol (Stockh)* 1987; 67: 85–8.

[310] Zackheim HS, Glogau RG, Fisher DA, Maibach HI. 6-Thioguanine treatment of psoriasis: experience in 81 patients. *J Am Acad Dermatol* 1994; 30: 452–8.

[311] Ramagosa R, Kerdel F, Shah N. Treatment of psoriasis with 6-thioguanine and hepatic veno-occlusive disease. *J Am Acad Dermatol* 2002; 47: 970–2.

[312] Mason C, Krueger GG. Thioguanine for refractory psoriasis: a 4-year experience. *J Am Acad Dermatol* 2001; 44: 67–72.

[313] Gerdes S, Shakey K, Mrowietz U. Dimethylfumarate inhibits nuclear binding of nuclear factor of kappaB but not of nuclear factor of activated T cells and CCAAT/enhancer binding protein beta in activated human T cells. *Br J Dermatol* 2007; 156: 838–42.

[314] Ockenfels HM, Schaltewolter T, Ockenfels G *et al*. The antipsoriatic agent dimethylfumarate immunomodulates T-cell cytokine secretion and inhibits cytokines of the psoriatic cytokine network. *Br J Dermatol* 1998; 139: 390–5.

[315] Altmeyer PJ, Matthes U, Pawlak F *et al*. Antipsoriatic effects of fumaric acid derivatives: results of a multicenter double-blind study in100 patients. *J Am Acad Dermatol* 1994; 30: 977–81.

[316] Nugteren-Huying WM, van der Schroeff JG, Hermans J, Saarmond D. Fumaric acid therapy for psoriasis: a randomized, double-blind, placebo-controlled study. *J Am Acad Dermatol* 1990; 22: 311–2.

[317] Mrowietz U, Christophers E, Altmeyer P. Treatment of psoriasis with fumaric acid esters: results of a prospective multicentre study. German Multicentre Study. *Br J Dermatol* 1998; 138: 456–60.

[318] Talamonti M, Spallone G, Di Stefani A, Costanzo A *et al*. Efalizumab. Expert Opin Drug Saf. 2011 Mar;10(2):239-51. Epub 2011 Jan 10.

[319] Kothary N, Diak IL, Brinker A, Bezabeh S, *et al*. Progressive multifocal leukoencephalopathy associated with efalizumab use in psoriasis patients. *J Am Acad Dermatol*. 2011 Apr 21; in press.

[320] van der Laken CJ, Voskuyl AE, Roos JC, Stigter van Walsum M, *et al*. Imaging and serum analysis of immune complex formation of radiolabeled infliximab and

antiinfliximab in responders and non-responders to therapy for rheumatoid arthritis. *Ann Rheum Dis* 2007;66:253-6.
[321] Lecluse LL, Driessen RJ, Spuls PI, deJong EM *et al.* Extent and Clinical Conseuences of Antibody Formation Against Adalimumab in Patients With Plaque Psoriasis. *Arch Dermatol* 2010; 146:127-32.
[322] Bartelds GM, Wijbrandts CA, Nurmohamed MT, Wolbink GJ et al. Anti-adalimumab antibodies in rheumatoid arthritis patients are associated with interleukin-10 gene polymorphism. Arthritis Rheum 2009; 60:2541-2.
[323] Gupta AK, Ellis CN, Siegel MT *et al.* Sulfasalazine improves psoriasis: a doubleblind analysis. *Arch Dermatol* 1990; 126: 487–93.
[324] Gupta AK, Grober JS, Hamilton TA, Ellis CN, *et al.* Sulfasalazine therapy for psoriatic arthritis: a double blind, placebo controlled trial. *J Rheumatol.* 1995 May ;22(5) :894-8.
[325] Greaves MW, Dawber R. Azathioprine in psoriasis. *BMJ* 1970; 2: 237–8.
[326] du Vivier A, Munro DD, Verbov J. Treatment of psoriasis with azathioprine.*BMJ* 1974; 1: 49–51
[327] Haufs MG, Beissert S, Grabbe S, Schütte B *et al.* Psoriasis vulgaris treated successfully with mycophenolate mofetil. *Br J Dermatol* 1998; 138: 179–81.
[328] Davison SC, Morris-Jones R, Powles AV, Fry L. Change of treatment from ciclosporin to mycophenolate mofetil in severe psoriasis. *Br J Dermatol* 2000; Gupta AK, Ellis CN, Siegel:405–7.
[329] Gellen CC, Arnold M, Orfanos CE. Mycophenolate mofetil as a systemic antipsoriatic agent: positive experiencve in 11 patients. *Br J Dermatol.* 2001 Marc;144(3):583-6.
[330] Asadullah K, Docke WD, Ebeling M, Friedrich M *et al.* Interleukin-10 treatment of psoriasis: clinical results of a phase 2 trial. *Arch Dermatol* 1999; 135: 187–92.
[331] Kimball AB, Kawamura T, Tejura K, Boss C *et al.* Clinical and immunologic assessment of patients with psoriasis in a randomized, double-blind, placebo-controlled trial using recombi nant human interleukin-10. *Arch Dermatol* 2002; 138: 1341–6.
[332] Ghureschi K, Thomas P, Breit S *et al.* Interleukin-4 therapy of psoriasis induces Th2 responses and improves human autoimmune disease. *Nat Med* 2003; 9:40–6.
[333] Duvic M, Crane MM, Conant M, Mahoney SE *et al.* Zidovudine improves psoriasis in human immunodefi ciency virus-positive males. *Arch Dermatol* 1994; 130: 447–51.
[334] Matt LH, Kingston TP, Lowe NJ. Treatment of severe psoriasis with intravenous somatostatin. *J Dermatolog Treat* 1989; 1: 3–4.
[335] Dockx P, Decree J, Degreef H. Inhibitor of the metabolism of endogenous retinoic acid as treatment for severe psoriasis: an open study with oral liarozole. *Br J Dermatol* 1995; 133: 426–32.
[336] Berth-Jones J, Todd G, Hutchinson PE. *et al.* Treatment of psoriasis with oral liarozole: a dose-ranging study. *Br J Dermatol* 2000; 143: 1170–6.
[337] Collins P, Robinson DJ, Stringer MR. *et al.* The variable response of plaque psoriasis after a single treatment with topical 5-amino/aevulinic acid photodynamic therapy. *Br J Dermatol* 1997; 137: 743–9.
[338] Robinson DJ, Collins P, Stringer M *et al.* Improved response of plaque psoriasis after multiple treatments with topical 5-amino/aevulinic acid photodynamic therapy. *Acta Derm Venereol* 1999; 79: 451–5.
[339] Asawanonda P, Anderson RR, Chang Y, Taylor CR. 308-nm excimer laser for the treatment of psoriasis: a dose–response study. *Arch Dermatol* 2000; 137:95–6.

[340] Feldman SR, Mellen BG, Housman TS, Fitzpatrick RE *et al.* Efficacy of the 308-nm excimer laser for treatment of psoriasis: results of a multicenter study. *J Am Acad Dermatol* 2002; 46: 900–6.

[341] Jegasothy BV, Ackerman CD, Todo S, Fung JJ *et al.* Tacrolimus (FK506): a new therapeutic agent for severe recalcitrant psoriasis. *Arch Dermatol* 1992; 128: 781–5.

[342] European FK506 Multicenter Psoriasis Study Group. Systemic tacrolimus (FK506) is effective for the treatment of psoriasis in a double-blind, placebo controlled study. *Arch Dermatol* 1996; 132: 419–23.

[343] Gottlieb AB, Griffiths CE, Ho VC, Lahfa M *et al.* Oral pimecrolimus in the treatment of moderate to severe plaque-type psoriasis: a double-blind, multicentre, randomized, dose-finding study. *Br J Dermatol* 2005; 152: 1219–27.

[344] Krueger GG, Papp KA, Stough DB, Loven KH. Et al. A randomized, double-blind, placebo-controlled, phase III study evaluating efficacy and tolerability of 2 courses of alefacept in patients with chronic plaque psoriasis. *J Am Acad Dermatol* 2002 Dec;47(6):821-33.

[345] Leonardi CL, Powers JL, Matheson RT, Goffe BS. *et al.* Etanercept as mponotherapy in patients with psoriasis. *N Engl J Med.* 2003 Nov 20; 349(21):2014-22.

[346] Gordon KB, Gottlieb AB, Leonardi CL, Elewski BE, *et al.* Clinical response in psoriasis patients discontinued from and then reinitiated on etanercept therapy. *J Dermatolog Treat* 2006; 17(1):9-17.

[347] Gottlieb AB, Evans R, Li S, Dooley LT, *et al.* Infliximab induction therapy for patients with severe plaque-type psoriasis: a randomized, double-blind, placebo-controlled trial. *J Am Acad Dermatol* 2004 Oct;51(4):534-42.

[348] Reich K, Nestle F, Papp K, et al. (EXPRESS study investigators). Infliximab induction and maintenance for moderate to severe psoriasis: a phase III, multicentre, double-blind trial. Lancet 2005: 366 (9494): 1367–1374.

[349] Gordon KB, Langley RG, Leonmardi C, Toth D. et al. Clinical response to adalimumab treatment in patients with moderate to severe psoriasis: Double-blind, randomized controlled trial and open-label extension study. *J Am Acad Dermatol* 2006 Oct;55(4):598-606.

[350] Menter A, Tyring SK, Gordon K, Kimball AB. *et al.* Adalimumab therapy for moderate to severe psoriasis: A randomized, controlled phase III trial. *J Am Acad Dermatol.* 2008 Jan;58(1):106-15.

[351] Menter A, Papp K, Crowley J, Gu Y et al. Long-term Outcomes of Interruption and Retreatment versus Continuous Therapy With Adalimumab for Psoriais: Subanalysis of REVEAL. Presented at the 19th European of Dermatology and Venereology in Gothenburg, Sweeden.October 6-10, 2010.

[352] Papp K, Crowley J, Ortonne J-P, Leu J. Adalimumab for moderate to severe chronic plaque psoriasis: efficacy and safety of retreatment and disease recurrence following withdrawal from therapy. *Br J Dermatol.*2011;164:434-41.

[353] Leonardi CL, Kimball AB, Papp KA, Yeilding N. et al. Efficacy and safety of ustekinumab, a human interleukin-12/23 monoclonal antibody, in patients with psoriasis: 76-week results from randomized, double-blind, placebo-conmtrolled trial (PHOENIX 1). *Lancet* 2008 May 17;371(9625):1665-74.

[354] Papp KA, Langley RG, Lebwohl M, Krueger GG et al. Efficacy and safety of ustekinumab, a human interleukin-12/23 monoclonal antibody, in patients with

psoriasis: 52 week results from a randomized, double-blind, placebo-controlled trial (PHOENIX 2). *Lancet* 2008 May 17;371(9625):1675-84.
[355] Abuakara K, Azfar RS, Shin DB, Neimann Al. *et al*. Cause-specific mortality in patients with severe psoriasis: a population based cohort study in the UK. *Br J Dermatol* 2010 Sep;163(3):586-92.
[356] Roth PE, Grosshans E, Bergoend H. Psoriasis: development and fatal complications. *Ann Dermatol Venereol* 1991;118(2):97-105.
[357] Suárez-Fariñas M, Fuentes-Duculan J, Lowes MA, Krueger JG. Resolved psoriasis lesions retain expression of a subset of disease-related genes. *J Invest Dermatol*. Epub 23 Sep 2010.
[358] Palatsi R, Hägg P. The immune response against microbial infections in the skin - weak in atopic dermatitis and strong in psoriasis. Duodecim. 2011; 127(2):127-34.